SENIOR STRENGTH TRAINING RESISTANCE AND CORE

DAVID O'CONNOR

FOREWORD

SCAN FOR AUDIO CHAPTER

Maintaining a strong body is essential to a healthy life. Without intervention, once you reach your 30s, you start to lose around 3% of your muscle tissue every decade. And it's all downhill from there because this muscle loss accelerates as you age. By the time you reach your 50s, around 10% of us will suffer from sarcopenia—less scarily known as muscle loss due to aging.

And that's not all! After 60, your muscles lose their strength even more rapidly, which can lead to a higher risk of injuries due to falls and increased frailty. In fact, the frailty we associate with old age stems from loss of muscle strength.

Therefore, it's time to turn back the clock with a combination of resistance and core-strengthening exercises that can reinvent a younger and stronger you. Exercising regularly will not only strengthen your muscles and improve your physique but also help you avoid injury, build resilience against falls, boost metabolism, and improve overall health. A stronger body will fortify your mental and emotional health so you can sleep better, feel younger, and foster a sense of well-being.

I'm sure you're no stranger to the symptoms of muscle loss: Walking more slowly, difficulty climbing stairs, decreased stamina, and constant fatigue. It just sounds like getting older, doesn't it? So, do you accept it as a natural part of aging—accept that you're stuck with a body that's getting frailer with each passing decade?

No! You CAN do something to prevent the unpleasant effects of muscle weakness. With the combination of resistance and core strength training, weakness will NOT be an inevitable part of your old age. Building muscle strength and avoiding frailty are within your control, and I'm here to help you.

We can apply the adage "use it or lose it" to muscle strength. If you don't keep exercising your muscles, they'll lose strength, it's as simple as that. The Centers for Disease Control and Prevention (CDC) recognizes this and recommends that all adults engage in muscle-strengthening activities at least two days a week (CDC, 2021).

How should we combat muscle weakness as we grow older?

Traditionally, weight training is the go-to activity to increase muscle strength. However, as a senior, you have a greater risk of injury, especially when exercising at home without the benefit of personal trainer to guide you. What you need is an inexpensive and safe way to strengthen your muscles from the comfort of your home.

That's where this book comes in! You'll be amazed at the effectiveness of our exercise regimens that strengthen your entire body with just two types of exercises: Training with inexpensive resistance bands and building core strength.

The exercises in this book build muscle, resilience and confidence reducing the effects of aging on your body.

The first book teaches you how to use resistance bands safely, whether you use them at home, in the park, or in the gym.

Resistance bands offer the same strength training benefits as free weights while being inexpensive, accessible, safe and are ideal for seniors. Studies show that regularly exercising with resistance bands can reduce the frailty associated with old age (Lopes et al., 2019). Moreover, resistance training adheres to the CDC's recommendation of two days a week of strength training. Put simply, you can give the boot to weakness from old age by regularly following the resistance band exercises in this book!

Another vital aspect of strength training for seniors is building core strength. While often associated with 25-year-old's striving for an elusive six-pack, core strengthening is actually not about vanity, has benefits for everyone and arguably seniors benefit most from.

Your core is involved in every movement you make—walking, getting out of a chair, climbing stairs, maintaining balance, and even picking up your grandchildren. If your core muscles are weak (which they often become with age), it can harm your well-being and make everyday activities more arduous.

Have you ever tried picking up your grandchild and struggled to get them off the floor? What about getting your groceries home? If you've ever found yourself muttering, "I'm getting too old for this," then this book is for you.

Engaging in core-strengthening exercises regularly will fortify your body and make you feel like a superhero the next time you scoop your grandchild up for a hug.

Other benefits to restoring core strength include a reduced risk of back pain and injury, improved balance, a reduced risk of falls, and an overall sense of vitality.

Each workout has been designed to suit the needs of seniors. With exercises and workouts separated by their level of difficulty. The book provides two tests you can perform at home to determine your current level. This ensures that you are not at risk of harming yourself by performing exercises that are too advanced for your abilities.

Following our dual strengthening program, you will strengthen muscles throughout your body and slow down or even stop muscle mass and strength loss, thus keeping frailty at arm's length and guaranteeing long-term health. The best part is you can gain all this from the comfort of your home—safely, inexpensively, and sustainably!

The two books dovetail perfectly to provide the ideal combination of exercises for effective strength training and a roadmap for safe, full-body, at-home workouts with minimum cost and maximum flexibility.

Audio:

For those that may on occasion prefer to listen rather than read, you can simply scan the QR code next to each chapter heading to listen to the audio without the need to download files.

Video:

The majority of the exercises are also accompanied by complimentary videos of my senior class members performing the exercise. If you are unsure how to correctly perform an exercise simply scan the QR code to watch the video

Trust me, muscle weakness is not something you HAVE to deal with as you get older.

No matter your current muscle strength, these simple exercises will help you build a strong body. Say "No, thanks" to the muscle weakness associated with aging and resolve to improve your health and quality of life by getting ahead of frailty before it's too late!

Strength Training for Seniors 50, 60 and Beyond: Resistance and Core Training is ideal for those primarily looking to regain strength and build muscle mass.

If you're more worried about falls, looking to avoid injury, or experiencing aches and pains, Strength Training for Seniors 50, 60 and Beyond: Balance and Stretching is a great addition to your library too!

TABLE OF CONTENTS

RESISTANCE BANDS FOR SENIORS 50, 60 AND BEYOND

CORE TRAINING FOR SENIORS 50, 60 AND BEYOND

RESISTANCE BANDS FOR SENIORS

50, 60 and Beyond

Home Strength Training, Improve Flexibility and Regain Muscle safely using inexpensive bands. Fully illustrated, 32 workouts + 80 videos

DAVID O'CONNOR

FREE BONUS
FITNESS MATERIAL TO HELP YOU ACHIEVE YOUR GOAL

To ensure you gain as much value as possible from Resistance Bands For Seniors, I've put together some additional free bonus materials to help you achieve your goals, including:

- **32 Workout Plans** provided as printable PDF documents (8 each for Beginners, Intermediate, Seated and Advanced).
- **4 fitness Word Puzzles**. As a bit of fun to help maintain brain fitness too.
- **Direct access to the exercise videos** from our members area (without scanning QR Codes)
- **Members Only Access** to videos showing the exercises contained in each of the 32 workout plans (not available from within the book via QR codes)
- **Monthly Newsletter** on topics to help you succeed on your fitness journey.

GET YOUR FREE BONUS MATERIAL

FOREWORD

Exercise is an effective way to maintain and improve physical and mental health, regardless of age.

It is important to recognize that seniors, like any other demographic, have varying fitness levels. You may be just starting out or a seasoned athlete with many years of training behind you. This book is written for all levels, from beginners to advanced.

If this is your first time exercising in a while, or if you're dealing with an illness, don't worry if you cannot do all the exercises in the book.

If you're a beginner, don't expect to be able to do all the exercises right away—take it slow, and work your way up.

The same goes for intermediates—look to the advanced exercises as motivation to continue your fitness journey, but only move on to them when you're ready.

If you're more advanced, use the full range of exercises in the book as a way to mix up your routine and stay motivated. When planning workouts do not feel obliged to only include advanced exercises.

Find a workout routine that works for you, and stick to it, consistency is the key. Above all, remember that your health is the most important thing, and any exercise you do is a step in the right direction.

If you enjoy this book and it helps you achieve your goals, as I most definitely trust it will, please take a minute to leave a short Amazon review. Your feedback will help others considering starting their fitness journey.

SCAN TO LEAVE AMAZON REVIEW

INTRODUCTION

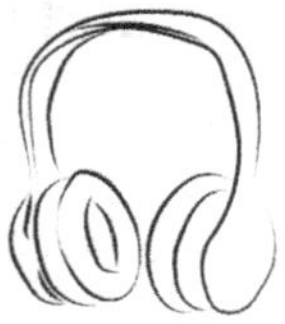

SCAN FOR AUDIO CHAPTER

Physical fitness is not only one of the most important keys to a healthy body, it is the basis of dynamic and creative intellectual activity.

John F. Kennedy

What if There Were a Way for You to Become Stronger?

With the recognition that physical fitness can equate with mental fitness, what if there were an enjoyable, effective way to build strength and endurance, resulting in an improvement to your overall health as you grow older; a convenient, inexpensive, simple form of exercise that:

- Has no need for dumbbells, barbells, kettlebell weights, or exercise machines?
- Does not require expensive equipment or a gym membership?
- Can be performed at home, at work, or just about anywhere?
- Is safe to perform at any age, yet provides the same benefits of weightlifting workouts without the risks?

Resistance Band Training

Resistance Bands are the new alternative to traditional weight training workouts. This method of exercise is quickly growing in popularity for good reason – these bands are easily accessible, portable, and cost effective. Resistance bands are made of stretchable rubber and/or latex materials and are readily available in varying levels of resistance; they are emerging in popularity as the new alternative to achieving optimal fitness levels, regaining lost muscle mass, building strength, and increasing endurance. Seniors are discovering they can become healthier as they attain physical fitness levels they once thought were out of reach.

Resistance bands are proving to be the preferred bodybuilding and strengthening option for anyone, but especially for seniors, because they can be performed at home or just about anywhere; they don't require a gym membership or expensive equipment, and best of all, they really give the results you want – with less risk of injury:

- Safety needs to be a priority when seniors are working out, because muscles and ligaments are less flexible, and more subject to pulls and strains.
- Balance is another concern, and working with heavy weights can cause falls as well as strains. Resistance bands reduce the potential for injury that is common in traditional weight workouts and those that involve a lot of jumping.

In the following 10 chapters, you'll be instructed on how to use these bands to their full advantage, with a comprehensive list of beginner to advanced exercises along with programs for every level of fitness, safety tips to prevent training injuries, and more.

In this book, you'll learn:

1. **How resistance bands work:** In Chapter 1, you will be introduced to the concept of using these stretchable bands to achieve the level of resistance appropriate for your level of fitness in order to challenge your muscles as effectively as possible. Just as lifting heavy weights puts a strain on various muscle groups, resistance bands can do the same, resulting in the positive type of cellular-level damage required to stimulate muscle tissues to rebuild bigger and stronger. Here you will learn why resistance bands are safer than traditional workouts for everyone, but especially for seniors whose muscles, joints, and connective tissues are more susceptible to strains, pulls, tears, and other injuries.
2. **The benefits of this style of training:** Chapter 2 will delve deeper into the benefits of resistance training, and why it's an essential part of preparing for your senior years. You may not realize that a good resistance training program goes beyond preventing injuries, helping to protect your joints and bones, and even improve balance, making you less susceptible to falls. You'll not only look and feel better, but you'll also enjoy a higher level of fitness, resulting in an overall improved quality of life.

3. **Resistance band basics:** In Chapter 3, the world of resistance bands will be opened up to you, so you can understand what types of bands you need, and for what each type is designed. These amazingly simple tools come in a variety of colors – usually to designate varying levels of resistance – and you'll be pleased to know that they are widely available online, and in the many retail stores where you can also find yoga mats and exercise balls. You'll also be impressed to learn just how inexpensive a set of these bands are!
4. **How to jumpstart your workout:** The first round of basic resistance band exercises will be presented in Chapter 4, which is devoted to beginners. I'm sure you're anxious to get going, and this is the best place to start, especially if you are new to working out, or have let a few too many years slip by since you last did any cardio, did a round of pushups and crunches, or hit the gym. Are you ready to make up for lost time? This chapter will be your jumpstart. Start light, and push the resistance levels as you feel able. Be careful not to overdo it; as a senior, your responses and recoveries will be slower. Take it easier than you feel like in the very beginning to avoid injury and avoid overly sore muscles, both of which will decrease motivation to stick with your new fitness routine in the long-term. Just Temper your ambition with patience, and you will reap the rewards.
5. **Intermediate level exercises:** In Chapter 5, we raise the level with some more challenging exercises. Are you ready to tighten those abdominals and bring back that lost six-pack? Or do your upper arms need some work to get those biceps and triceps in better shape? Maybe you need to strengthen your core and back muscles to improve your posture, and there's a good chance your lower body—quadriceps, hamstrings, shins, calves, and ankles—could use some constructive work.
6. **Advanced resistance training:** When you are ready to face the challenge, Chapter 6 will familiarize you with the more advanced resistance band exercises. Use sound judgment, and wait to try the advanced movements until you are comfortable with the beginner and intermediate level movements, and are able to safely and comfortably perform 2 to 3 sets of each of those with at least a medium level of resistance.
7. **Tips for those with special conditions:** Many of you may have certain conditions that require more customized resistance training. These are the specialized resistance exercises for when you are recovering from injury, or if you can't comfortably perform resistance training while standing; alternatives that are done while you are seated, and which offer

the same benefits of muscle development and increased strength and mobility as their standing versions.

8. **Calisthenics and aerobics:** To round out your complete fitness program, you can supplement your resistance band training with bodyweight calisthenics and aerobics. These are two forms of exercise that will increase your overall level of physical fitness, both improving cardiovascular conditioning and increasing strength. Plus, adding variation to your workouts can help prevent boredom, reduce the risk of injuries, and potentially increase the frequency and consistency of your workouts over the long term.
9. **A top athlete's routine:** Discover a highly effective resistance band routine that you can easily learn and practice. This is the workout that Tom Brady uses to maintain the peak level of fitness that allows him to still be a winning National Football League quarterback well into his 40s. This routine works for Tom, and will also work for you.
10. **Extras including safety tips and diet:** Chapter 10 will cover how to protect and strengthen your joints, and reduce pain throughout your body. Then, in the spirit of the *Hippocratic Oath's* 'First, do no harm,' (North, 2012), there will be a summary of safety tips that will help prevent injuries, and enable you to make your fitness program a part of your daily routine, putting more years in your life, and more life in your years.

What about diet?

Yes, what you eat (and how much) is essential to health and fitness, and we'll give you the lowdown on some healthy foods that most experts agree on. I'll be recommending healthy, delicious foods, so you can ignore all those fad diets, and go with the one that will help you live the longest and, most importantly, enjoy the best quality of life possible, so you can feel and perform at peak levels even during your later years.

Meet the Author

Who am I? Well, I'm a Personal Trainer and proud to say I've been studying and practicing physical training for most of my life and can appreciate the benefits this conditioning has done for my own health, not to mention many others whom I have trained so they were able to benefit from this same training and health information. Following are a few notes and quotes to give you a quick overview of my background and experiences, so I can let you know how to start, improve, and finally become an expert in order to achieve a better quality of life, benefiting from my knowledge, and this new exercise method, the benefits of which numerous academic studies have verified, that continues to grow in popularity.

- A fitness nut since my days at UCLA, cross-fit, trail running, and skiing are still my passions. During the last 25 years as a Ski Instructor and Personal Trainer, I've trained people of all ages and abilities to achieve their fitness goals. A couple of years ago my father required assistance to improve his health, having become increasingly sedentary with each passing year. It took a sustained effort to get him to accept that it's never too late to get fit, certainly not at just 65 years of age!
- I guided my father through a simple yet progressively challenging home exercise program, and introduced him to healthier eating habits appropriate for his stage of life and individual body type, also taking into account his specific needs due to a medical condition. Today, he lives a fulfilling, active Californian lifestyle, regularly beating me on the golf course.
- Another source of inspiration for me is George Jedenoff. He's the oldest living graduate of Stanford Graduate School of Business (GSB) and was still skiing Snowbird at the age of 103. George attributes a daily exercise program and a positive mindset for this vitality, "***That's why I'm still here because I've been adaptable and optimistic all my life".*** If you get a moment, watch George's video it is inspirational. He celebrated his 105th birthday in July 2023, and hopes to get at least a couple of days skiing this season at a lower altitude resort than Snowbird. The link and QR code below are to George's video where he shows his daily workout routine. Please take a look, I'm sure you will find it inspirational!

SCAN FOR VIDEO

- Through extensive research, teaching many different forms of exercise over my 25-year coaching career, and working with trainers and specialists both in the USA and Europe, I've become an authority on the latest workouts and lifestyle habits that will allow anyone, especially seniors, to learn and adopt effective, efficient, and safe fitness routines. Routines that will give positive results, both mentally and physically, building slowly to ensure you can follow a sustainable and consistent fitness routine that can be continued for life.

What sets this book apart from other strength and fitness guides is that I use my expertise and experience to describe each exercise in detail, so you can easily understand them and follow along at your own pace. I promise to keep it simple, but I also carefully explain the movements and positions with sufficient detail so you can perform each exercise correctly and avoid injury. As part of my promise to you, each exercise in the book is not only illustrated but accompanied by a QR Code, scan it on your mobile to see a video clip of that specific exercise being performed correctly.

My goal is to make complex subjects easy for the rest of us to understand.

Imagine your life with fewer injuries or pain, greater strength, increased endurance, and better overall health. Imagine how good you will look and feel, knowing you are in the best shape you can achieve. I'm excited to share this knowledge with you now, and help you improve your quality of life. Let's get started with Chapter 1!

CHAPTER 1

Resistance Band Basic Workouts

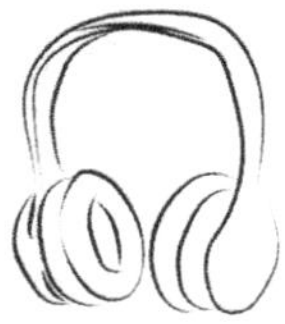

SCAN FOR AUDIO CHAPTER

I think exercise tests us in so many ways: Our skills, our hearts, our ability to bounce back after setbacks, and it can serve us all well as adult athletes.

Peggy Fleming
Olympic Champion Skater

Safely Benefitting and Building Every Part of Your Body

It's all about resistance—physical resistance, that is—when it comes to building muscles, strengthening joints, protecting your bones from breaking, improving your posture and balance, and overall, making you look and feel better about yourself. There are other important components to being able to achieve your state of fitness; notably bodyweight calisthenics, cardiovascular (aerobic) conditioning, and following a healthy diet. We'll get to those subjects later on, but the focus now is on resistance training with stretchable bands and tubes.

This is your orientation to learning how to correctly, safely, and effectively use various types of stretchable bands and tubes to achieve the resistance you need to challenge your muscles. Resistance bands have a few terms—you may also hear the terms 'exercise bands' or 'fitness bands.'

As mentioned in the Introduction, just as lifting heavy weights puts a strain on various muscle groups, resistance bands can be used to achieve a similar effect, resulting in the same tearing down of muscle tissues at the microscopic cellular level, followed by a period of rest to permit the amino acids, peptides, and proteins present in your body to rebuild the damaged muscles, making them bigger and stronger. Your muscles don't care how you achieve the resistance, as long as it's performed correctly, and increases gradually in intensity, allowing them sufficient time to rebuild.

Importantly, using resistance bands is safer than weightlifting, *especially for seniors*, whose muscles, joints, and connective tissues have less strength and flexibility and are therefore more susceptible to strains, pulls, tears, and other injuries.

The Basics

Resistance bands are an easy way to introduce yourself to strength training. You can start at a very low resistance level (if desired) and gradually increase the resistance as you build your strength. Whether you are recovering from injury or building muscle strength, there are bands for every level of physical strength.

Resistance bands are pieces of rubber that form flat loops or thin tubes with handles on each end. Personally I find loop bands are easier to use for total body exercises, but regular flat bands can be just as effective, and may be less expensive than tubes which generally have handles to grip. When it comes to flat bands, you simply grasp them, or wind the ends around your hands for an improved grip. You may also connect one end of a resistance band or tube to a fixed object; we'll get to that in a moment.

Resistance bands and tubes are generally sold in sets and are available in increasing levels of resistance depending on the thickness of the band, and its length. Some sports specialty stores may have long lengths of the flat bands on rollers, which can be cut to customized lengths.

"Using resistance bands helps you build your muscle strength and lowers your risk of injury," advises WebMD 2022, citing the versatility of the bands, which can be used to target any desired body part. They help target weight loss, build leg and core strength, and open up your range of movement to advance to other forms of exercise.

How the Bands Are Used

You will typically be using flat resistance bands in several ways; don't be concerned about the following simple examples, because all resistance exercises will be explained, step-by-step, in later chapters:

- **Using only your hands:** the bands are stretched apart, then slowly returned to the starting position. Imagine a simple overhead stretch where you pull the band apart over your head while gripping the right and left ends of the band. Pause for a moment in this position, then allow the band to contract back to the starting position, for 1 repetition in a series. Now think of doing the same thing across your chest—do you see the similarity in movement to working out with weights and machines?
- **Using one of your hands plus a stationary (unmoving) object:** that the band is attached to, so that you are able to pull and stretch the band away from the object, which might be a doorknob or the leg of a heavy table that you've tied one end of the band to. Imagine standing at a right angle to the doorknob, and stretching the band across your chest as far as you are able, pausing, then letting the band contract back to its starting position. This is similar to pulling on the cables of an exercise machine.
- **Using both of your hands plus a stationary object:** that the band is dependent upon; so for example, you can pull up or pull down with both hands at the same time. Picture looping the band over the *top of a door,* so that you can pull down on the bands to create the kind of resistance you'd experience doing pull-ups, chin-ups, or on a pull-down machine at a gym. Similarly, the band can be looped *under the door* to allow you to pull and stretch it upwards, mimicking the movements of barbell or dumbbell curls to build your biceps. *Variation:* Instead of looping the band under a door, you can stand on the middle of the band to hold it as you pull and stretch it upwards with both arms. It's the same effect: Your biceps will strengthen just as they would with dumbbells!

"You can hold a band in one hand, two hands, loop it around a pole, tie it around your knees or ankles, step on one side, and more," according to a conditioning and strength specialist at New York City's Hospital for Special Surgery. This method is *even better* than using free weights (dumbbells, for example). Jason, a trainer from *Silver Sneakers* (2022) says, "Resistance bands provide more and more resistance as you progress through any given movement. The tighter you pull it, the 'heavier' it gets."

A note of caution: Before we go further, let's pause for a moment to underscore the importance of not allowing the resistance bands or tubes to come loose or slip off whatever they are attached to, or are dependent upon, as in the above examples. Be careful as well not to damage the bands by looping them over rough or sharp objects.

How do you determine which kinds of resistance bands or tubes to purchase and use? Since each of us has our preferences, it's best if you try out the different types of bands and tubes before deciding which type to go with, in order to determine which is the most comfortable for you. Flat stretch bands are found to be more versatile than tubes for some people, while others prefer the handles that the tubes usually have, making gripping easier.

In Chapter 3, we'll go much deeper into the various types of resistance bands and tubes you can select.

Benefits of Resistance Bands

The benefits of resistance band training extend to the gains you'd expect from more traditional forms of resistance workouts, so you should not feel that you're missing out, or that resistance bands are a poor substitute. Consider this:

Tom Brady, the legendary quarterback whose professional football career continued into his 40s, retiring for the second and final time in February 2023, advocates a full body workout routine based entirely on resistance bands. His basic resistance band exercises will be shared with you later in the book.

A quick overview of the benefits which I'll elaborate on further in the next chapter:

- **Increased overall physical strength**, from your neck and shoulders down through your arms, chest, abs and core, legs, ankles, and feet. These gains will be accompanied by an increase in muscle mass if the exercises are sufficiently challenging to your muscles, and if you continue your resistance training over time.
- **Improved posture and balance**, as your back and central body core muscles are stretched and strengthened. These muscles are often weakened by the bad posture we assume by leaning over our smartphones, tablets, and laptops, from sitting too long, and not exercising or walking enough.
- **Increased blood flow and circulation**, resulting from the demands made on your tensioned muscles, requiring your heart to pump more oxygen-rich blood to meet the needs of every muscle cell, and the needs of connective ligaments and tendons. We associate improved circulation with aerobic exercises, but resistance workouts also contribute a meaningful addition.

- **Increased joint and bone strength and health**. Your joints can be the weak or strong point in your body; you have the opportunity with resistance training to strengthen the muscles and connective tissues that will prevent your joints from weakening as you age. The same goes for your entire skeletal system: Strong muscles and connective tissues give your bones the support they need to reduce porosity and prevent breakage.
- **Enhanced mental health and mood** comes from knowing you are taking the effort to be strong and physically healthy, and that you are consciously being proactive in your self-protection. You further benefit from the release of the 'feel good' beta endorphins, which are hormones that come into play following a good resistance or cardiovascular workout. You'll enjoy what's often known as the 'runner's high' for hours.

Inevitably, the question of *increased longevity* arises—will a long-term resistance training program add more years to your life? The answer depends on the combined effect of other factors: cardiovascular conditioning, a healthy diet, abstention from smoking, maintaining a normal weight, management of stress, and lifestyle activities including social interaction are among the most frequently identified factors.

Your genetic profile will have influence, of course, but the most positive approach is to do the best you can with what you have. Of all the actions you have control over, beginning and sustaining a good resistance training program is one of the easiest to take, and one of the most beneficial. Resistance bands and tubes are what makes it easy.

Best for Seniors

When given a choice of resistance training alternatives, age plays a definite role in the selection. Among young adults, generally anything goes, because there's greater flexibility, faster response times to grow muscles, and faster recovery times when there's a strain or pull. So weightlifting, which is potentially the most demanding—and most risky—is a viable option for them.

But once we're out of our 20s and 30s, our bodies' needs and abilities start to change, and our response and recovery times are not as fast or assured as when we were younger. Naturally, as we enter our 50s and 60s, it's a new ballgame altogether, with aches and pains showing up uninvited; that is, even without the challenges and stresses of resistance training.

These are the times to become more careful. And if you are already into your 70s or beyond, your cautions must be even greater. Try doing more repetitions with lighter resistance levels, rather than a few reps of a level that may cause strains. Don't be discouraged; you have every right to perform resistance exercises at any age, but recognize the risks, and don't take unnecessary chances.

In other words, focus on resistance bands as your go-to form of resistance training. You can begin your training with minimal resistance, and there's no chance of dropping a heavy weight on yourself.

There's also an opportunity to improve your balance as you learn the correct form and posture for resistance band exercises. Compare that to the increased risks of losing your balance and falling while lifting weights.

Finally, as a senior, you probably have little interest in having to go to a gym or fitness center, and paying for it! Nor do you want to invest in a set of weights and have them cluttering up your home. Resistance bands are inexpensive, and you can put the entire set in a dresser drawer and still have room for your socks and underwear.

Get Checked Out

This chapter, and most others, include a recommendation to see your doctor or medical professional before beginning an exercise program, especially if you are new to this, and have not worked out in some time.

This applies whether you are planning to conduct resistance or cardiovascular exercises, or ideally, both. You may feel okay, and think you're up to any physical challenge, but you never know what surprises your body may have waiting for you. Let the doctor check you out and clear you for whatever level of working out is medically appropriate for your particular condition.

- If you can't see the doctor before you begin training, play it safe and go slowly using minimal resistance at first. You'll not only benefit by preventing strains or injuries, but you will also find the exercises enjoyable, rather than difficult and enduring. As suggested above, doing more reps with low resistance is less risky than a few reps with greater resistance levels.

- Remember, resistance and other forms of physical training are for the long haul; they are marathons, not sprints. So resist the temptation to push hard and fast. It will pay off generously down the road. And don't forget to see your doctor!

What About Pain?

Any pain that occurs while you are exercising should be taken seriously, especially if it's chest pain. If you feel pain, slow down and see if it goes away; if so, you can continue the exercise at a slower pace, or with less resistance. If the pain persists, stop the exercise, and let your doctor know.

Sometimes it's hard to distinguish pain that's concerning from the discomfort you may feel when you've maximized an exercise, and your muscles are letting you know 'hey, that's enough.' A sharp pain is generally an indication that something's not right and you need to stop immediately. This is different from that feeling your muscles give you when they've been maxed out, and signal that you're reaching your limit of exhaustion.

Don't be influenced by the outdated maxim, "No pain, no gain." Pain is a warning that you need to be attentive to.

The Benefits

We've given you an overview on the benefits of resistance training; now in Chapter 2, you will take a deep dive into the science of resistance band training, gain an understanding of the amazing things your body can do, and how your workouts will transform you.

CHAPTER 2

Benefits of Resistance Band Workouts

SCAN FOR AUDIO CHAPTER

Take care of your body. It's the only place you have to live.

Jim Rohn
entrepreneur and motivationalist

Look Better, Feel Better, Be Better

Let's take a dive into the science and facts behind the benefits of resistance training, and why you as a senior (or soon-to-be senior) should make your workout program an essential part of preparing for your body's currently changing needs, as well as for what's to come.

You may not realize that an effective resistance band training program goes beyond building and strengthening your muscles; it can also aid in preventing injuries, and actually improve your skeletal structure by increasing bone density through firming up the support of your bones as it also strengthens your joints.

Training with resistance bands will also increase your stamina and endurance, help you lose weight, and even help increase your sense of balance so you'll be less susceptible to falls.

Become the best you can be! You'll not only look better and feel better, but you'll also experience the ultimate—a better overall quality of life in your senior years.

How Resistance Bands Protect Your Skeleton

Strength training with resistance bands has been found to help keep your bones strong by increasing calcium and magnesium levels in the body, thus making these essential structural elements for our bones. As a result, these weight-bearing activities contribute to increased bone density, thus preventing or reducing osteoporosis, a leading cause of broken bones among both senior men and women.

As health and fitness editor Robert A. Lyon reports in *Senior Fitness* (2022), workouts with bands can isolate and target every muscle in your body. They're portable so you can do them at home or anywhere else you have enough space, making them ideal for "inclusion into your fitness routine on the go," thus making resistance bands a practical, readily available tool for combating bone loss, bone porosity, and bone breakage.

About Osteoporosis

Osteoporosis is a serious health condition that can cause bones to become weak and porous over time. This condition is characterized by bone loss, and increasing porosity of the bones, making them more fragile and subject to breakage. Although there is no cure for osteoporosis, treatments and lifestyle changes can help improve bone density and decrease the risk of fractures.

Why Does It Happen?

Osteoporosis is caused by a number of factors that lead to bone loss such as age, exercise practices, genetics, diet composition, and an inability (or unwillingness) to carry out daily activities that engage the muscles.

Bone density tests are generally used to diagnose the symptoms of osteoporosis, notably fragile or broken bones.

Orthopedists often recommend lifestyle modifications that can supplement medications through helping to reduce bone loss in patients with osteoporosis. Along with diet and weight management, those lifestyle changes often include recommendations to begin a safe exercise routine, and resistance bands tend to be part of that regimen.

Furthermore, by strengthening the muscles that support the skeletal structure, the risk of the injured or broken bones is reduced. Consider your muscles as the brick-and-mortar of your body, supporting and protecting the steel girders and rebars that form the structure. The stronger and more energized your muscles are, the better they can hold your bones in place, protect them from strains, and giving them much-needed flexibility.

Practicing strengthening exercises with resistance bands can also improve joint mobility by improving the flexibility and strength of the ligaments and tendons that connect your muscles to your bones.

Resistance bands are a great choice for people who want to add more variety and intensity to their workouts, as well as those with joint pain or other medical conditions that preclude them from performing traditional weight-bearing exercises.

- Furthermore, the National Osteoporosis Foundation advises, "Exercise and a nutritious diet are important for reversing osteoporosis." They recommend that "People with osteoporosis should aim to engage in weight bearing exercise (ideally using resistance bands) three times per week for at least 20 minutes each time" (Lyon, 2022).

Research Confirms the Efficacy of Resistance Bands

In response to the question of whether training with resistance bands effectively builds muscle and increases strength and endurance, the Cleveland Clinic (2022) cites a 2019 research report by the National Institutes of Health (NIH) that confirmed training with resistance bands creates virtually the same gains in strength as when using conventional gym machines and free weights.

This report is convincing, so if you've ever doubted whether resistance bands are equal to free weights and weight machines, the following should give you confidence:

Methodology

- To answer the question of just how effective resistance bands and tubes are, the NIH determined that a "Systematic review with meta-analysis, comparing resistance bands and tubes with conventional (weightlifting) devices could clarify and quantify the benefits provided by both modes."
- The objective of these studies was to measure the effects of resistance band training compared to weightlifting training on muscular strength, in varying population groups.

- Participants who used bands were matched with those who used weights; this precaution was to prevent bias due to demographics such as gender, age, where they lived, as well as health, and physical condition. This assured that the results, and any differences between resistance techniques, would be due to the type of equipment used, and not be influenced by other factors.
- A total of eight separate studies were selected to be included in the analyses; each compared resistance training using only tubes and bands with resistance training using only weight machines and dumbbells, finding the results were similar "Regardless of complementary training performed concomitantly, provided it was similar for both groups." The single key measurement of the results were the effects on muscular strength as the outcome.
- In total, the eight studies involved 224 individuals of varying ages up to 88 years, located in diverse regions: The studies were conducted in separate locations, including the U.S., France, Brazil, Spain, and Australia.
- All studies were among people who were already in the habit of performing some form of strength training, but whose health varied. "Regarding health, the samples varied from physically active individuals and athletes to individuals with coronary heart disease and moderate COPD (Chronic obstructive pulmonary disease). The duration of training ranged from 4 to 12 weeks, two to five times a week."

The Results of the Analyses

In summary, the NIH states that "The outcomes of this systematic review and meta-analysis demonstrated that training with elastic resistance provides strength gains similar to training with conventional resistance." In other words, the studies confirmed with statistical confidence that there is "No superiority between training performed with elastic resistance and training with weight machines and/or free weights on strength gain."

Other studies verify these findings:

- "Systematic reviews with meta-analysis ... demonstrated positive effects on muscular strength gained from the use of elastic resistance when compared with a control group in the elderly and individuals with osteoarthritis and fibromyalgia."

Conclusion:

"Evidence from this study suggests that resistance training with elastic devices provides similar strength gains when compared to resistance training performed with conventional weightlifting devices" (Cleveland Clinic, 2022).

The NIH recommended that these results should encourage physiotherapists, coaches, and trainers to recommend using resistance bands and tubes, which are safe and easy to handle, relatively low in cost, and can be used in the home or workplace to effectively build muscle mass and gain muscular strength and endurance.

Additional Advantages to Resistance Bands

Cited by the Cleveland Clinic (2022), exercise physiologist Christopher Travers, MS says that "No matter what your fitness level, resistance bands are a great piece of equipment to use. Resistance bands might not look like much, but they can strengthen your muscles as effectively as more traditional weights," he affirms. The bands may even have an advantage in terms of their effectiveness. As Christopher suggests: "In many ways, bands put more tension on your muscles and work them longer during movements."

Many Weight Lifters Give Up

Weight lifting does not appear to have good staying power among its participants; possibly less continuity than resistance band usage. This suggests there are advantages to the conveniences and unique benefits of resistance bands and tubes. The researchers who conducted the analyses have offered explanations as to why resistance band training may have further advantages over traditional weight lifting practices:

- "Despite the widespread use of conventional devices, such as weight machines and dumbbells, and their results regarding strength gains, it is believed that, on average, 50% of people who adopt this type of training give up during the first year of practice" (NIH, cited by Cleveland Clinic, 2022). No resistance technique can be considered effective if its adherents don't stay with it for the long term.
- This behavior by those who begin resistance training by lifting weights and using weight machines may be traced to factors such as logistical difficulties, financial costs, and

the lack of time to head out to the gym, which make the use of weights impractical in many situations.

- Therefore, because resistance band training does not impose these kinds of difficulties, the use of portable bands and tubes allows for greater accessibility, leading to better adherence, at no loss in the quality and results of the exercises!

So, based on these findings, you can confidently begin resistance training with bands and tubes, and stick with these devices over the long term.

Why Resistance Bands Are So Effective

There's an actual physiological advantage to using stretchable bands and tubes, compared with lifting weights. It's called 'accommodating resistance'. This means the farther you pull a resistance band, the greater the degree of resistance it exerts. This is a different and potentially more beneficial form of resistance compared to a dumbbell or barbell, or a machine with cables and weights.

For example, consider when you perform bicep curls:

- As you curl the dumbbells upwards towards your shoulders, "There comes a point where the curl actually gets 'easy' for your biceps, near the top of the motion." The length of the lever that challenges your biceps decreases as you finish the exercise.
- Therefore, the downward pull of gravity is no longer able to challenge your bicep with the dumbbell, and as a consequence "Your muscle no longer needs to create as much force to fight that challenge." What should be the area of peak resistance – the top of the curl – ends up as a moment of minimal resistance.

In contrast, when you perform a similar upward curling movement with a resistance band, the reverse effect occurs:

- "As you near the top, it doesn't get easier; instead, you have to work to earn the squeeze at the top of the curl." As the band stretches, it fights harder, tensing your bicep increasingly throughout the full range of motion, challenging your muscle fibers via a continuous increase in tension.
- *Men's Health* concludes: You'll be sure to feel the optimal resistance at the top of the curl; there's no "slacking off" as with the dumbbell. "You'll have to squeeze your muscles extra-hard to fight banded resistance" (2022).

Physical Changes You Can Expect

Resistance bands are cited by *BodyGym* (2022) for their effectiveness in improving your posture, increasing blood circulation, reducing the risk of disease, improving mental health including elevating your mood, decreasing the chances of injury during training, and improving balance and mobility.

This is, of course, in addition to helping increase your physical strength and endurance, given that consistent resistance training builds muscle mass.

As confirmed in the NIH meta-analysis discussed above, resistance bands provide similar increases in strength compared to traditional resistance training like weight lifting, with the added benefit of causing increased muscle activation in the ancillary muscles:

- In weight training, and especially for powerlifting, 'ancillary' refers to muscles that support and interact with other muscle groups, including those that help support the main muscles when doing heavy duty lifting during squats (which engage the quadriceps), bench presses (for the chest), and deadlifts (to strengthen the lower back). Training with resistance bands and tubes helps engage these ancillary muscles without using weights.

"Due to the nature of the resistance bands, you will force your muscles to contract faster," reports *BodyGym*, emphasizing that "The constant resistance that you have to work against increases your muscle control when done correctly. The effect is more muscle mass and more significant stability."

Consistency Is Key to Results

It may be tempting to think that you can perform resistance exercises for a brief time, then coast for a while. Perhaps you become satisfied with your physical progress after a month of training, and feel you've earned some time off. But it doesn't work that way.

Unlike the flu and pandemic vaccinations we're all receiving, resistance training is not a one-time shot that will protect you for months or even longer. If you want to continue to grow stronger and increase your endurance, you will need to invest your physical efforts on a continuing, consistent basis. If you don't, your gains will be lost, and the benefits you've earned will diminish.

This does not imply that you should not rest—quite the contrary—since rest is an essential component of effective resistance training. But the rest you need is in days, not weeks or months:

- We've mentioned the process of 'hypertrophy', which occurs when you damage the cells of your muscle fibers during an effective resistance workout, whether it's done with bands or weights. In the 24 to 48 hours that follow, your body undergoes a repair process, with infusions of proteins sent to the damaged muscle fibers. In performing these repairs, there is a small amount of protein overbuilding, which accumulates over time to increase muscle mass, and strength potential.

This is why you do not want to perform resistance exercises using the same muscle groups on consecutive days. If you are a senior, allow at least two days for your muscles to rebuild; possibly even a third day if you feel it's needed. Therefore, you only need three days of resistance training each week to experience maximum benefits.

So what happens when you stop your resistance training, or let too much time pass between workouts? Your muscles will gradually atrophy or diminish in size and strength. Whatever progress you made will be lost. In addition, the psychological benefits from working out—the sense of satisfaction that comes from the feeling of toned and strengthened muscles, and the feel-good post-workout beta endorphins—will not occur.

It's okay if you miss a day from time to time, but try to get in at least two good workouts with your resistance bands every week.

Finally, be sure to get a *full body workout*, rather than limiting your total conditioning to a limited group of muscles, like arms and shoulders, or your chest and abdominals. Optimal health and fitness is dependent on overall conditioning.

You can achieve this by doing full body workouts, with days of rest in between, or you can work different muscle groups on different days. It's okay, for example, to exercise your upper body on one day, and your lower body the next day. You'll learn more about all of these resistance band exercises in subsequent chapters.

Equipment: Let's move on to the types of resistance bands and tubes that you can choose from.

CHAPTER 3

An Introduction to Resistance Bands

SCAN FOR AUDIO CHAPTER

Age is no barrier. It's a limitation you put on your mind.

Jackie Joyner-Kersee
Olympic track athlete

Knowing What to Buy and How to Use

It is time to learn about resistance bands and tubes, so you can determine what you need, and what they will do for you. Despite their basic simplicity, bands and tubes come in a variety of colors to indicate levels of resistance, which range from low level beginner's strength to resistance levels that can challenge even the most serious weight lifters. This chapter will help you understand the advantages of the various types, so you won't be overwhelmed by their many advertising and product displays.

Finding where to buy resistance bands and tubes needn't be difficult; there are loads of offers online, from Amazon to smaller suppliers. Many different types of bands and tubes can also be found at sporting goods stores like Dicks, at specialized retailers that also offer other types of exercise equipment such as yoga mats and exercise balls, and even mass retailers like Target, Walmart, and Bed, Bath & Beyond.

Finding the bands and tubes won't be hard, but selecting the ones that best fit your needs may take some research, and searching a few local or online stores. The objective of this chapter is to help with your decision-making.

Low Cost and Compact

You'll appreciate how inexpensive a set of these bands is, especially compared to the monthly costs of a gym or fitness center membership. And as we've mentioned, you can pack them away easily, bring them with you to work, or when traveling.

How much will you pay? As a quick guideline, you can purchase a set of three resistance bands of varying strengths (that is, resistance levels) for about $15, or a single resistance tube with handles for $10-$15. You may want to consider the many kits and more elaborate sets of bands and tubes available at higher prices. These can range in cost from $25-$50 or more, but that's still nowhere near the cost of a full set of weights, benches and racks, which can add up to hundreds of dollars or more.

Consider too the compact size and portability of resistance bands and tubes, compared to the bulk of weights and related equipment. Would you really want to clutter up your home or office with all that bulky iron and steel?

Bands, Tubes, or Both? Different Types of Resistance Bands

There are really just two distinct types of stretchable resistance devices: flat bands, and cylindrical tubes with handles. But there are variations within these two categories, resulting in a total of nine types of bands. For example, flat stretch bands may be straight or looped; the loop makes certain exercises easier to perform but may also limit other uses. Which type you will choose will depend on how you plan to use them, and with which style you are most comfortable.

Following, you'll find the nine band styles described by fitness authority and editor Evan Porter in *Trusty Spotter* (2020). See if you can relate to the types of bands that seem right for you; they range from very low resistance levels for rehab from injuries, to intense resistance for those who are serious about building big muscles and getting much stronger.

As you review these descriptions, and subsequently 'shop' the options online or at retail, you will realize that the bands are mostly interchangeable; that is, a few basic bands can be used to perform a wide range of exercises. One of the most important considerations is being sure you obtain a range of resistance ranges: low, medium, and high.

1. **Therapy bands:** As the name implies, therapy bands are typically used for rehabilitation. Therapy bands are generally lighter in resistance than other bands. If you are recovering from an injury, especially to a limb or a joint, your doctor may recommend these minimal resistance bands to gradually work and strengthen your muscles without the risk of straining the injured area, or making the injury worse. According to personal trainer Allan Misner in Trusty Spotter (2020), who specializes in training seniors, "These are straight thin elastic bands that provide mild resistance. These are useful for rehabbing an injury as you work to begin rebuilding some basic strength and stability." As with most other bands, you may hold an end in each hand, or attach one end to a sturdy object, or even stand on the band for certain movements. Note that instructions for all types of bands will be coming in subsequent chapters.
2. **Compact bands:** These are bands that are tubular in shape, available either individually, or in a set with varying levels of resistance. These consist of a set of cord-like bands available in varying colors and resistance levels. As with all types of tube-shaped bands, they generally have handles at both ends, or just a handle at one end, plus clips or other anchoring mechanisms that allow you to attach the band to a door or other sturdy object; compact bands may also come with wrist or ankle cuffs. Tubes tend to be longer than flat stretch bands, extending to up to four feet in length. Tubes with plastic handles at one or each end are recommended for training your arms, and upper and lower body. This form of resistance band provides a wide variety of uses, and due to its versatility, is recommended by many trainers and rehab specialists.
3. **Mini loop resistance bands:** These are comparatively small bands, typically nine to 12 inches in length, that are looped around your thighs, knees, ankles or calves. The idea is to provide resistance as you separate your limbs, creating tension between them. They are cited as the best for tensing the glutes and hips, among other lower body muscle groups. Personal trainer Monica Straight says in Trusty Spotter (2020) that "Mini Bands are my current favorite! They're great for lateral workouts, for maintaining form, and intensifying common exercises like squats." When we perform squats, there's a tendency to let the knees come together, but by using a mini loop, you can remain conscious of the need to keep the knees apart. Another advantage of mini loops is their ease of use compared to holding on to the ends of a flat, straight resistance band.

4. **Figure-eight bands:** As the name says, this is a looped band that is connected in the center to form the shape of a number eight, with handles you can grip. This type of band is reminiscent of spring-based stretchable exercise devices that were once popular. The popularity of figure-eight bands is their ease of assisting you in performing many functional exercises. For example, they help to isolate specific muscle groups to increase the effectiveness of strength conditioning. You can also find ways to incorporate this type of band into physical therapy, or pilates exercises. For example, to use a figure-eight band to strengthen your abdominal muscles, you would lie back on a mat in a crunch position, and insert one foot into a loop of the band, holding the other loop with the opposite hand. As you pull with your hand and push with your foot, you will feel your abs tensing. You would perform this exercise for a certain number of stretches, then reverse the position to repeat on the other side. Despite their small, compact size and portability, figure-eight bands can be used to work different muscle groups, and they're great for working different muscle groups. I find these particularly useful when traveling, or if time only permits a quick home workout.
5. **Ring resistance bands:** This type of band resembles a chain with links; it's designed to let you alter the width of your grip, which allows you to easily increase or decrease the degree of resistance. Users of ring bands find them extremely versatile, allowing them to target their hands and arms, neck and shoulders, core and abdominals, joints, thighs, calves, ankles and feet, depending on where they grip the band, and which body part or muscle group they choose to exercise.
6. **Lateral resistance bands:** These are long, flat bands with cuffs on each end that are particularly useful when performing leg exercises. For example, the cuffs facilitate being able to wrap the band around your ankles to perform a movement called 'lateral walk' strength training. This, and other walking exercises with a resistance band, can help you target your hip abductors, and your gluteus maximus and medius (bum) muscles. As an alternative, longer loop bands can also be used for these effects. For example, with the bands attached to your ankles, you can dip down into a half-squat by bending your knees and taking side steps (being careful to not lose your balance!) Walking with bands that constrain your legs can provide a good warmup routine before beginning challenging

cardiovascular exercises. The bands help improve stabilization of your knee joints, and increase ankle stability early in your workouts to help prevent strains and injuries.

7. **Pull up bands:** Here is an excellent example of how resistance bands can be used in place of traditional resistance band exercises: in this case the pull up, which normally requires an elevated horizontal bar. Resistance bands can be used to replicate the full motion and exertion of a real set of pull ups, or can be used at a lower resistance level, to train you to be able to do pull ups later on, as your strength increases. As you will learn, pull up bands can be stretched over a door, enabling you to pull down, providing the equivalent effectivity of a traditional pull up, if the resistance level is sufficient; otherwise, you'll be underachieving the effort. Alternatively, you can use them to assist in a traditional pull up: In a gym or fitness center, you may see a trainer or spotter helping someone do pull ups with a helping upward shove; the resistance bands can play this same role. To perform this function, the resistance band has to be quite long so you can stand on it and extend it to the bar.

8. **Flat resistance bands:** As the name implies, these are simple, flat stretchable bands, without any cuffs, clips or handles. They are simply longer, higher resistance versions of Therapy Bands. They may be purchased in pre-cut lengths, or cut to order from a large roll. If you are cutting to order, be sure the band is long enough for all of the movements you'll be making. Also be sure to get several bands with differing levels of resistance. Exercises that can be performed with these long flat bands include the chest press, lateral raise, lunges, standing or seated curl, and the standing high row. Using your imagination, most weight lifting movements can be replicated with flat bands, and many bodyweight exercises can be intensified (like squats, pull-ups, and push-ups).

9. **Tube bands:** Unlike flat stretchable bands, tube bands are cylindrical, with the further distinction of having handles at each end, or at least a handle at one end, and a clip for an attachment at the other end. At first look, the tube band with handles may look like a jump rope, but don't underestimate its potential. It makes holding on to the band a cinch, and may potentially facilitate your ability to handle greater resistance than you could with a flat band that doesn't have any grip except for the band itself. Tube bands possess the advantage of acting like a cable pulley you'd find at the gym and dumbbells combined.

They are one of the most versatile and useful types of resistance bands available. My advice, if you can only buy one type of resistance band for home use, a set with handles is a great choice. Tube bands with handles may be a bit more expensive than their flat counterparts, but you may find them easier and more effective to use. As noted earlier, you can acquire a basic set of three flat resistance bands for $15 or less, or to get a complete set of bands and tubes with handles, the costs can range from $25-$50 or more.

Now that you know more about the types of bands available, let's take a look at how and where to purchase them.

Where to Purchase

Online: The selection of resistance bands and tubes online is awesome, with hundreds of selections from major retailers like Target and Walmart, to online stores like Amazon, plus many other smaller suppliers.

The upside to buying them online is that you can get information about each offer with a click, and be able to find the best prices.

The downside is the absence of personalized assistance and advice, and having to wait for delivery. Many suppliers offer free, expedited shipping, but make sure you are meeting their minimum payment to qualify. Another downside of online shopping for resistance bands and tubes is the overwhelming selection, making it hard to choose.

Be sure the online vendor offers a satisfaction guarantee, so you can return or exchange your purchase if the resistance bands don't meet your expectations.

Retail: If you live or work near a Target, Walmart, Bed, Bath & Beyond or other mass retailer, chances are good their sporting goods section will have a limited supply of resistance bands to choose from. It will be limited because they don't have the room for as extensive selection as they have online, where they can draw from large warehouse inventories.

The good news is you can see and even test the equipment, and hopefully get some advice from store personnel. And there's no waiting for delivery!

If you can get to sports-focused retailers such as Dick's, Big 5, or Paragon, you will find a larger selection, and will most likely have access to more knowledgeable staff to guide you better in your search.

Using Your Bands: Some Safety Tips

You will use your bands or tubes in essentially two ways: holding one end of the band in each hand, or holding one end while the other end is anchored to an immovable object.

When anchoring: It's important to be attentive in order to prevent injury to yourself, or damage to the band or tube. If an end is clipped or tied to a doorknob or the leg of a dresser or heavy table, ensure it will not detach under the strain you'll be subjecting it to. You do not want the band snapping back and hitting you, especially in the face!

Similarly, be careful if you are attaching the band to a doorknob or are inserting one end into a dresser drawer. Before starting your workout, double check by pulling hard on the band to ensure it's well-anchored.

If your exercise requires draping or looping the band over a door so you can perform variations of pull ups or chest pull downs, be sure the band is far enough from the edge that it won't slip off. And be sure the top of the door isn't rough enough to cut or abrade the rubber material the band is composed of. You can place a small towel under the band to protect it from abrasion.

Note that it's not advised to try to anchor a tube by hooking one handle on a doorknob or other object, because it can slip off during the movement. This can be even more dangerous than the rubber band hitting you!

When gripping both ends of the band or tube: The handles of a tube band make it reasonably sure that you can hang on without trouble, but when you are using a flat band where you're holding onto the rubber stretch band itself, it's a good idea to wrap each end around your hands rather than attempting to clench or squeeze it. Just be aware that wrapping the band like that shortens it and increases its resistance—a good thing to remember when increased tension is desired.

Getting Started

Once you've selected your resistance training bands, you are ready to go! The following chapter will give you a good start with some basic exercises for beginners.

CHAPTER 4

Beginner Resistance Band Exercises

Scan for Audio Chapter

First, do no harm.

Hippocratic Oath

Enthusiasm Tempered by Caution

If you are a beginner or completely new to working out, and want to start getting bigger, stronger muscles and improving your overall well-being, we'll help you get started in achieving results that will make your investment of time and effort worthwhile.

We especially don't want you to either underachieve and end up discouraged, or to overdo it and injure yourself. Too many well-intended seniors start working out enthusiastically, only to become disappointed waiting for results, or sustaining injuries, leading to a lack of motivation and becoming tempted to quit instead of developing a healthy, positive lifelong exercise habit.

You're now ready for a set of basic exercises that will help you become familiar with using resistance bands. You're probably excited to begin, and this is a good place to start, especially if you are new to working out, or haven't done resistance training with weights, calisthenics, or bands in recent years.

Know your limits: As a senior, your responses and recoveries will be slower, so it's recommended that you exercise patience at this point, controlling your ambition to build muscles and grow stronger, so you avoid overdoing it, or causing injuries. As the Hippocratic

Oath taken by new doctors reminds us, caution is the best course. While your risks of injury are less than with weight lifting, you can still cause strains, pulls, and tears, or just over-exhaust yourself if you force your body to exceed your current level of ability.

Preparation

Minimal equipment: Apart from the resistance bands and tubes, there isn't much equipment needed. Wear sweats, or any light stretchable clothing, so you don't constrain movement or range of motion. If there's any kneeling or lying down involved, use a yoga mat or carpet to protect your joints and back.

The way resistance bands can be used is almost limitless. They can be held in one hand, tied around your knees for side-steps, as mentioned earlier, or securely looped around a pole. These are only some of the possibilities available.

Unique advantages: Another advantage compared to free weights, resistance bands provide increasing resistance as you progress through each movement. The tighter you pull it, the greater the bands' resistance and the 'heavier' the movement becomes. This was mentioned previously: A free weight, such as a dumbbell or barbell, gets light at the top of a movement, while resistance bands keep on intensifying the resistance!

Another important benefit unique to resistance bands is enabling you to challenge your muscles from many different angles, which helps you to perform everyday tasks. As you proceed through your day's activities, "You don't just move your arms side to side or your legs up and down. You want to be able to move in a variety of directions," notes Alisha Fetters, C.S.C.S., in *Silver Sneakers*.

Warm Up and Breathing

Warming up: Before beginning even a resistance workout, give your body some preliminary exercise and stretching to get your circulation going, helping your heart to start pumping more blood throughout your body:

- Ideally, you will perform a cardiovascular workout before resistance training, for the most complete oxygenation of all your muscles. 5 to 10 minutes on the treadmill or elliptical, or, if working out at home and time is limited, you can do some brisk walking for five to ten minutes, or climb a few flights of stairs.

- Next do some light stretching and yoga movements, such as the cat-cow, sphinx and cobra, pelvic tilt, downward dog, child's pose, seated leg extensions, and some side stretches (if you're not familiar with these yoga moves and poses, a quick lookup online will show you how to perform each pose). Throw in a few squats and a plank for 30 seconds, and you should be ready to go.
- Perform the movements you plan to make with the resistance bands, but without any resistance initially. This will help loosen your muscles and lubricate the joints that will be involved.
- Give your sense of balance a warmup too; this will help reduce the risk of falling. Stand erect, and raise the knee of your right leg until your thigh is parallel to the floor, or as high as you feel comfortable with. You may wish to gently hold the back of a chair or place one hand against a wall. Hold for 10-15 seconds, then lower and repeat with your left leg.

Breathing: During the warmup, begin to concentrate on your breathing, since managed breathing will improve the quality of your resistance training, as well as improving your state of mindfulness and inner peace:

- Inhale slowly and deeply, extending your gut outwards. This will expand your diaphragm, enable your lungs to fill with more air, and hence, be able to deliver more oxygen to the blood, and onward to your muscles.
- As you perform each move, exhale slowly and fully, pulling in your gut to contract your diaphragm. It should feel like you are pulling your abs towards your spine. More air will be expelled, and with it, more CO_2 and metabolic waste.
- Remain conscious of these deep inhales and exhales, since they will focus your concentration and divert any distressing thoughts—this type of breathing is practiced during yoga, as well as many types of meditation.
- As you perform each resistance exercise, exhale during the harder part of the movement, and inhale during the easier part. For example, exhale as you raise your hands and forearms in a curl (when the resistance increases), and inhale as you lower (as the resistance decreases).

Reps and Sets

Reps: All forms of resistance training are based on doing a certain number of 'reps', also known as repetitions; the consecutive reps are called a 'set'. So if you do 10 reps without stopping to rest, that's one set of 10 reps.

How many reps you perform in a set depends on the resistance of the bands or weight being lifted. Logically, the lighter the resistance, the more reps you can do and vice-versa; heavier weights or resistance will reduce the number of reps you can perform.

For most situations, there is a consensus among trainers and physiologists that the level of resistance should be what you can lift or pull for 8 to 12 reps in a set before finding it difficult to do more:

- Of course, how much you can lift is entirely a function of your personal condition, so no one should dictate to you to curl 10 reps of a 20 lb weight (or its resistance equivalent).
- Through some testing, you should be able to determine what your starting resistance should be to get to that 8 to 12 rep range.
- If your supply of varying resistance bands is limited, you may find that one level is too low, and the next is too high. In that case, opt for the *lower level* of resistance and do more reps to get to the point of *enough!* In time, you'll grow stronger and be able to move up to the next level of resistance to achieve your 8 to 12 reps.

Sets: The standard among noted physiologists is two to three sets of reps per muscle group workout, with a 40 to 60 second rest between each set. This brief rest period gives your muscles some recovery time, so even though the previous set may have exhausted your muscles, they will bounce back enough for you to start another round:

- Don't be surprised if you find it difficult to do the same number of reps in sets two and three that you performed in the first set. This is a positive sign that you are giving yourself an effective, challenging workout. Try to tough it out, knowing the harder you work, the greater the muscle and strength increases you'll experience. (If you need to, extend your rest time between sets to increase recovery time as is individually necessary.)

- Later in your training, when you have been working out regularly for at least one month, you may also want to try increasing the resistance in the latter sets to further work each muscle group; just be prepared to do fewer reps than in the previous set.
- Finally, remember not to perform resistance workouts with the same muscle groups on consecutive days. Give yourself at least one, or ideally two rest days, to allow for the protein-adding hypertrophy process to rebuild and strengthen your muscle fibers and tissues.

Beginner Resistance Band Exercises

These are a group of resistance exercises which are relatively simple and few in number but can give you a full body workout. These moves come together to form a good starter kit if you are new to resistance training with bands, or if you want a short, manageable group of exercises to begin with.

Always remember to keep good form, since bad posture and slouching will reinforce any tendencies to be bent over (which often happens as we age).

Chest Pull Apart #1

This move opens your chest and strengthens your pectoral and shoulder muscles, as well as your arms and wrists. Your posture benefits too:

- Stand upright, holding one end of the band or tube in each hand. Raise your hands to chest height and about six inches out from your chest. Begin the exercise by pulling the bands apart, keeping your elbows close to your body. The resistance level should be sufficient to feel the tension, but not enough to cause strain or extreme difficulty.
- Try to stretch the band until your hands and forearms are perpendicular to your body, that is, pointing to the sides. If you can, extend the movement by reaching out further to the sides; this will engage your lats and upper back muscles.
- As you reach the peak of the stretch, try to force your shoulder blades apart. Pause then slowly return to the starting position. Perform 10 to 12 reps, rest, and repeat for one or two more sets.

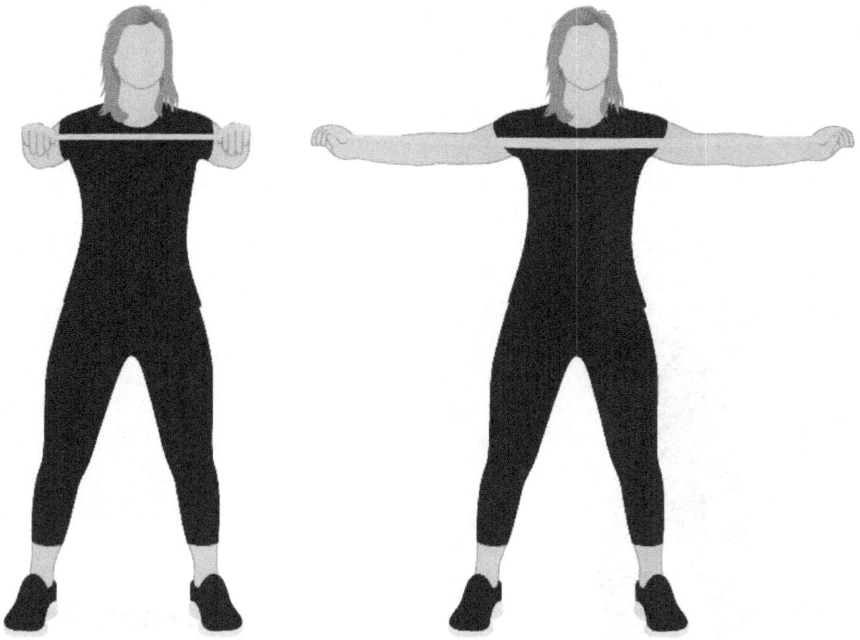

SCAN FOR VIDEO

Lat Pulldown #2

Muscles engaged: The lats (latissimus) that are the muscles just beneath your shoulders and that connect your chest, shoulders, and upper back. This simulates the lat and chest pulldown machine in fitness centers.

- Hold a straight (not looped) flat exercise band or tubular band in both hands. Stand erect with your arms raised directly overhead and held shoulder-width apart. Your palms should face forward.
- Create tension in the band by pulling it until it is fully extended, but not yet stretched. Keep the left arm elevated as you slowly lower your right arm, and pull the band apart until your right hand until it's in line with your shoulder.
- Slowly raise your right arm to the starting position and repeat the exercise with your left arm. That makes 1 rep. Or you may do all of the reps with one arm before repeating with the other arm.
- Perform a first set of 8 to 12 reps with each or both arms. Rest for up to 60 seconds, then perform a second set, and a third if you are able.

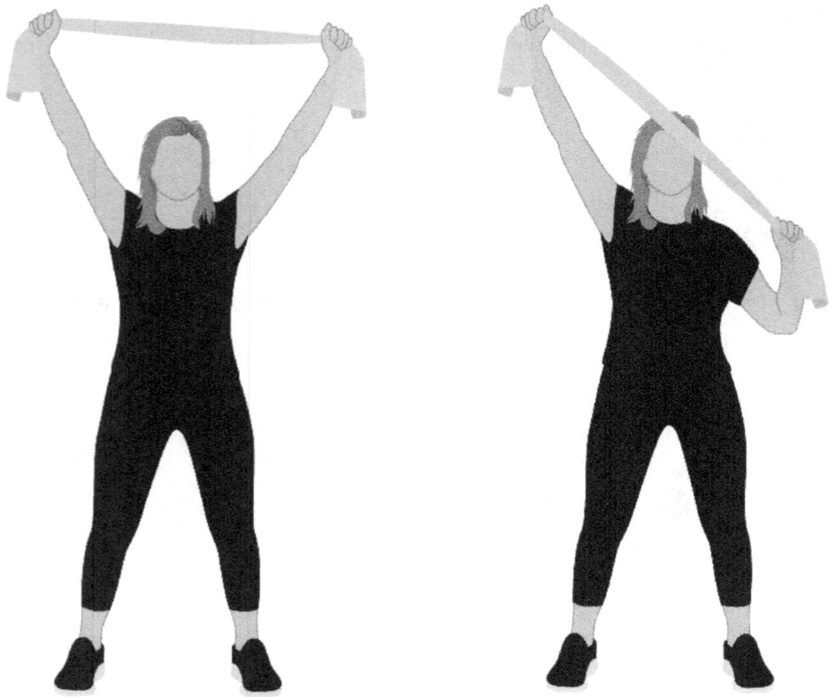

SCAN FOR VIDEO

Seated Row #3

Rowing machines are used to exercise the upper and lower back, the core, and the shoulders. You will like the feeling of this nearly full body exercise.

- Sit in a chair or on a bench with both legs extended, and extend the center of a long band or tube behind the middle of your feet. Hold the ends of the band with each hand, and extend your arms, turned so your palms are facing each other.
- Sit upright (making sure not to bend at the waist), bend your elbows, and pull the band inward, towards your gut. As you reach the peak of the stretch, squeeze your shoulder blades together.
- Return slowly to the starting position and repeat for 10 to 12 reps. Rest for up to 60 seconds, then do a second set.

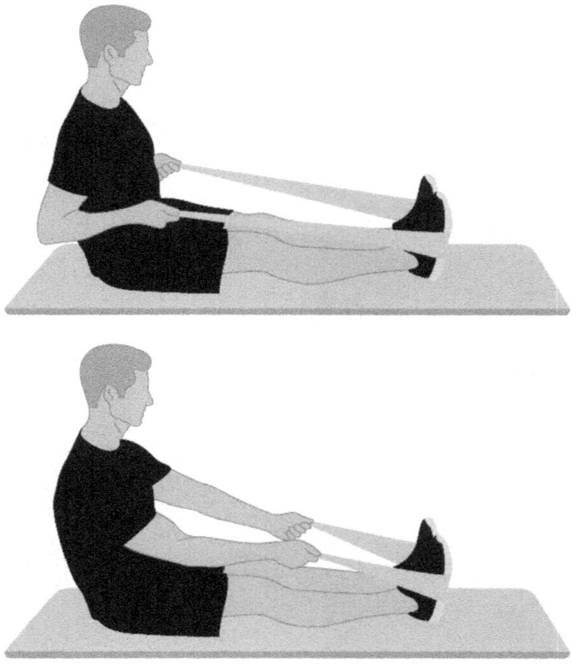

SCAN FOR VIDEO

Modified Seated Row

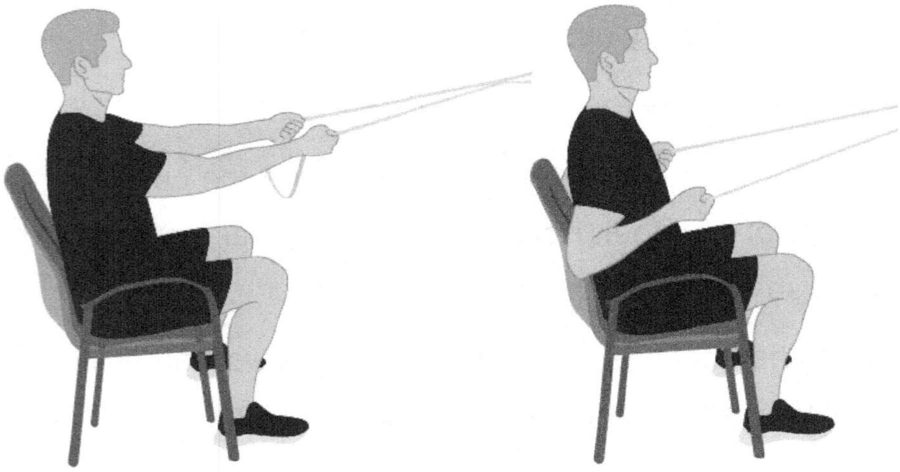

SCAN FOR VIDEO

Pallof Press #4

This is an effective way to improve core stability and help relieve back pain.

- Securely wrap the resistance band around a doorknob or other immovable object. Hold the other end of the band with both hands, raised to chest height. Stand facing the object.
- Step backwards (carefully, so as not to trip) until the band is taut. Then turn your body 90 degrees from the object, so it's on your side. Using both arms, push the band or tube directly forward and hold for 15 seconds, making sure to keep your body straight throughout the movement.
- Return slowly to the starting position. Repeat the exercise on the other side. You may do a second round if comfortable.

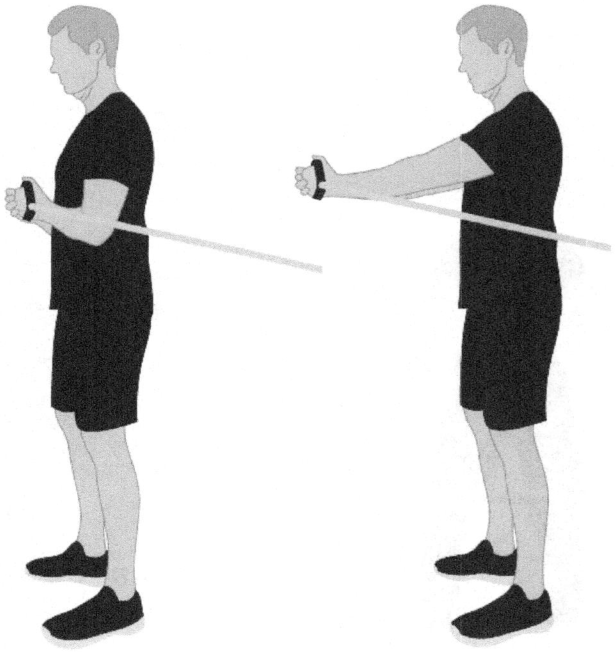

SCAN FOR VIDEO

Band Side Step #5

Walking sideways is good for balance training, but does not build strength, unless, that is, there is some serious resistance involved. Your hip flexors will benefit, as will your glutes, quads and hamstrings, when a looped resistance band gets involved.

- Loop an exercise band around your knees, with the option of (1) above your knees for the least resistance; (2) below your knees for medium resistance; or (3) closer to your ankles for the most resistance.
- Bend your knees slightly and place your feet hip-width apart. Now begin to walk sideways by stepping to one side until the band gives you resistance, then slide your rear foot back over to its starting position. Continue this sidestepping movement for about 10 to 15 feet in one direction, then go back the same way, for the same distance, in the opposite direction.
- Rest for 40 seconds or so, and repeat the back-and-forth one more time.

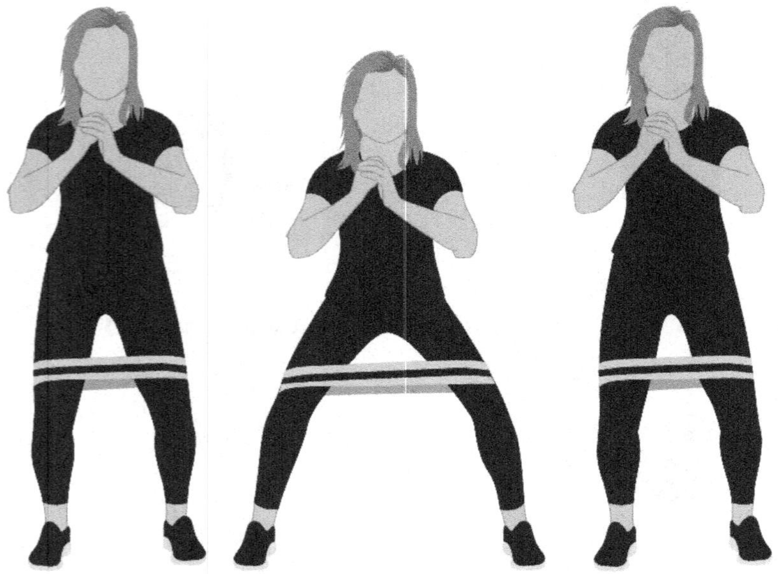

SCAN FOR VIDEO

Clamshell #6

This will engage your glutes while it strengthens your hips muscles and hip flexors.

- Begin by lying down on one side, with a resistance band or tube looped or tied just above your knees. Lie on one side with one leg on top of the other—stacked with your knees bent at a 45-degree angle. Keep your top foot down as you raise your top knee as high as you can, creating tension in the looped band.
- Hold for 5 seconds, then lower your top knee back down. Perform 8 to 10 reps, then roll over to repeat the exercise on the other side.

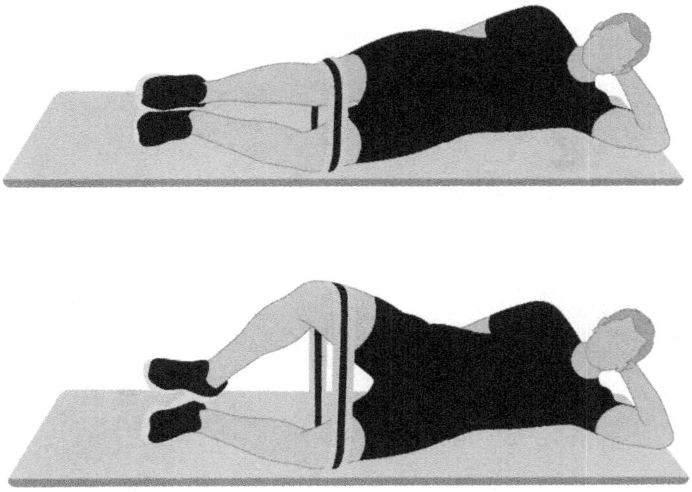

SCAN FOR VIDEO

Side Leg Lift #7

This is similar to the clamshell, but with your legs fully extended. It benefits your hip joints and flexors, and your quadriceps.

- Again, lie on your side with an exercise band or tube looped or tied just above your ankles. Place your head on your lower arm as you place your other hand on the floor in front of your chest; this will help you keep your balance. Keep your legs straight with your upper leg on top of the lower leg.
- While keeping your body steady, slowly raise your upper leg as high as you are able, extending the band as you push against its resistance.
- Hold for 5 seconds and lower your upper leg back down. Perform 8 to 10 reps, then roll over to repeat the exercise on the other side.

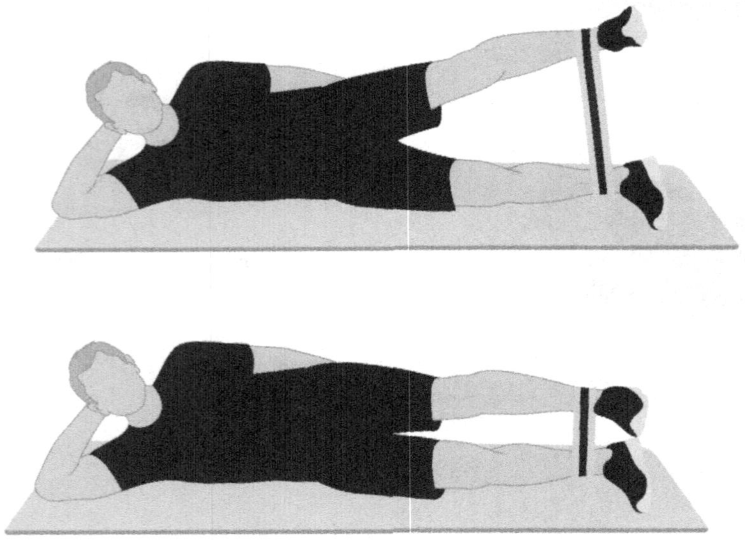

SCAN FOR VIDEO

Chest Press #8

Consider this exercise to be like a standing push up. It will help strengthen your arms, shoulders, and upper back, improving your posture.

- Wrap the band around your back and pull it up so it's directly under your armpits. Hold each end of the band with your hands by your armpits and ensure there's no slack in the band.
- Reach out and extend your arms directly in front of you, keeping your hands and the ends of the band at chest level. Extend your arms fully, pause, then slowly return to the starting position, bringing your hands back, close to your body.
- Perform 10 to 12 repetitions, rest for 20 to 30 seconds, then do a second set. If you are able, perform a third set after another brief rest.

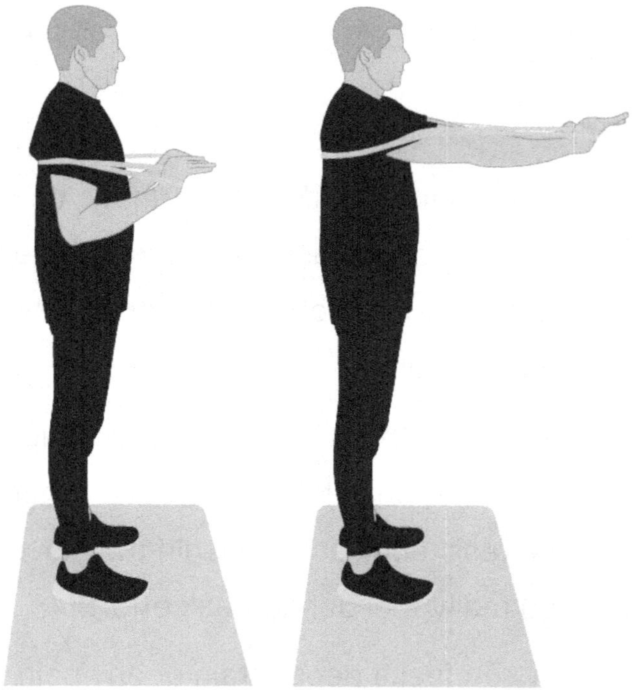

SCAN FOR VIDEO

Onward!

You're now underway, and you've learned some of the best basic starter exercises; now let's advance to more intermediate movements that you can use to focus on your own specific developmental needs.

CHAPTER 5

Intermediate Resistance Band Exercises

SCAN FOR AUDIO CHAPTER

It's going to be a journey. It's not a sprint to get in shape.

Kerri Walsh Jennings

three-time Olympic gold medalist volleyball champion

Moving up and Getting Stronger

With the basic resistance band exercises under your belt, it's time to move up a notch to learn a range of intermediate level movements. These exercises are more challenging than the basics, so practice them carefully by following the instructions, and go slowly at first, so that you are able to keep good form and correct posture.

Another important consideration for intermediate level resistance training is to be sure to have adequate tension (or resistance) as you perform the movements. What does this mean? You should be able to feel at least some resistance as you begin the movement, and that tension should increase to a level that you really feel during peak effort.

Make sure the effort is not so difficult that you feel a deep strain or any pain. If you do, stop, and lower the resistance level of the band, or reduce the degree or length of the stretch.

Remember the Hippocratic edict "First, do no harm," which becomes more relevant as the intensity of your workouts increase. Don't strain or injure yourself; the goal is to stay healthy and fit enough to keep on a consistent resistance training schedule.

Lower Body Intermediates

Hip Thrust #9

This variation of the popular hip thrust will further strengthen and improve your hips through improving their connecting muscles' range of motion.

- After placing your feet in the end loops and placing the center of the band in your lap, slide your hips down to the floor, and slide your feet forward about two feet from your bottom. Begin the movement by raising your hips up off the floor—as high as you can without straining.
- Hold this position for 5 to 10 seconds, then lower your hips to the floor to complete 1 rep.

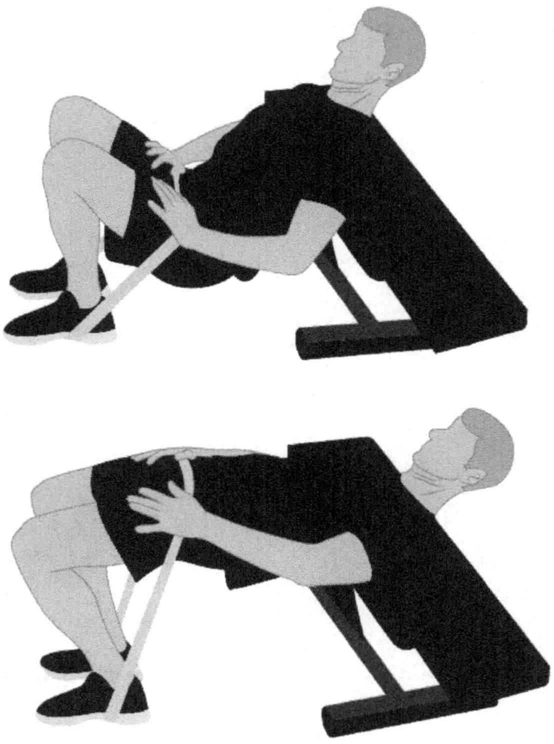

SCAN FOR VIDEO

Bulgarian Split Squat #10

While all squat exercises can benefit the upper thighs, especially the quadriceps, this version adds additional resistance, so the strengthening effect is increased.

- Stand with your back to a sturdy chair or sofa. Take a long looped resistance band that can reach from head to toe; if necessary, tie two shorter bands together to create a larger loop.
- Stand on one end of the looped band with your right foot, placed about 18 to 24 inches forward of your left foot. Place the upper end of the loop around the back of your neck. Lift your left foot backward and place it on the chair or sofa.
- *Be careful:* you may want to have a table or counter next to you to hold on to for balance.
- Begin the squat by bending your right knee and lowering your body, being careful to maintain an upright posture—no bending your back! Dip down as far as you can without causing knee pain, pause, then slowly rise back up to complete 1 rep.
- Perform 8 to 12 reps, then lower your left foot to the floor to step forward on the band, placing your right foot behind you on the chair or sofa, and repeating the exercise on the other side by bending your left knee.

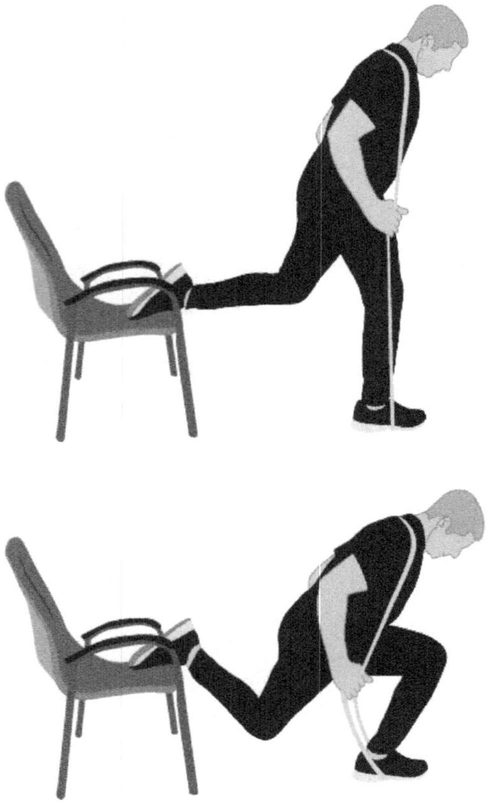

SCAN FOR VIDEO

Upper Body Intermediates

Pull Down #11

Your arms and shoulders will benefit from this exercise, which also strengthens your lats, upper back, and chest.

- Use a long looped resistance band (or tie together the ends of a long straight band to form a loop), and fold it in half. Or use a smaller looped band which needs no folding. Insert your hands into the center of the loop, and lightly press your wrists outward, holding the looped band in place.
- Raise your arms up towards the ceiling, keeping the loop open with your wrists pressed lightly outward. Begin the movement by first spreading your arms outward so that they're at a 45-degree angle (or as far as you are able to go without straining).
- Continue the movement by pulling your arms directly downward until your elbows are pointing toward the floor and the band is either close to or touching your chest. Pause for 1 second, then raise your arms back up and release the tension, making sure to maintain light pressure with the wrists to hold the band in place). This completes 1 rep.
- Do a total of 10 to 20 reps, rest for 30 to 40 seconds, then do a second, and if able, a third set.

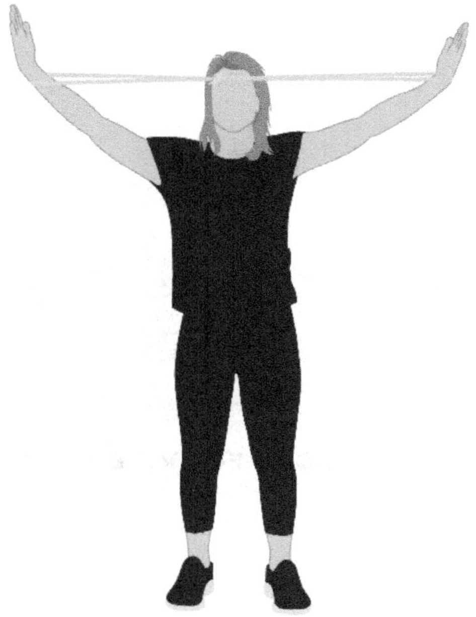

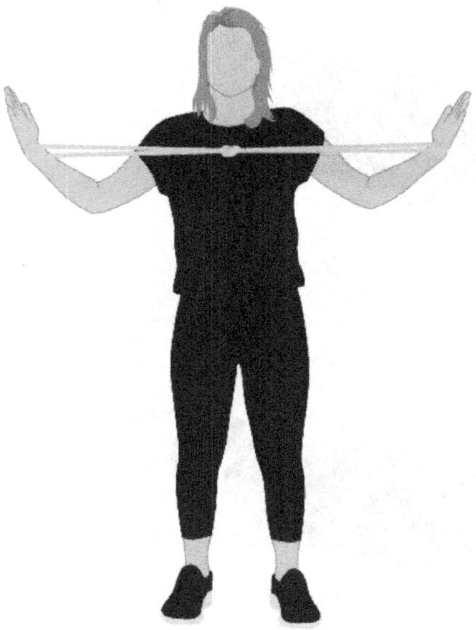

SCAN FOR VIDEO

Banded Push Up #12

Here's how to use a resistance band or tube to make traditional push-ups more challenging. This movement will strengthen your shoulders, upper arms, upper back, and midbody core muscles.

- Take a resistance band or tube; it can be a single length or a large looped band. Place the band behind your shoulders and place your hands—which are grasping the band—in front of your shoulders. Get down on all fours, slide your feet backwards to straighten your legs, and lay your chest on the floor, with your hands (holding the band) beneath your shoulders. Tighten the band so there's no slack.
- Begin the exercise by pushing up and fully extending your arms. You should feel the resistance of the band, making the upward movement harder than without a band. Slowly lower back down to complete 1 rep.
- Do 10 reps, pause for 30 seconds, then continue to do a second set. Once you are conditioned, you may do a third set, and/or increase the level of resistance of the band you are using, or use two bands.

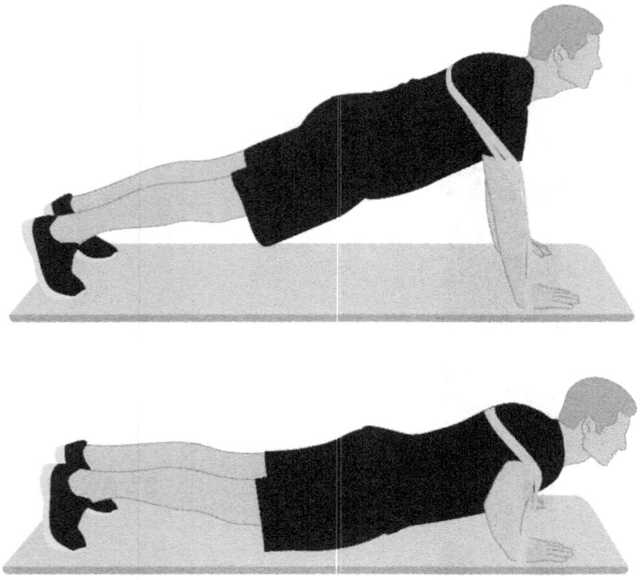

SCAN FOR VIDEO

One Arm Shoulder Press #13

Your shoulders and lats are the primary beneficiaries of this simple but effective movement.

- Stand on a large looped band with your right foot, or use a single (or pair) of straight flat bands. Place your right hand into the upper end of the loop or wrap the upper end of the straight band around your right hand. Raise your right hand to your right shoulder.
- Begin the press by pushing your right hand directly upward towards the ceiling, fully extending your arm. Pause for a moment, then slowly lower your right hand back to your right shoulder. Perform 8 to 12 reps, then repeat with your left side. Do two or three sets, with 20 seconds rest between sets.
- You can increase the intensity of the press by tightening the band or using a higher resistance level.

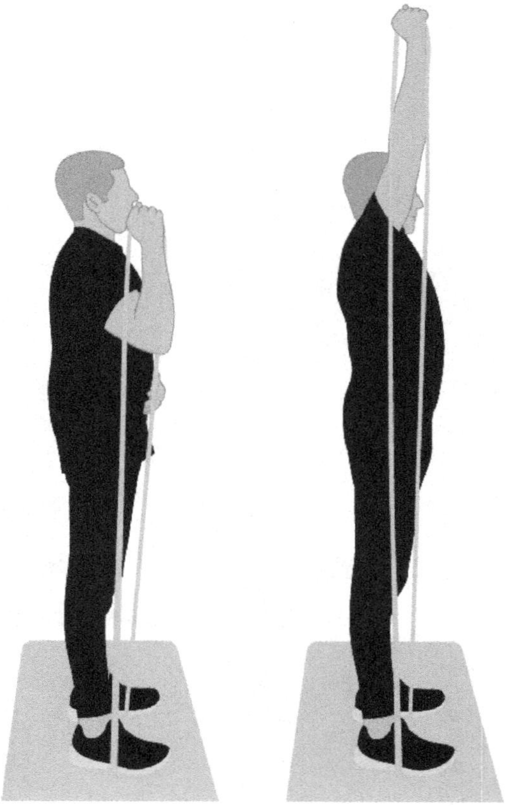

SCAN FOR VIDEO

One Arm Row #14

This is a fundamental shoulder and chest exercise that is typically performed with weights or cable machines; this version uses your resistance bands without the need for weights.

- Stand upright with your feet shoulder-width apart, and your left foot about 24 inches forward of your right. Place a looped resistance band or tube under *both feet* to hold the band in place and partially stretch it.
- With your right hand, bend forward at the waist and grasp *both sections* of the looped band at the center, and extend your right arm downward. If the band seems loose and without tension with your arm fully extended, spread your feet to stretch the band slightly.
- Begin the exercise by pulling your right hand straight up, and try to point your right elbow towards the ceiling. Pause when you've gone as far up as you can, then slowly lower your right hand to the starting position.
- Perform 10 to 12 reps, and switch the position so you can repeat the one arm row with your left arm. A second set is recommended after a 20 to 30 second rest.

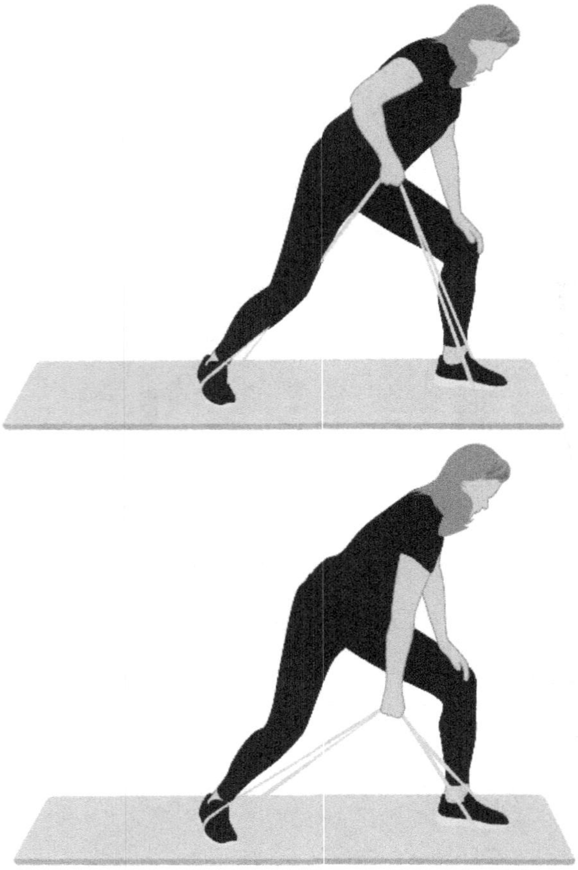

SCAN FOR VIDEO

Mid Body Intermediates

Bend Over #15

You will both loosen and strengthen your lower back, and the rest of the core muscles which surround your body, including the sides, and front abdominals.

- Stand upright and step on a large looped resistance band with both feet. Wrap the upper end of the loop over your head, onto the back of your neck. You should feel a good amount of resistance in this position; if needed, grasp the band and push it out to both sides to increase the stretch.
- Begin the movement by leaning forward from the waist, keeping your back straight, and your knees slightly flexed. Extend forward until your upper body is parallel to the floor, then pause, and slowly rise back up to the erect position. (It is during the upward movement that you should feel the resistance).
- Continue bending up and down for 10 to 15 reps. Rest for 30 seconds, then repeat for a second, and if able, a third set.

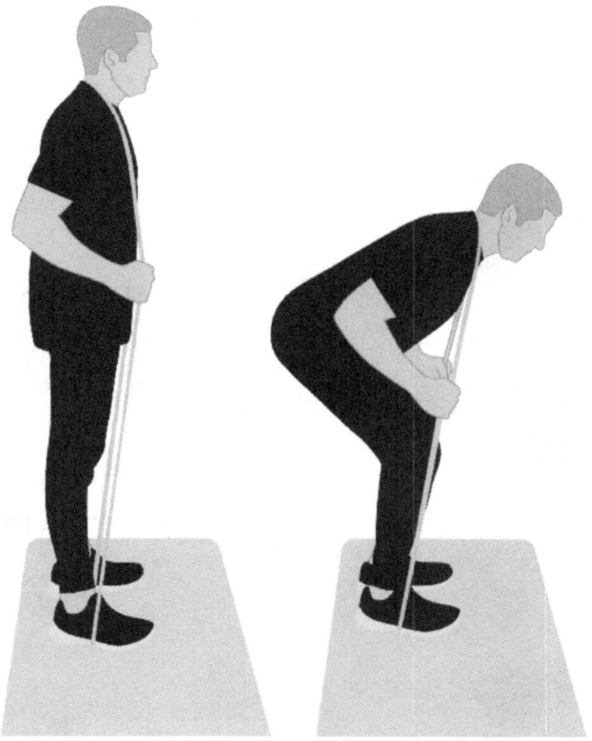

SCAN FOR VIDEO

Banded Dead Bug #16

Your core will be strengthened by this exercise, which is performed lying on a yoga mat or carpet to protect your back. Using your legs to extend the band will also help stretch and strengthen your legs, especially the hamstrings.

- Use a loop mini-band, or tie a straight band into a loop about 12 to 18 inches long. While lying on your back, loop the band over your right foot and hold the other end of the band in your right hand. For the starting position, raise both knees and point them upward, while extending your right hand upward.
- Begin the movement by extending your right leg forward, and pulling back on the band with your right hand; you can adjust the level of band resistance by the degree that you pull back. Return your right leg and right arm to the starting position to complete 1 rep. (in the video clip a very strong band is being used, therefore the arm didn't pull back however, as you can see the arm muscles were still fully engaged to maintain it's position, this is perfectly fine)
- Do about 12 reps on the right side, then switch and do 12 on the left side. Be sure not to go too fast, and to maintain a good amount of tension on the band for resistance.

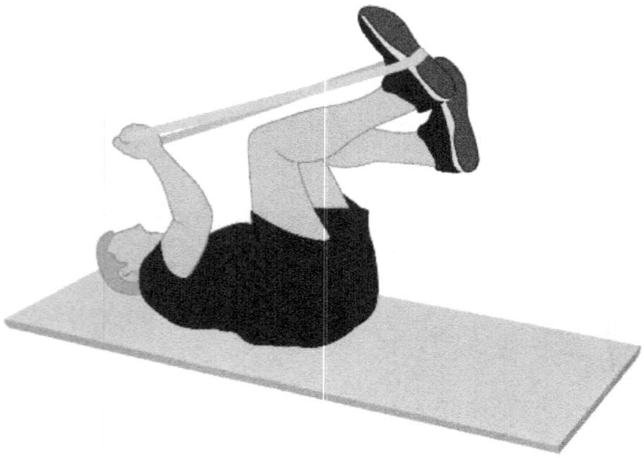

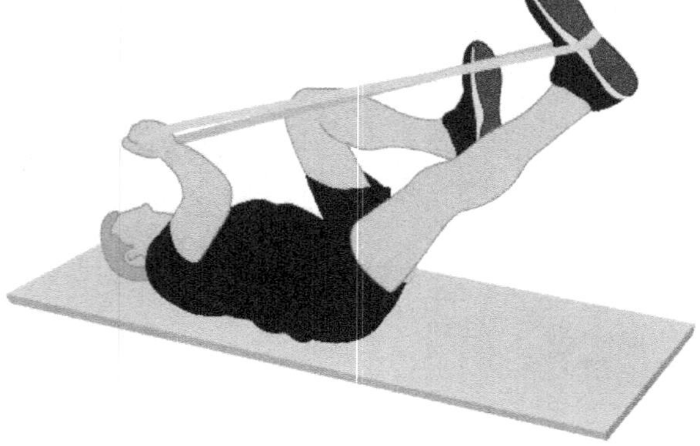

SCAN FOR VIDEO

Banded Plank Walk #17

The upper and lower abdominals and the entire core will gain strength and endurance from the exercise, and it will also be of benefit to your legs and shoulders.

- Place a mini loop band around your legs, just above your knees. Assume the push up or straight arm plank starting position with both arms fully extended, your back straight, and your lower body supported on your toes.
- Begin by pulling your right knee forward towards your chest and placing your right foot on the floor. Now pull your left leg forward in the same manner, so both knees are now in the same forward position. Continue by first returning your right leg to the starting, fully extended position, then follow with the left leg. You should now be back to the original plank position.
- Repeat the right-then-left movements for 8 to 10 reps, pause for 30 seconds, then do a second set.

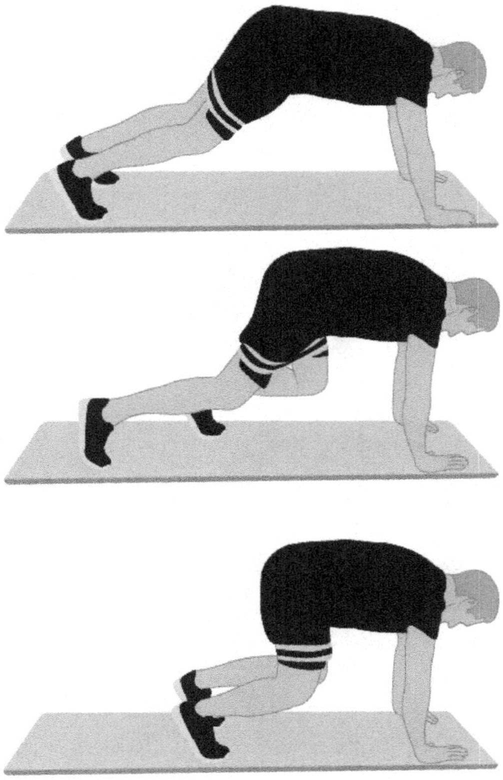

SCAN FOR VIDEO

Special Exercises

Before moving forward to Advanced exercises, we're going to cover special exercises for when you are recovering from injury, and when circumstances require you to perform movements while seated.

CHAPTER 6

Resistance Training for Special Conditions

SCAN FOR AUDIO CHAPTER

I just knew if it could be done, it had to be done, and I did it.

Gertrude Ederle
Olympic swimming champion;
world record holder

Injury Recovery and Seated Workouts

This group of specialized resistance exercises is for when you are recovering from injury, or if you can't comfortably perform resistance training while standing; alternatives that are done while you are seated, and which offer the same benefits of strengthening and muscle development as their standing versions.

Seated resistance exercises are not limited to those who have difficulty standing, or with keeping their balance. Anyone can use these seated movements to perform a full body workout, or to focus on specific muscle groups, for example the upper body, core, and lower body.

Recovery Band Exercises for Injuries

No matter how much you think that injuries are what happen to other people, a day may come when you get hurt during a workout or develop an injury through an accumulation of small injuries from many workouts. It may be a slight strain that will go away in a matter of days, or more often, it can be a more serious tear or pull that will take some time and attention in order to fully heal.

Immediate Action

If you feel pain from a pull, strain, or other exercise-induced discomfort, there is a set of actions abbreviated as 'RICE', which stands for Rest, Ice, Compression, and Elevation.

- Whether this is effective is under debate among doctors and trainers, but it's worth trying. Whenever I suffer any minor pulls or strains, I've found the RICE method to reduce the symptoms, especially if applied immediately after the problem occurs.
- Apply ice wrapped in a protective cloth as soon as possible after the injury to help reduce swelling; similarly, elevation may limit swelling if this is done soon after the injury has been sustained.
- Be careful that any compression does not aggravate the injury, especially if there is any risk of a broken bone.

Get It Checked

Any injury that lasts more than a few days needs medical attention, so if you're hurting, head to the doctor and get it checked out. X-rays or a scan may be necessary to get an inside look at what's going on, and the prognosis may require treatment.

If the injury isn't too serious, there's a good chance you can manage the recovery through healing practices such as outlined by a professional, and some rest. Below, you'll find tips on the basics of what to do and when to do it in order to minimize trauma, and get you back to working out as quickly as possible.

You might think that rest is the only way to treat injuries, but it's actually a combination of rest plus light exercise that often works best. The key is to select exercises that encourage flexibility without straining or aggravating the injury. Bands can be safely used at low resistance levels, and given their portability, can be carried most anywhere, and used when needed.

According to *GND Fitness* (2022), resistance bands can support recovery from "Tennis elbow, IT band injury, ankle sprain, knee strain, dislocated shoulder, and hip bursitis." As noted earlier, resistance bands can strengthen weak, porous bones to prevent the progression of osteoporosis, and reduce the risks of broken bones.

Go Lighter in Resistance

Recovery requires a reversal of the training to build and strengthen muscles; instead of doing, say, 8 to 12 reps in a set, to recover safely you should be able to perform 20 or even 30 reps. And even then, you should stop as soon as it starts to become difficult, resisting the temptation to push on.

Assuming you'll be using very light resistance, you can perform many of the resistance band exercises we've already covered in previous chapters, especially those introduced in the chapter for beginners, such as:

- Chest pull aparts, seated rows, lat pull downs, leg extensions, pallof press, side leg lifts, clamshells, and banded side-steps.
- You may also try some of the intermediate exercises, as long as you are careful to keep the resistance at the lowest levels possible.

"Be patient, make gradual improvement and let your body guide you to full recovery and you will soon be back to your pre-injury condition," *GND Fitness* (2022) counsels.

Seated Resistance Band Exercises

Take a seat, literally. For the following exercises, you'll simply need a regular chair that is sturdy, and not likely to tip over easily. The chair should be without arms, which may constrain your movements or range of motion.

Alternatively, you can sit on a bench, whether it's in a fitness center, a park, or your office. You can be seated anywhere you'd like to do these convenient and safe resistance band workouts:

- Why be seated? As we mature, our balance can diminish, and certain standing movements may become harder to do without the risk of falling.
- Some seniors experience difficulty standing or walking, may be in a wheelchair, or need a walker or rollator to get around. For those with any of these challenges, being able to have a complete resistance training workout while seated is an extremely valuable option.

Even if you are fully mobile, doing your workout while seated can provide a variation in your routine, and maybe work some muscle groups differently. So, I invite you to give the following a try, with the pleasant discovery that they're as beneficial as fitness experts say they are.

Pointed Toes #18

This fairly simple yet effective movement, performed one leg at a time, will work your lower leg muscles, calves, ankles, and feet.

- Sit upright and face forward, holding one end of a long resistance band or tube in each hand. Place your right foot on the center of the band so it's up against the ball of your foot. Pull the band to create tension as you extend your right leg fully outward and up to hip height, or as high as you can.
- Flex your foot by tilting your toes back towards your knee, pausing, then bending your foot in the opposite direction, forward then downward. Return your foot to the starting position to complete 1 rep. Be sure there is tension throughout the entire movement.
- Do 5 slow, deliberate reps with the right foot, and 5 with the left. Pause, then do a second set of 5 reps with each foot.

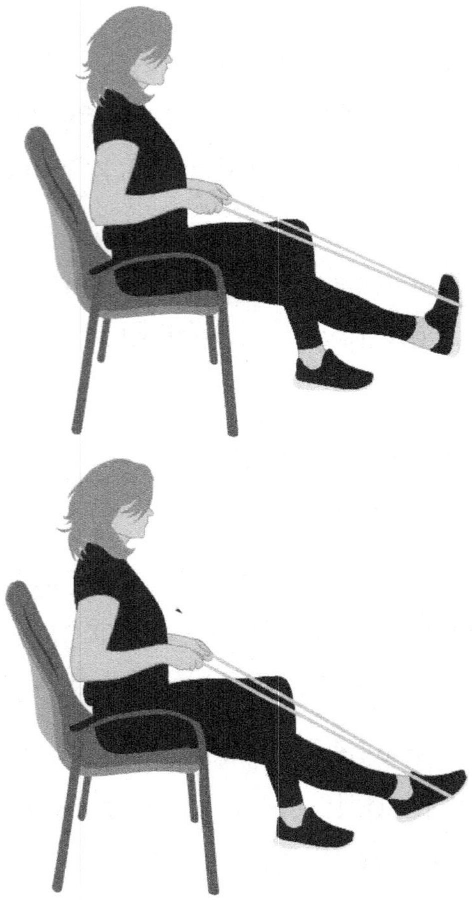

SCAN FOR VIDEO

Leg Lift #19

Your quadriceps—the strong, large muscles in the front of your thighs—are the primary beneficiary of this move.

- Begin as in the previous exercise, seated upright, with one foot on the center of the band so it's up against the ball of your foot, while holding the ends of the band in each hand. Fully extend your leg, taking up any slack, and pull on the band to create tension.
- Slowly raise your leg so your toes are pointing toward the ceiling; take it up to hip-level or as close as you can, being sure to keep the band tense so your leg has to work hard. Hold your leg up for 5 to 10 seconds.
- Lower your leg to the starting position, pause for a second or two, then repeat for a total of 5 reps. Switch, and do the same with the other leg. You may do a second, and possibly a third set if you are up to it.

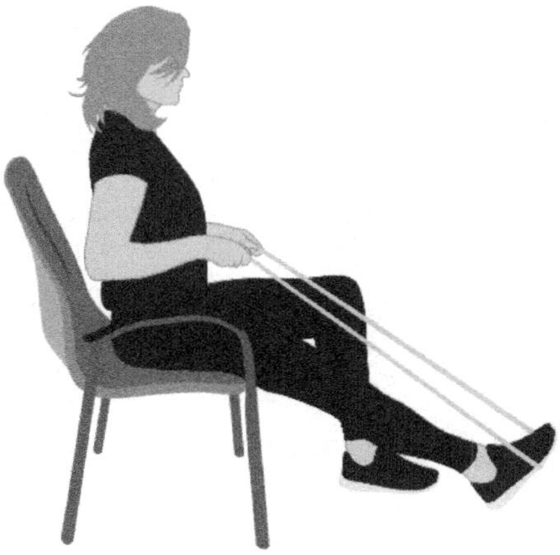

SCAN FOR VIDEO

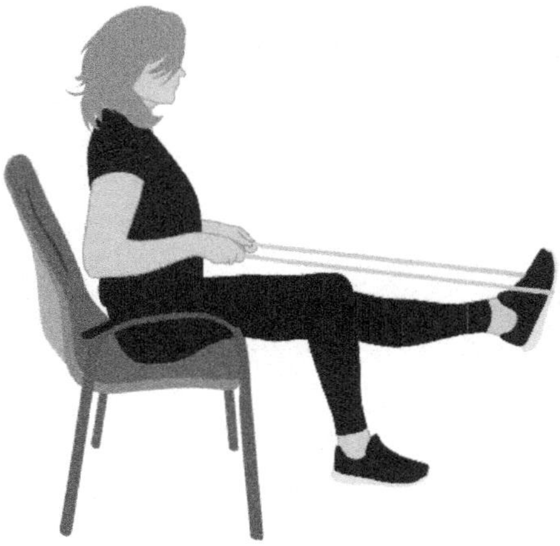

Modified Leg Lift

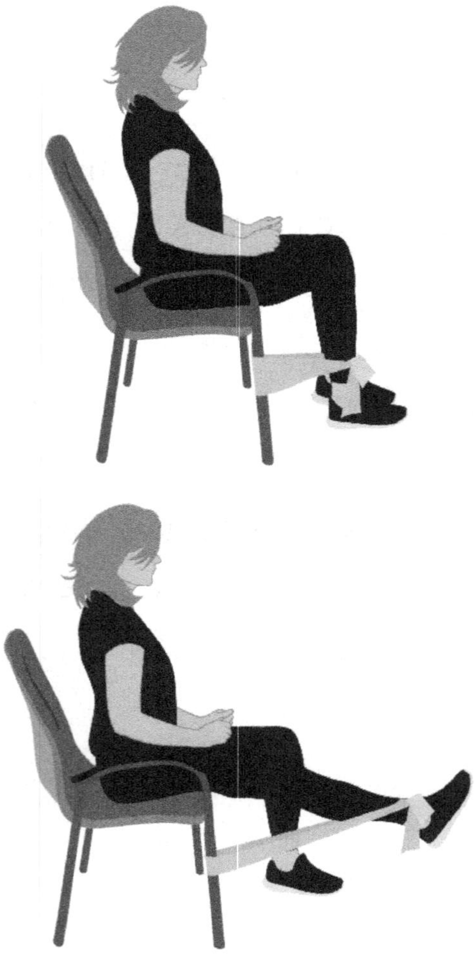

SCAN FOR VIDEO

Leg Press #20

This third leg exercise benefits the quads, hamstrings, glutes, and hips.

- This also begins in the same position as the previous two exercises; you should be seated upright with the band against the ball of the foot, with your leg extended and raised.
- Holding the band with each hand, pull as you bend the knee of the raised leg, pulling it back towards your chest. Continue pulling on the resistance band as you then extend your leg back to its starting position. You should feel a good amount of tension as your leg straightens and your foot moves forward.
- Do a total of 5 to 10 reps with each leg, pausing for 20 to 30 seconds before performing a second set. Depending on how much resistance is involved, you may be able to do a third set.

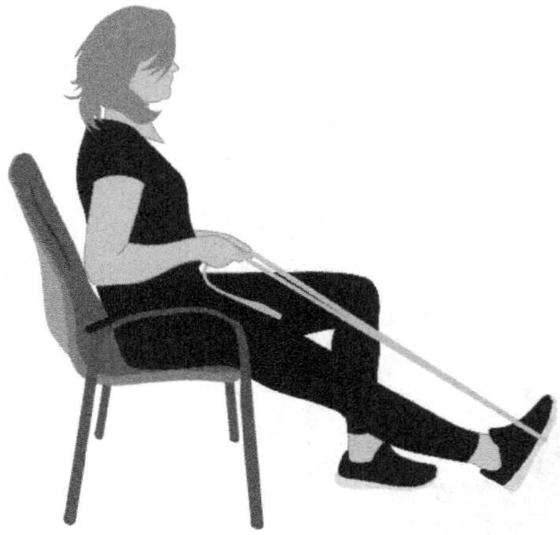

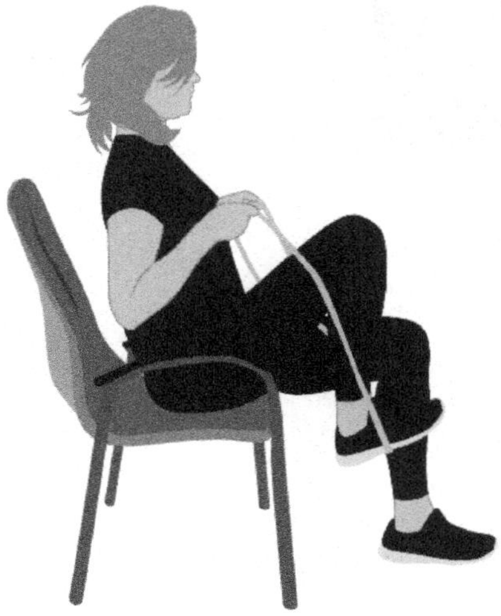

SCAN FOR VIDEO

Hip Opening #21

This is the last of the moderate level leg exercises; it tenses and strengthens the muscles of the hip joints and thighs, with the secondary benefit of strengthening the glutes.

- While seated, take a long resistance band and lay it across your thighs, just behind your knees. Now wrap the band around your thighs by folding each end under your thighs and pulling the ends directly upward. You should have now formed a loop that extends completely around your thighs. Maintain tension by holding the bands upward.
- Lift your right foot slightly, and swing your right leg out to the side, increasing the resistance and feeling the tension in your right thigh and hip. Hold for 2 or 3 seconds before returning to the center position.
- Do a total of 5 to 8 reps, then repeat with your left leg. You may do additional sets if able.

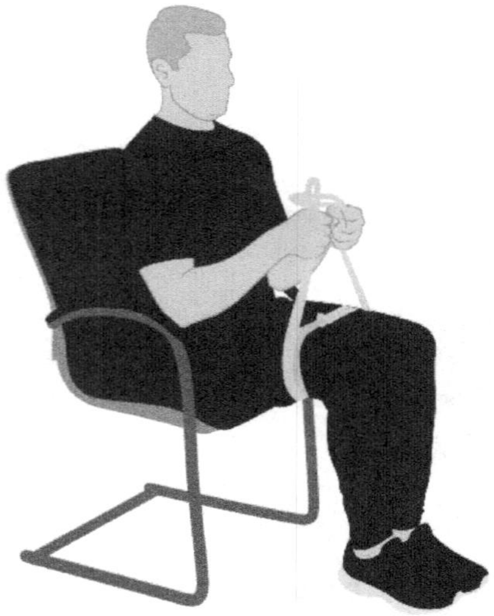

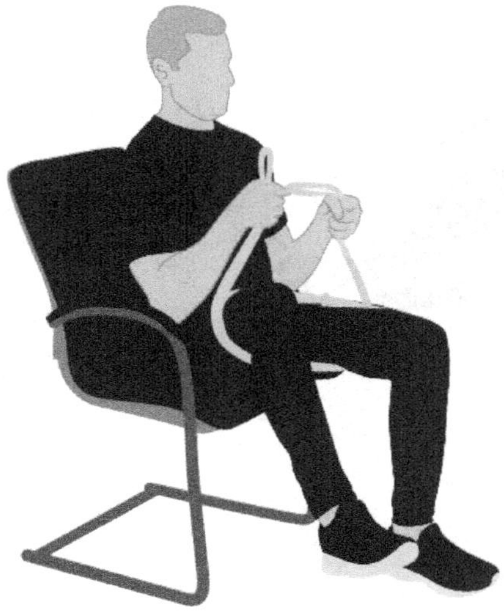

SCAN FOR VIDEO

Abdominal Lean #22

Moving on to our core, the abdominal muscles are extremely important; they support our trunk, allow for better movement and less chance of back injuries, and hold our organs in place. The following move is deceptively simple, but its efficacy depends on your keeping tension on the resistance band throughout the movement.

- Seat yourself in the middle of the chair to leave space behind you, and place your feet flat on the floor, about hip-distance apart. Hold the resistance band or tube at shoulder level, stretched sufficiently to create a good amount of tension.
- Sit up straight, keeping your head, neck, and spine in vertical alignment; tighten your abdominals to engage your core.
- Begin the exercise by leaning as far back as you can to feel tension in the abdominals. Hold for 5 seconds, then rise back up to the upright position to complete 1 rep.
- Perform 10 reps, being careful to go back and forward slowly to fully benefit from the exercise. Rest for 20 seconds, then do a second set.

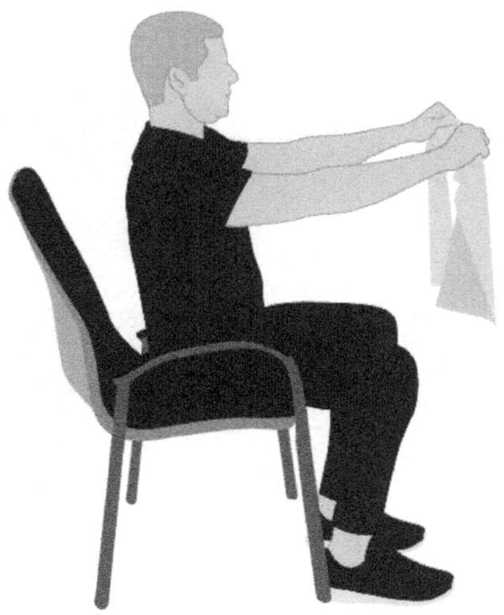

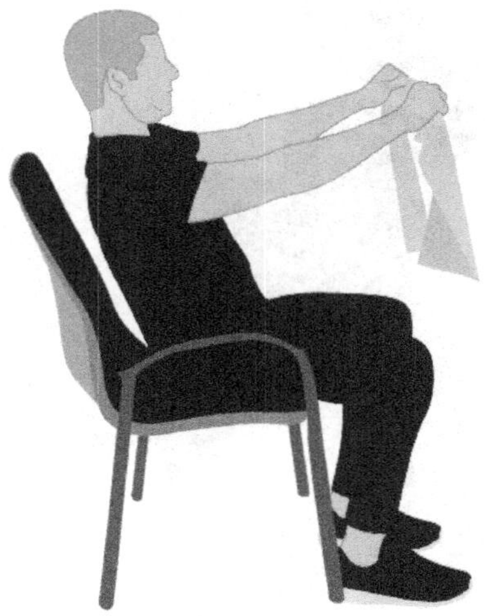

SCAN FOR VIDEO

Chest Press #23

You'll recognize this exercise from the previous chapter, but now you'll see how the same exercise, with the same strengthening and postural benefits as a traditional Chest Press, can be performed while sitting instead of standing.

- While seated in an upright position, wrap the resistance band or tube behind your back and place it just below your armpits. Hold each end of the band and pull enough to ensure there's no slack in the band.
- Extend your arms forward at chest height. Pause when your arms are fully straightened, then slowly return them to the starting position, bringing your hands close to your body.
- Perform 10 to 12 reps; the resistance level should be enough for these reps to be challenging. Rest for 20 to 30 seconds, then do a second set. If you are able, a third set can follow another brief rest period.

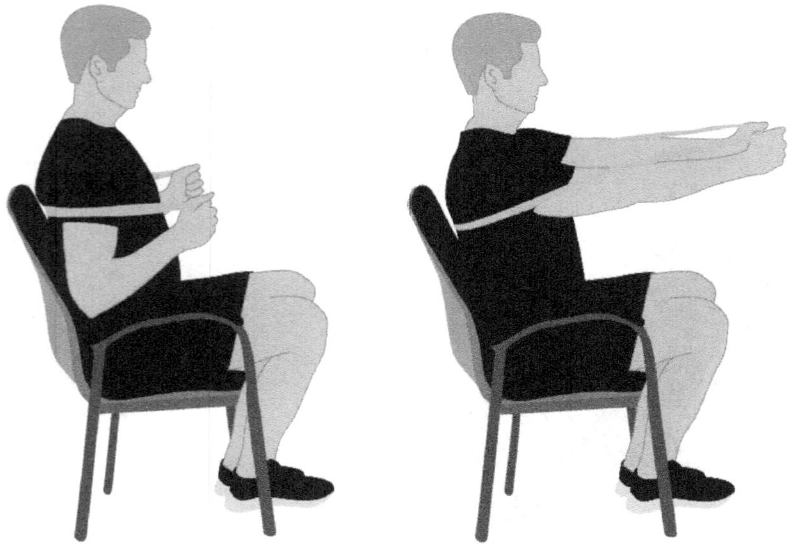

SCAN FOR VIDEO

Shoulder Press (Upwards) #24

This exercise will isolate the shoulder's rotator cuff muscles, and also strengthen the muscles of your arms, especially the triceps in the rear of your upper arms.

- While seated, hold a long resistance band in your right hand, and lower the other end of the band to the floor. Step on the band with your right foot, and reach up with your right hand to your right shoulder.
- At this point, there should be light tension in the band; if it's not tense enough, shorten the length between your hand and foot, and if it's too tense, lift your right foot and release some slack.
- Begin the exercise by lifting your right hand directly upward, pressing it towards the ceiling, and extend until your arm is straight. (Be sure to keep your right foot firmly in the band—don't let it slip out).
- Pause for 2 seconds, then slowly lower your hand back to the starting position. Repeat 10 to 12 times, then switch sides.

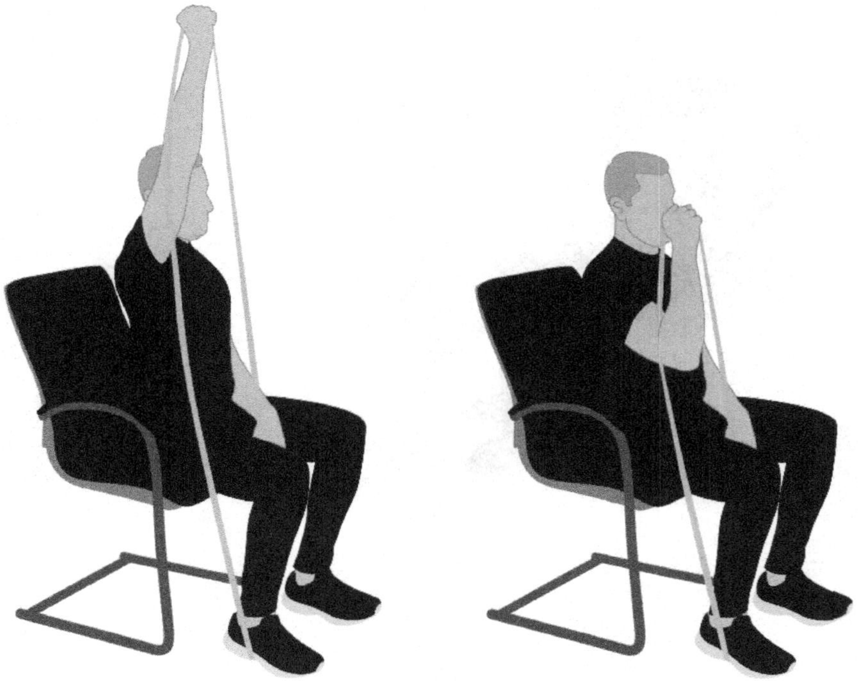

SCAN FOR VIDEO

Triceps Extension (v.1) #25

If the previous exercise works your triceps, this one will do so even more. It will also help strengthen your shoulders and wrists.

- Be seated, and hold one end of a long resistance band in your right hand, and rest the other end on the floor. Step on that end with your right foot to hold it in place.
- Starting with your right hand by your right hip, pull your right hand up to your shoulder with your elbow pointing to the rear, and make sure there is a moderate amount of tension—not too much.
- Continue the movement by straightening your right arm as you swing it back, so your right hand is now pointing to the rear. Be sure to fully extend your right arm. Pause, then rotate your right hand to return it to your shoulder, and point your right elbow to the rear. This completes 1 rep.
- Do a total of 8 to 10 reps, then switch to the left side and repeat. Do a second and third set if you are able.

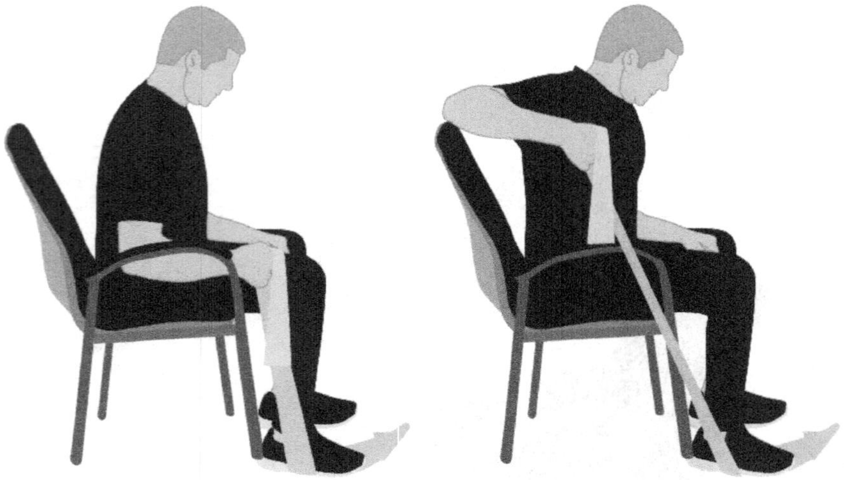

SCAN FOR VIDEO

Triceps Extension (v.2) #26

If the previous triceps press seems complicated, here is a simpler alternative with equally effective results.

- Be seated, and as in v.1, hold one end of a long resistance band in your right hand, and rest the other end on the floor. Step on that end with your right foot to hold it in place.
- Raise your right hand to your right shoulder, and ensure there is resistance in the band at this stage. Raise your upper arm until it is parallel to the floor; your elbow is pointing forward, and your right hand is pointing rearward. You should already feel some tightness in your triceps.
- Begin the movement by pulling the band upward and forward at about a 45-degree angle. Pause for 2 to 3 seconds, then return your hand and arm to the starting position. This completes 1 rep.
- Perform 8 to 10 reps, then switch to the left side and repeat. Do a second and third set if you are able.

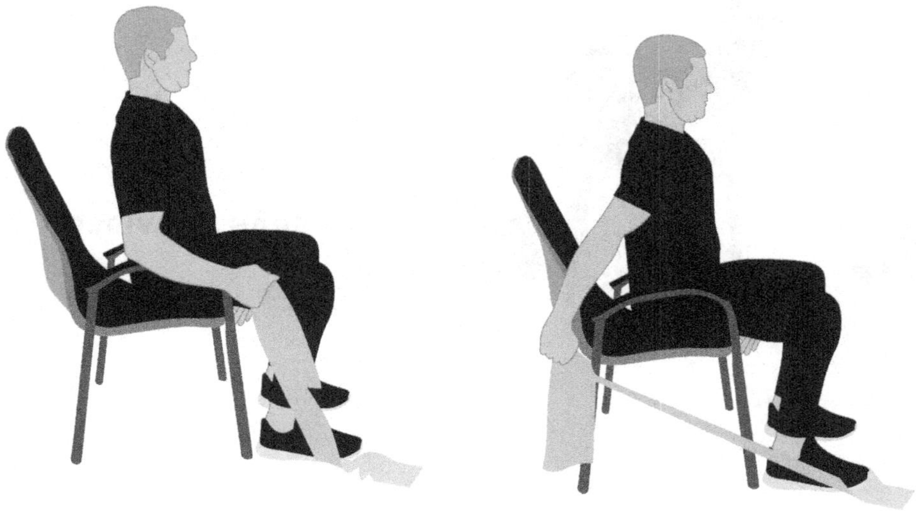

SCAN FOR VIDEO

Biceps Curl (v.1) #27

This classic is often performed by weightlifters in a seated position on a bench with a backrest; you can do the same in a chair using your resistance bands, and with equal benefits.

While seated, hold the band in your right hand, and step on the other end with your right foot. To achieve the correct resistance, hold your arm fully extended downward, with your hand at the level of your hip; the band should be without any slack.

Begin by curling your right hand upward, keeping your elbow tight to your side, and raise your hand until it is close to your right shoulder. Pause, then curl your arm and hand downward to the starting position to complete 1 rep.

Do 10 reps, then switch to the left side. Ideally, you should perform a total of three sets; it's okay with this move if you find it hard to do the full number of reps by the third set.

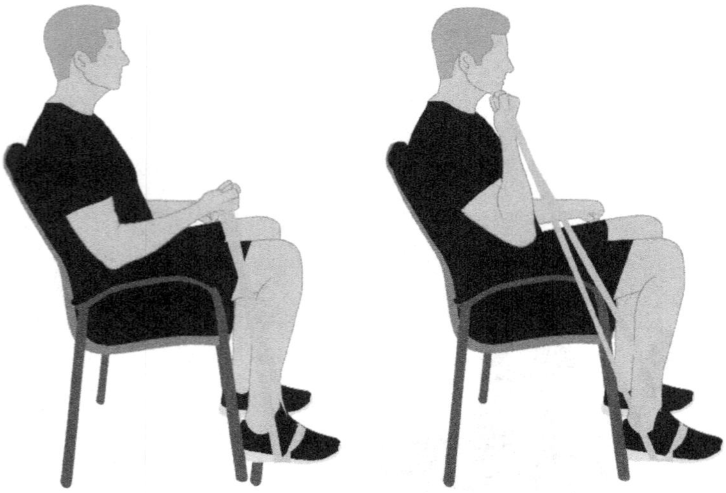

SCAN FOR VIDEO

Biceps Curl (v.2) #28

You can save time by curling with both arms at the same time. This can be done with two resistance bands or tubes, except in this version, you would set up both arms, but in the same manner as with the one-arm option.

Or you can use one long band: Hold each end of the band in each hand, and slide the center of the band beneath both of your feet. As above, eliminate any slack in the band so there's slight tension when your hands are at your hips, before curling upward.

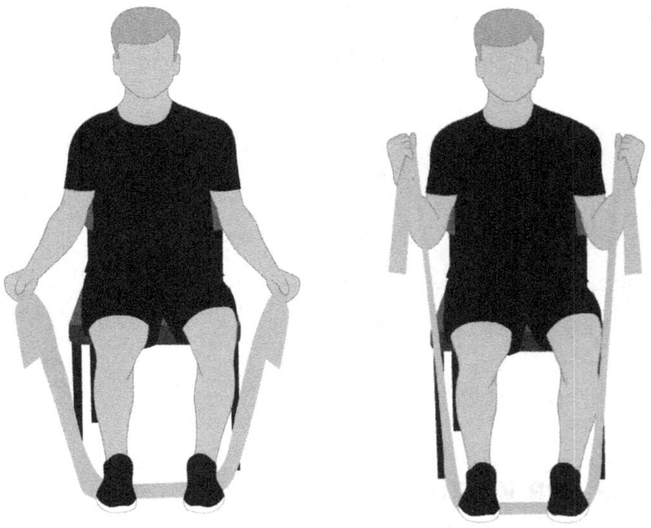

Chest Stretch #29

You will build strength and endurance in your pectorals (chest muscles), as well as your shoulders and upper arms with this simple yet effective seated upper body exercise.

- Hold a resistance band or tube with both hands, spaced shoulder-width apart, extended straight ahead, at shoulder height. Be sure there's no slack in the band, and there's enough resistance to make you work to pull the band apart.
- Begin the movement by stretching the band to both sides, while at the same time pulling your elbows back so they are pointing to the rear. Pull your elbows back until the band reaches your chest (or close to it). Be sure that you are keeping the band stretched apart.
- Slowly return your arms and hands to the starting position to complete 1 rep. Continue until you reach 10 reps, then pause for 20 to 30 seconds, and repeat for one or two more sets.

SCAN FOR VIDEO

Advancing: Now onto the more challenging set of resistance band exercises, when your strength and balance are ready.

CHAPTER 7

Advanced Resistance Band Exercises

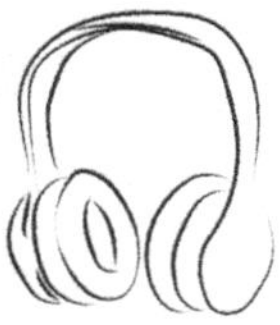

SCAN FOR AUDIO CHAPTER

If something stands between you and your success, move it. Never be denied.

Dwayne 'The Rock' Johnson

Stepping up to the Challenge

If you feel ready, this is where you can become familiar with the more advanced resistance band exercises. The assumption is that, at this point in your exercise journey, you now feel comfortable with the beginner and intermediate level movements, and are able to perform two to three sets of those exercises with at least a medium level of resistance.

A Few Cautions

Be careful: As is customary, it's a good practice to heed a few words of caution. Don't push yourself to overachieve and end up causing injury or excessive fatigue. Remember, resistance training is a marathon, not a sprint; it requires pacing for the long-term benefits you are working towards. Also, stay attentive to your balance, and use these exercises to improve it, continuing to focus on good form and posture.

Rest: This is an important yet often overlooked factor in building muscle, no matter how strong and conditioned you feel. Remember to allow at least one day of rest between resistance workouts so your muscles have the necessary time to recover and rebuild. You can work out every day if you wish, but not with the same muscle groups. The alternative is to do full body resistance workouts no more than three times a week.

The following exercises can be combined to give you a rigorous, 20-minute full body workout. "It includes compound movements that work multiple muscle groups at once; the exercises also challenge your core stability and balance," reports physiologist and sports performance coach D'Annette Stephens, ISSA-CPT, in *Livestrong* (2022).

She recommends using two mini bands, plus one long-looped resistance band at levels of resistance that feel hard, rather than easy, "but not too hard that you can't do the moves with good form." (You may also use flat bands or tubes as noted below).

Eight Advanced Movements

Pull To Face #30

Your shoulders and upper back are the principal beneficiaries of this exercise.

- Attach one end of a long-looped resistance band to an immovable, sturdy object close to head height. Pick up the opposite end of the band with both hands—palms facing out— with your arms extended in front of you. Step back far enough that there's some tension in the band when your arms are fully extended.
- Bend your knees, and lower your body to a quarter squat with your feet placed hip-width apart. Pull the band back to your forehead, focusing on pulling your shoulder blades together, and making sure your elbows are at shoulder height and pointing outwards to the sides when you reach the peak of the movement. Slowly return your hands to the starting position by extending your arms fully forward.
- This makes 1 rep; perform 10 to 15 reps for 1 set, rest for 20 to 30 seconds, then repeat a second set, and, if able, a third set.
- *Note: You can use a flat band or a tube if you are able to safely attach the far end to a sturdy object and can get a good grip on the end of the band you'll be pulling, or the handles if the tube has them.*

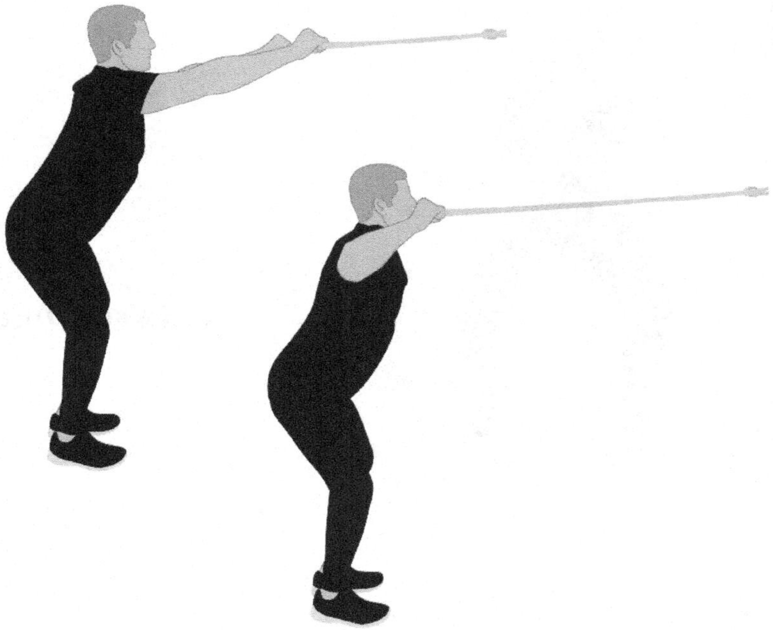

SCAN FOR VIDEO

Front Squat #31

This move will increase strength primarily in your bum and shoulders, and will also work your thighs, especially the quadriceps.

- Stand solidly in the center of the band with your feet placed about shoulder-width apart. Take an end of the band in each of your hands and raise them to shoulder height, with your palms facing up. This is the point of maximum resistance in this exercise, so be sure you're feeling a good amount of tension here.
- Keep your back straight and brace (tighten) your core, then force your hips back and bend your knees, to lower your hips until your thighs are parallel with the floor, or as low as you can go without hurting your knees. Remember to keep your back straight, to minimize any bending at the waist.
- Slowly stand back up to the upright position to complete 1 rep. Do three sets of 12 to 15 reps, with a 30 to 40 second rest between sets.

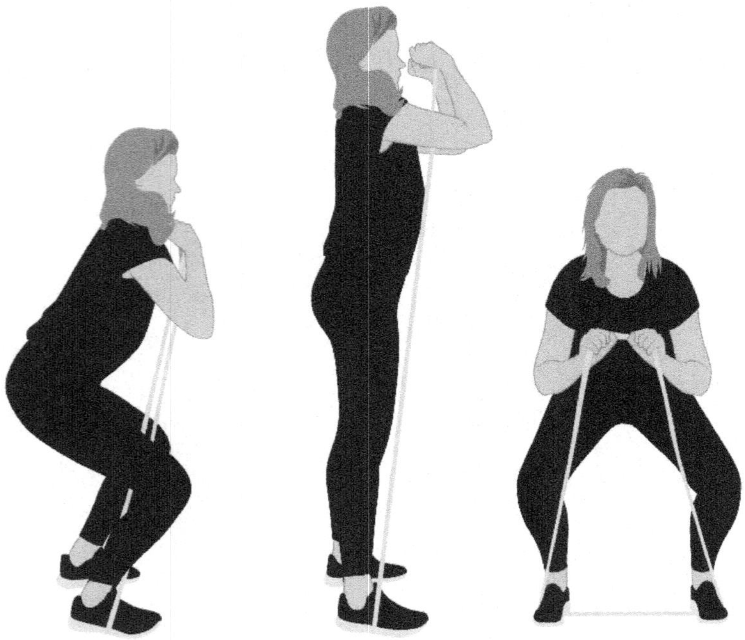

SCAN FOR VIDEO

Single Leg Deadlift #32

You will flex and strengthen your hamstring muscles, your glutes in the butt, as well as your shoulders, making this a 'compound exercise', meaning it works both the upper body and lower body at the same time.

- Place a looped band under your left foot, and hold the other end in your right hand, at hip level. There should be a good amount of resistance tension in the band, since this will be the farthest point of its stretch; slide your hand down the band to shorten it, if needed.
- Begin the movement by bending over at the waist, and at the same time, raising your right leg up to the rear, and lowering your right hand towards your right foot, letting the band pull your hand downward. Be sure to keep your back straight as you bend—this is very important in order to prevent back injuries. If you can achieve it, your body and right leg should form a straight, horizontal line.
- Hold this position for a moment, then raise your body back to an upright position, lower your right foot to the floor, and raise your right hand to your right hip. Feel the tension as the resistance in the band increases. This constitutes 1 rep.
- Continue for a total of 15 to 20 reps, then switch sides, bending forward, raising your left leg back and up, and lowering your left hand to your left foot. Do 10 to 12 reps. If you're up to it, do a second set on each side, and once you're conditioned, a third set.

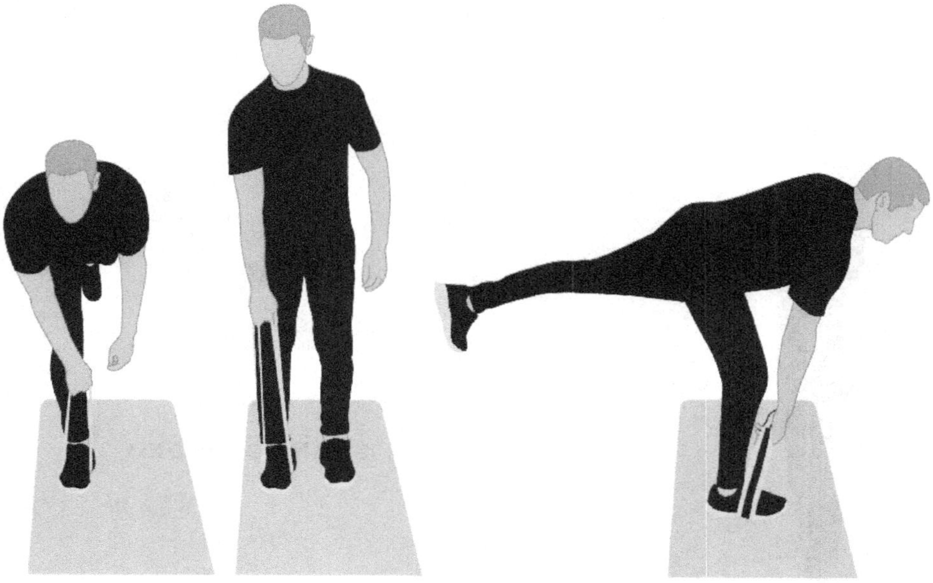

SCAN FOR VIDEO

Clean and Press #33

This is another upper and lower body compound exercise that strengthens the quadricep muscles in your legs, along with other supporting leg muscles, your hip joints, the glutes in your bum, and your shoulders.

- Stand upright with your left foot forward and with the right leg to the rear. Step into a long looped resistance band with your leading left foot, and stand on it. Hold the opposite end of the band at waist-height, with both hands spread shoulder-width apart, palms facing downward in an overhand grip.
- Begin the movement by squatting down into a sitting position, while simultaneously raising the band to your shoulders and pointing your elbows downward. Continue the movement by standing upright to come out of the squat, and as you rise up, press the band upward towards the ceiling, and fully extend your arms.
- Return to the starting position by lowering both your hands and the resistance band back to waist height. This completes 1 rep. Do 10 reps, then switch positions with the right foot forward stepping on the band. Do 10 reps to complete a full set. Do a second set, and when you are conditioned and able, do a third set.
- *Note: If you don't have a long looped band, you can perform this exercise with a long flat band, holding each end of the band in each hand, held shoulder-width apart, ensuring you have enough resistance to make the exercise productive.*

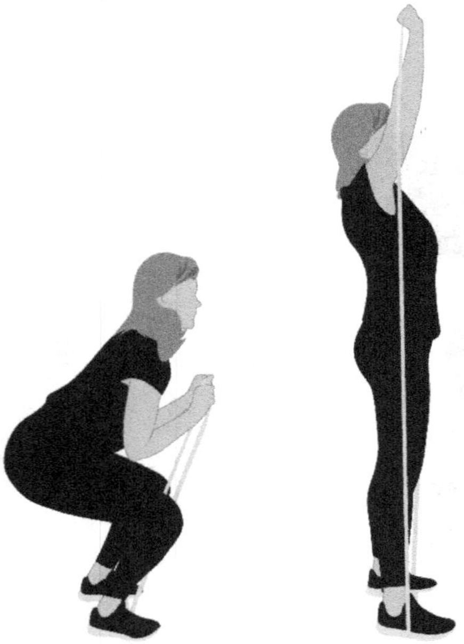

SCAN FOR VIDEO

Bear Crawl #34

Here is yet another compound resistance exercise; this move helps to develop your legs and hips, and especially your core, arms, and shoulders.

- You will need two small-to-medium sized looped resistance bands, or you can use flat bands or tubes that are tied to make the loops. Step into one loop with both feet so the band is around your ankles; place both hands inside the other loop so it is around your wrists. On a mat or carpet, go down on all fours, with your hands beneath your shoulders, arms fully extended. Raise your knees off the floor so your lower body is supported by your toes. There should be little or no slack in the looped bands to ensure at least a moderate amount of resistance during each movement.
- Begin the exercise by proceeding sideways, advancing your right hand and right foot about six inches (more or less) to the right, then catching up with your left hand and left foot. Immediately continue the movement with the right hand and foot, followed by the left hand and foot. If space permits, take about 10 right advances and left catch-ups.
- Then, reverse the movement so you're now moving to the left, leading with your left hand and foot, and catching up the right hand and foot. Return to the original starting point to complete 1 rep.
- You may be fatigued after one complete set of 10 reps, but if you are able, do a second set after resting for about 20 seconds. A third set can be done when your training has prepared you for it and you can get through it—even with fewer reps, if that's all you can do.
- *Note: If you find this exercise too difficult initially, perform it with only the band around your wrists. You then have the option of taking the 10 steps in each direction, or simply extending your right hand to the side, then returning it to beneath your shoulder, then repeating the same movement with your left hand.*

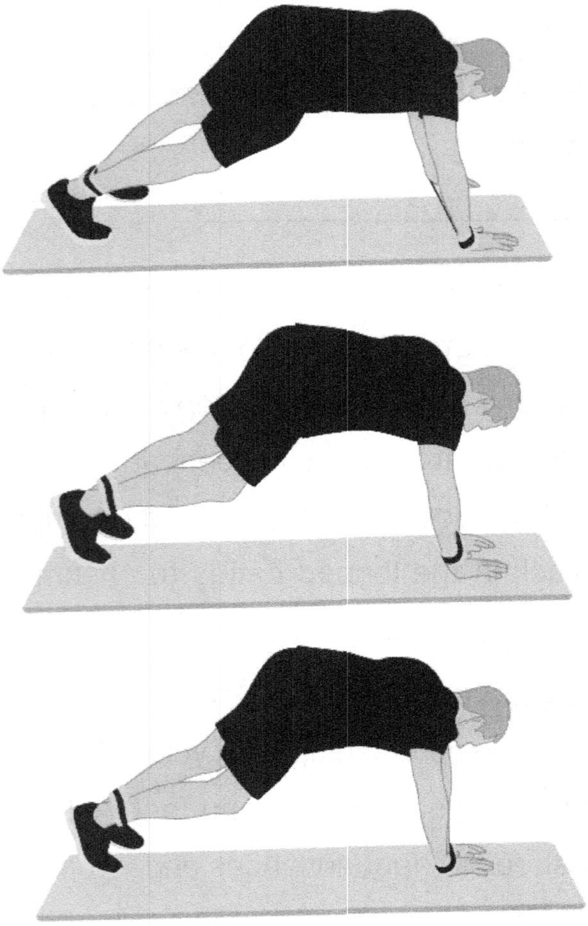

SCAN FOR VIDEO

Chest Crossover #35

This is a classic movement that is traditionally performed with weights (lying on a bench) or cables; you can do it with equal effectiveness with resistance bands or tubes in a standing position. Your chest's pectoral muscles, commonly referred to as 'pecs' and your latissimus dorsi muscles, referred to as 'lats', which extend from your upper back to your sides, will be the primary beneficiaries, along with your shoulders.

- Connect two medium length bands or tubes to a stationary post, or wrap one long band or tube around the post. To assume the starting position, stand with your back to the post and hold each end of the band (or handles of the tube), and raise your arms out to the sides, parallel to the floor at shoulder height. Step forward if needed to create some tension in the band. Your arms should be extended with a slight bend at the elbows, with your palms facing forward.
- Begin the movement by bringing your arms across your chest, keeping your arms straight as your hands form an arc as you bring them together, pointing outward in front of you. Flex your pecs and hold them contracted as you maintain the position for 2 or 3 seconds, then slowly return your arms to the starting position, keeping them extended throughout the movement. This constitutes 1 rep.
- Repeat, slowly and deliberately, for 10 reps, then relax, wait 30 seconds, then do a second set, and, if you're up to it, a third. If necessary, you can do fewer reps in the later sets, as long as you can do so without compromising your form and upright posture.

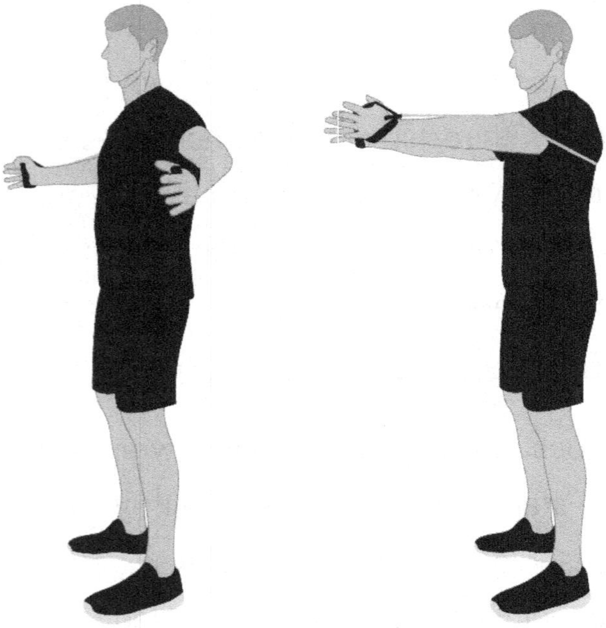

SCAN FOR VIDEO

Resistance Crunch #36

The crunch has replaced the sit-up as the favorite abdominals builder; it's the most popular move done by most people who want defined, flat abs, without risking the back strain that sit-ups often cause. But over time, 12 or so reps of crunches can become too easy. That's where weighted crunches come in useful, and you can achieve the same positive results with resistance bands.

There are at least two ways to achieve the needed resistance to intensify your crunches:

- **The first way:** Lie on a bench with your head flat and your knees partially raised. Place a resistance band or tube under the bench, below where your head and shoulders are resting. Hold the resistance band in each hand and pull your hands up to the sides of your head, being sure there is some resistance before beginning the movement.
- Start by raising your head, shoulders, and upper back off the bench to perform a crunch, with your head and shoulders only rising about 10 to 12 inches, unlike the sit-up, which takes your elbows all the way to your knees. As you rise upward, if you feel pain in your back, stop, and place a small, folded towel under your lower back for support then continue.
- Hold the crunch position for at least 3 seconds, tightening your core muscles, then slowly lower your head and shoulders to the bench to complete 1 rep.
- **A second method:** Add resistance by lying on a mat or carpet, with the resistance band attached securely to a post or the leg of a heavy table or dresser, positioned just beyond your head. As described above, hold the resistance band in each hand, and pull your hands up to the sides of your head, being sure there is some resistance before beginning the movement.
- Perform the crunch, feeling the resistance as you rise upward and away from the post or table leg. Be sure to tighten your core, and lower back down slowly.
- Regardless of which method you prefer, perform 12 reps, rest for 20 to 30 seconds, then repeat for a second, and possibly a third set.
- *Note: You may need to adjust the tension in the band so that about 12 crunches are just enough to wear you out.*

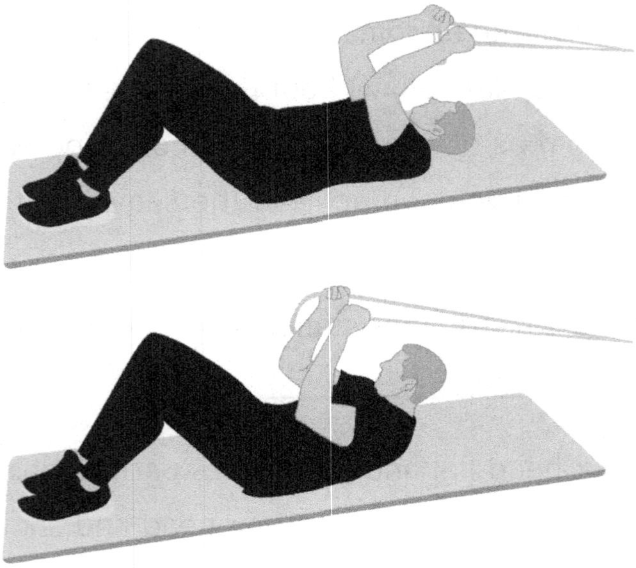

SCAN FOR VIDEO

Lateral Raise #37

This is a simple but highly effective exercise for your shoulders, and secondarily for your arms, wrists, and upper back muscles. It's a standard move, whether done with weights or resistance bands and tubes.

- Stand upright with your legs and feet close together (or slightly apart, if needed for balance). Place the center of a long resistance band or tube under your feet and grasp each end with your right and left hands. Hold your hands at your sides, with arms fully extended downward, and your palms facing backwards.
- Raise both hands up at a 45-degree angle, keeping your arms fully extended throughout the movement. Bring your hands up to shoulder level, or just above.
- Hold for a moment, then slowly lower your arms to the starting position. This is 1 rep. Do 10 to 12 reps, rest for 20 to 30 seconds, and follow with a second set.

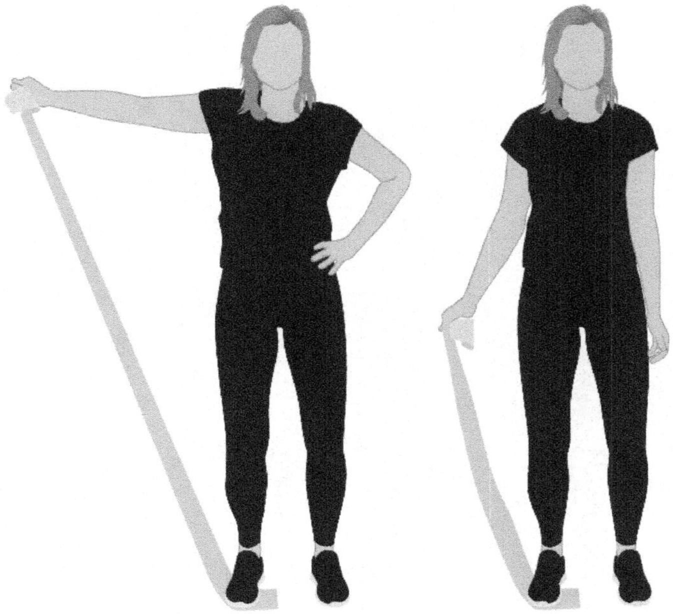

SCAN FOR VIDEO

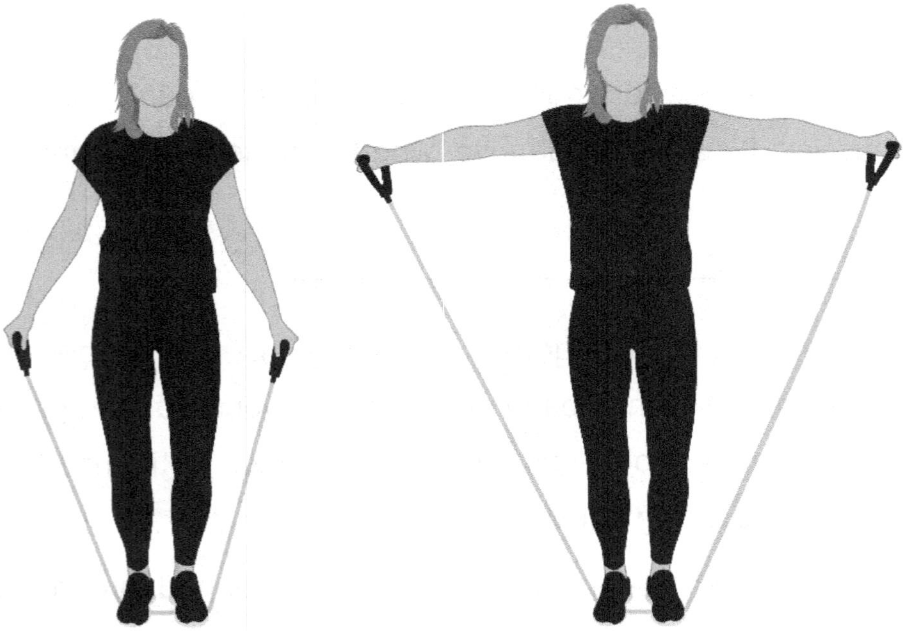

SCAN FOR VIDEO

Next: You'll learn how your bodyweight can create an extremely effective force of resistance with an increase in intensity when supplemented with resistance bands.

CHAPTER 8

Bodyweight Calisthenics and Aerobics

SCAN FOR AUDIO CHAPTER

Champions aren't made in the gyms. Champions are made from something they have deep inside them—a desire, a dream, a vision.

Muhammad Ali

Getting Even Stronger and Conditioned

You are encouraged to supplement your resistance band training with bodyweight calisthenics and aerobics; two other important forms of exercise that will increase your overall level of physical fitness, make you stronger, and increase your cardiovascular conditioning.

This is not to suggest that a full resistance band exercise program cannot make you as strong as calisthenics, nor does it imply that you can't intensify your resistance band workouts to achieve aerobic conditioning. It's important to note here that it is definitely possible to 'max out' your workouts with continual, vigorous rounds of reps and sets with resistance bands and tubes as your only form of exercise.

Variation in your workouts can help prevent boredom, reduce the risk of injury, and potentially increase your frequency and consistency of working out over the long term.

- You may find 20 to 30 minutes of aerobic jogging, fast walking, cycling, or swimming, for example, to be preferable to hustling through your resistance band workout in an effort to keep your heart pumping at the pace you desire, but now that you're in advanced shape, that could easily cause you to perform the movements too fast, forgetting proper form and posture, which is a recipe for injury.

- Adding some calisthenics without resistance bands is a good way to ensure all your muscle groups are being strengthened, while at the same time getting the best of both techniques by doing calisthenics supplemented with the bands, as noted in previous chapters.

Bodyweight Calisthenics

Push Ups #38

Push-ups build your shoulders, upper arms, chest, upper back, and core, making them one of the most productive resistance exercises.

- We all know this one, but for review, a push up is performed by first getting down on your hands and knees, then extending your legs to the rear, so your weight is suspended solely on your hands and toes. Keep your back straight as you bend your elbows to lower your chest towards the floor. Get as low as you are able to before slowly pushing back up to the starting position, with your arms straight; this completes 1 rep.
- Do as many as you can, working up over time to at least 10 to 12 reps. Rest for 30 to 40 seconds, then do a second set. If your shoulders are holding out, rest again, and do a third set. Remember to keep your back straight—no sagging!
- *Note: If you find that 12 reps are too easy, instead of increasing the reps, slow down the upward and downward movements. For example, take 5 or 10 seconds going down, pause for 5 seconds, then slowly rise back up; you'll feel the difference.*

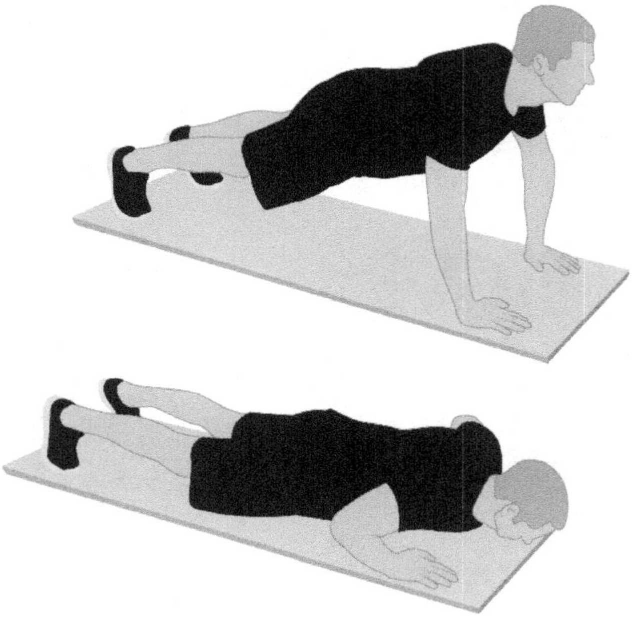

SCAN FOR VIDEO

Modified Push Up

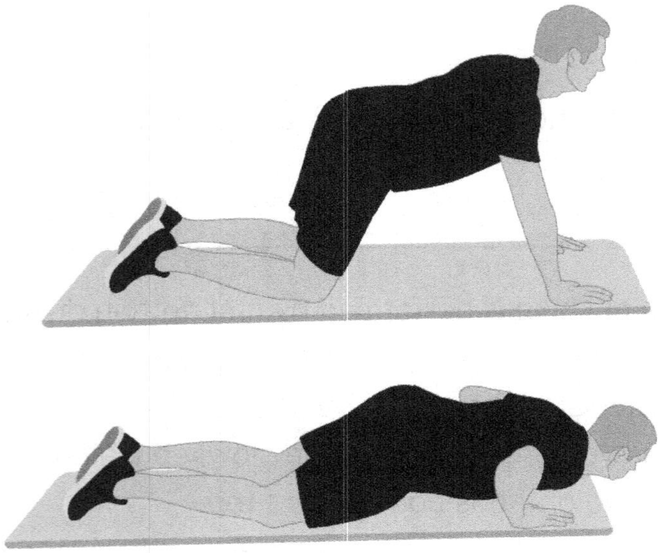

SCAN FOR VIDEO

Planks #39

This close cousin of the push up benefits the same muscle groups, but is a holding exercise, rather than a movement. There are two versions:

- **Version 1:** Assume the same starting position as the push up, with arms fully extended. Face downward (not forward) and hold this pose for at least 10 seconds, ideally being able to work up to 30 seconds, or even a full minute, as you become conditioned. Do a second plank after a 30 second rest.
- **Version 2:** The alternative plank pose is to rest your upper body on your forearms, with elbows bent and placed beneath your shoulders. Hold as with the version 1 arms-extended pose, and repeat after a 30 second rest.
- *Note: Be sure to keep your back from sagging or drooping, as this will reduce the benefits to your core. It's imperative with this move that you keep your back straight, all the way up to your shoulders, for it to be effective and to prevent lower back strain.*

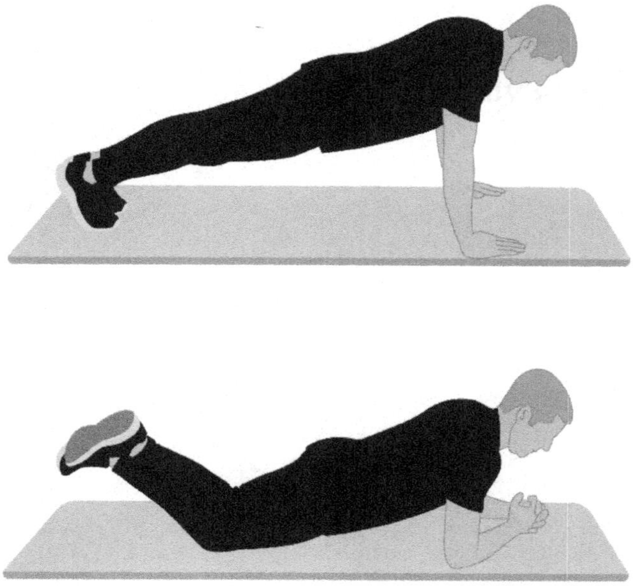

SCAN FOR VIDEO

Crunch #40

As you learned in Chapter 7, the crunch has replaced the sit up as the safer way to work those abs and the rest of the core muscles.

- Lie on a mat or carpet with your head flat and your knees partially raised.
- Begin the crunch by raising your head, shoulders, and upper back 10 to 12 inches off the floor (unlike the sit-up, which reaches to your knees). As you rise, if you feel pain in your back, stop, and place a small folded towel under your lower back for support, then continue.
- Hold the crunch position for at least 2 to 3 seconds, tightening your core muscles, then slowly lower your head and shoulders to the bench to complete 1 rep. Do a total of 12 reps in the first set, rest for 30 seconds, and repeat for one more set.

SCAN FOR VIDEO

Leg Raises #41

Despite the name, it's your core muscles—especially the abdominals—that benefit from leg raises.

- Lie on your back on a mat or carpet, with your legs fully extended. Slowly raise both legs with your knees slightly bent and continue raising until your feet are pointing to the ceiling. Pause, then slowly lower your legs to the mat for 1 rep. Continue raising and lowering your legs for a total of 10 reps.
- Tighten your abdominals to increase the effectiveness of the exercise.

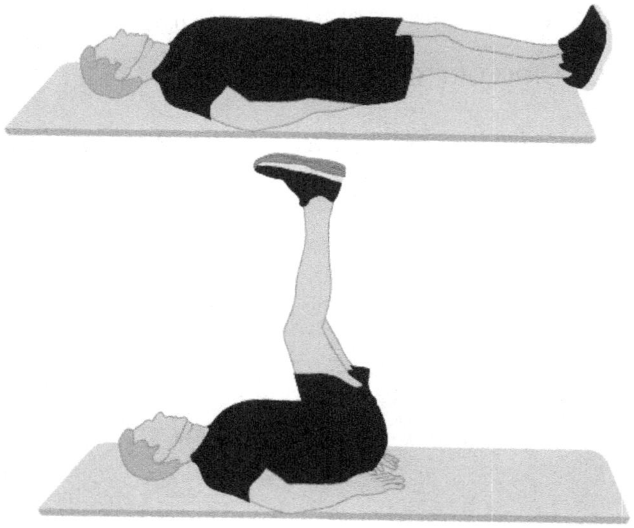

SCAN FOR VIDEO

Modified Leg Raises

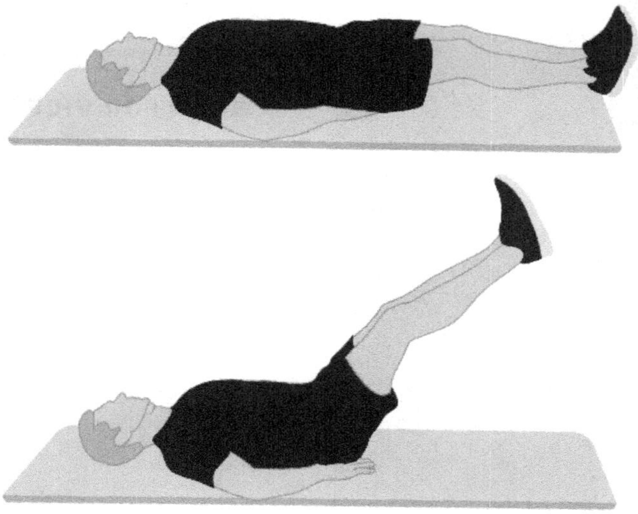

SCAN FOR VIDEO

Squats #42

The thighs, especially your quadriceps, are the primary beneficiaries of squats, with some added effort attributed to your hamstrings, hip flexors, glutes, and calves.

- Stand upright with your feet about 12 to 14 inches apart and place your right hand on your left shoulder and left hand on the right shoulder. Begin by pushing your hips back as you bend your knees to lower your body, as if you are going to sit in a chair.
- Lean your body slightly forward from the hips, while keeping your back straight, without bending it. Be careful not to let your knees go forward past your toes.
- Pause for a moment, then rise back up to the standing position to complete 1 rep. Do 8 to 12 reps for one set; rest for 30 seconds, then perform a second set.
- *Note: It may be easier if you do the squats with your back against a wall, sliding down and back up.*

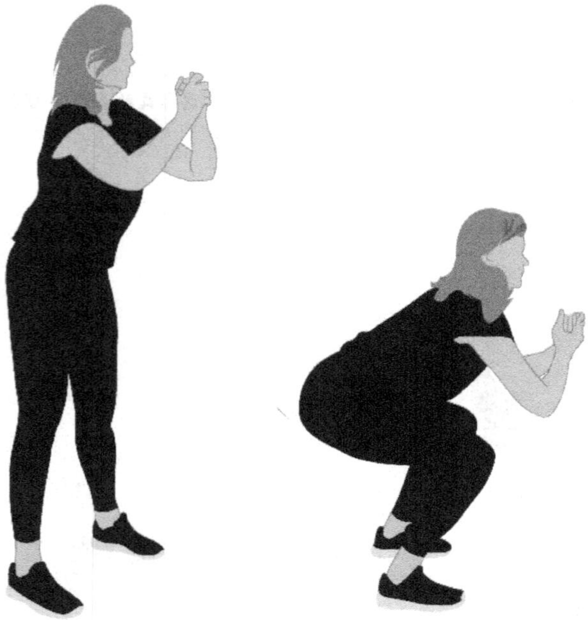

SCAN FOR VIDEO

Aerobic Exercises

This is what all those joggers and cyclists are doing because it's great for heart health, and disease prevention overall. Your heart is a muscle, and aerobic or cardio training is how that muscle gets its exercise. It's also a good way to burn a good number of calories and help with weight control. Following a good aerobic workout, you'll often experience the rush of beta endorphin hormones, which are the cause of the so-called 'runner's high.'

Aerobic Selection

In selecting which aerobic exercise to perform, keep in mind that these are for the long-term benefit of your health and well-being, so choose methods that you can stay with; in other words, don't take up jogging if you hate to run. And for that matter, if you are a senior, you'll be better off avoiding running on hard surfaces, or participating in any other high impact sport; your knees and joints will thank you.

- An aerobic workout can be achieved with a range of alternative activities, some of which can be done indoors on a treadmill, elliptical machine, or stair climber. You can also jump rope, and use an indoor stationary cycle. Or you can cycle outdoors, preferably in safe areas, and not in traffic with the danger of cars, and polluted air.
- If you have access to a pool, swimming is considered one of the most effective, risk-free forms of exercise. But this means doing laps, not splashing around.
- What about walking? Absolutely! It is low impact and can provide a good aerobic workout as long as it's done at a brisk pace, so that you are breathing deeply and your heart is pumping at a good rate—a subject we'll cover next.

Your Aerobic Heart Rate

Extensive studies of cardiovascular conditioning have identified target heart rates based on age and your 'VO2 Max', the maximum heart rate you can achieve. Here's how it works:

Your estimated VO2 Max is the number 220 minus your age; you then take 65% of that to determine an ideal 'cruising pace' that you can comfortably sustain for most of your workout. Here's an example for a 50 year old person in normal health:

220 - 50 = 170 X 0.65 = 110

Now let's do this for someone who has reached age 70:

220 - 70 = 150 X 0.65 = 98

These calculations are approximate and are based on averages. If you are age 50, a steady workout pulse of 110 may feel easy, or you may find it too intense, and need to slow down. How you react is largely dependent on your level of conditioning; you must be the judge of how you feel.

- You can easily check your pulse by pressing your fingers into the left side of your neck, where the carotid artery can easily be found. Take a reading for 10 seconds, then multiply that by 6 to calculate your beats per minute, or 'BPM's.
- If you have a smartwatch or other wrist-monitor, it will give you a continuous reading, and show you the ideal rate range for your age.

Another guideline is to be able to speak and hold a conversation as you proceed through your aerobic workout. If you can speak, your breathing rate is in the safe range, but if you're nearly out of breath, and breathing with difficulty, ease up until your breathing is manageable. At the other extreme is when your pulse and breathing rates are too low, and you are not working hard enough, in which case it's time to pick up the pace.

Meeting a top athlete: He is playing at top performance levels despite being a senior, as far as pro sports go. His secret: A total-body resistance band workout, and it's coming up next.

CHAPTER 9

A Top Athlete Tells You How

SCAN FOR AUDIO CHAPTER

The real glory is being knocked to your knees and then coming back. That's the essence of it.

Vince Lombardi
football legend

Learn From a Senior Who's Still Playing Tough

Consider this chapter a bonus; an extra, highly effective resistance band routine that you can easily learn and practice. This is the workout that Tom Brady uses to keep the top shape that allows him to still be a winning National Football League quarterback, well into his 40s.

Tom recently decided to retire, and then changed his mind, deciding to stay in the game. Why? His reasons may be personal, but one thing is for sure: He knew he could do it; that he was physically able to step onto the playing field and compete successfully among much younger players.

Tom Brady and I have a common goal: To help as many people as possible, especially seniors, to become stronger and healthier with more endurance and reliance, by staying physically active throughout their lives.

Warming Up

As you've already read, it's important not to jump right into your resistance band workout without getting your heart to pump some extra oxygen-rich blood throughout your body, especially to your muscles.

If you can do a 10 minute cardio workout first, that's great, but if time or motivation is short, spend at least 5 minutes on a treadmill, stationary cycle, elliptical, or stair climber. If you're at home without access to those machines, do some running or hopping in place, interspersed with some yoga stretching, a few squats, some calf raises, maybe a few jumping jacks; anything that will warm you up. There are more instructions on warmups in Chapter 4's coverage for Beginners.

A Full-Body Workout

Tom Brady and You

These eight exercises, all performed with resistance bands, are the essentials of Tom Brady's full-body routine. He found that as he got older, his risks of injury with weights were increasing, and that he could stay in great shape with resistance bands. So can you!

You can choose to perform all of these exercises in one session, and assuming you've used sufficient resistance to really challenge your muscles, you should then rest for at least one day, or preferably two if you are a senior. So a Monday morning full-body workout should not be repeated before Wednesday or Thursday morning.

Alternatively, you can work your upper body including your arms, shoulders, and upper back on Monday; your midbody (abs and core) on Tuesday; and your lower body, from the hips, glutes, and thighs to calves and ankles on Wednesday. You'd then be ready to return to the upper body workout on Thursday.

As you perform this routine, the same guideline of two or three sets of 8 to 12 reps applies, with the last 1 or 2 reps in each set feeling challenging.

Standing Row #43

This is a good way to wake up your upper body, and get your back, shoulder and arm muscles into gear, as you keep your lower body stable.

- Take a long looped band, and anchor one end to a door, or a pole, at about chest height. If you have tubes with handles, anchor an end of each. Take the other end of the band, or the handles in each hand, and step back with your arms extended forward until you feel tension in the band.
- Stand with your feet shoulder-width apart and bend your knees slightly; keep your upper body upright. Tighten your core and glutes, keeping your elbows close to your body, and begin the movement by pulling your hands to the sides of your chest in a rowing motion, pausing, then slowly extending your arms to return to the starting position.

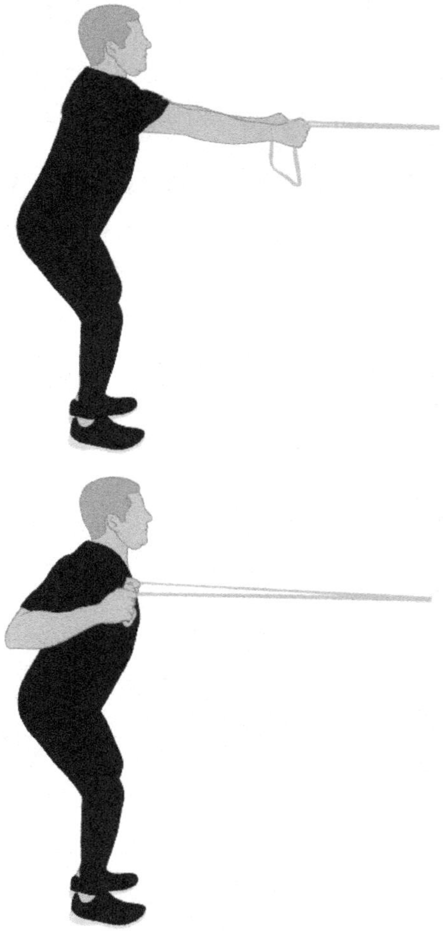

SCAN FOR VIDEO

Banded Push Ups #44

Banded push-ups are great exercise for your chest muscles, shoulders, and triceps.

- Make sure to keep your back straight. Complete the first rep of the exercise by lowering your chest to the floor. Pause, then slowly rise back up to the starting position.
- The idea is to make the push up harder, so be sure to have a good amount of resistance in the band before you lower yourself. If you don't feel enough resistance, pull the band tighter.

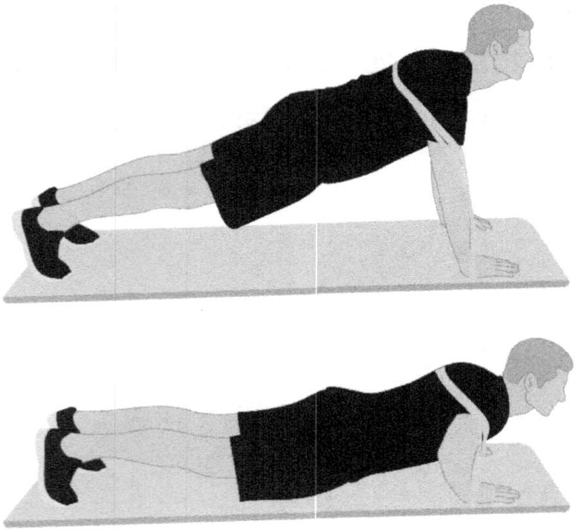

SCAN FOR VIDEO

Core Rotations #45

This exercise will strengthen your abdominals and the side and back muscles of your core; it helps Tom to gain torque when he throws.

- Take the same stance as in the standing row, but now turn 45-degrees so you are holding the anchored band with your arms extended across your chest; your hands and arms should be pointing towards the anchor. Take a few side steps away from the anchor to make sure there's resistance in the bands.
- Begin by pulling the bands across your chest, and at the same time, turn your body away from the anchor, trying to have your back facing the anchor. Slowly turn back to the starting position, with your arms extended and pointing towards the anchor.

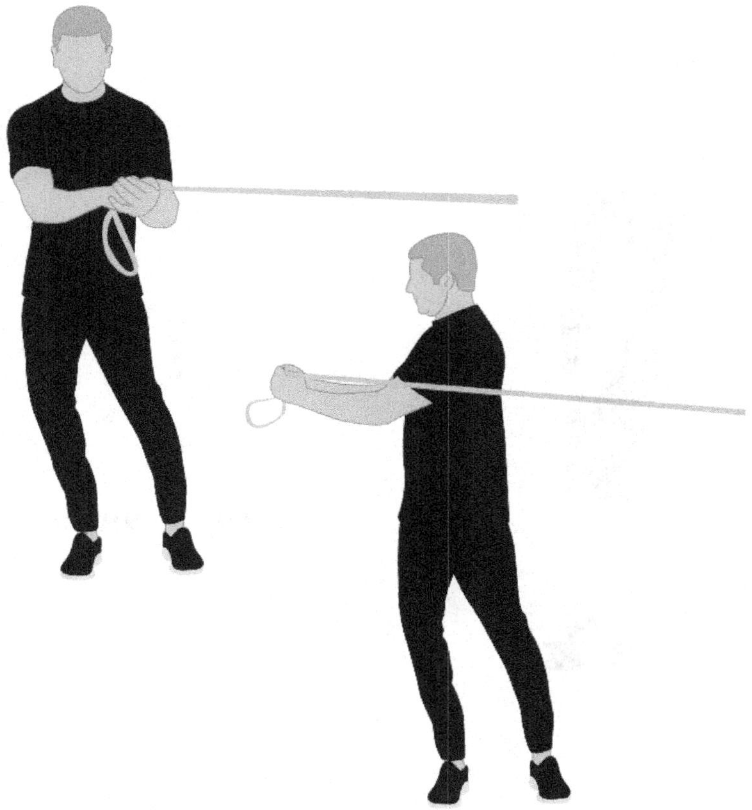

SCAN FOR VIDEO

Biceps Curl #46

This is the definitive builder of your upper arm biceps muscles; the band's resistance takes the place of a traditional pair of dumbbells or a barbell. (This version offers the same benefits as the seated version in Chapter 6).

- Stand upright, keeping your back straight as you step on the center of a loop band, or, you may place each foot on the end of a flat band or tube. With your arms extended and pointing downward, there should be some light resistance felt in the bands; if not, adjust your grip and placement under your foot to tighten the band.
- Begin by raising both hands to your shoulders, keeping your elbow close to your body. Pause at the top of the movement, then slowly lower your hands and fully extend your arms downward; this completes your first rep. Remember to keep your back straight.

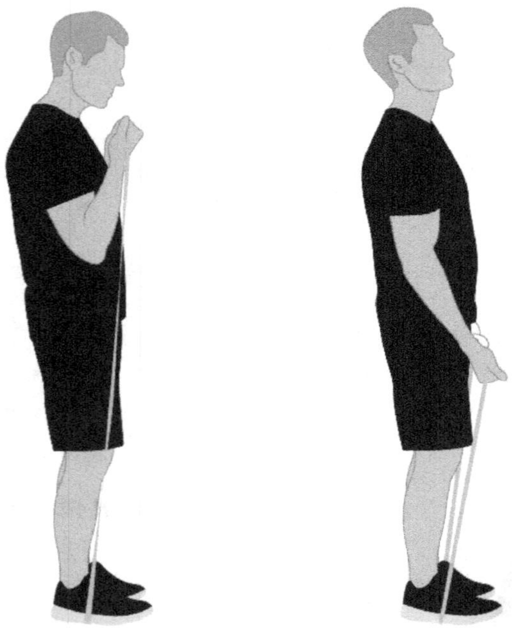

SCAN FOR VIDEO

Triceps Extension #47

This exercise isolates and develops the triceps muscles at the rear of your upper arms; your shoulders will benefit as well.

- You'll need one long loop or two flat bands or tubes. Stand on the center of the loop or on the ends of the single bands or tubes and raise your hands behind your head. You should feel some, but not too much, resistance at this stage.
- Begin by raising your hands upwards, and *just behind your head*, with your elbows pointing forward. Extend your arms upward as fully as you are able. Pause at the top of the movement, then slowly lower your hands behind your head to complete 1 rep.

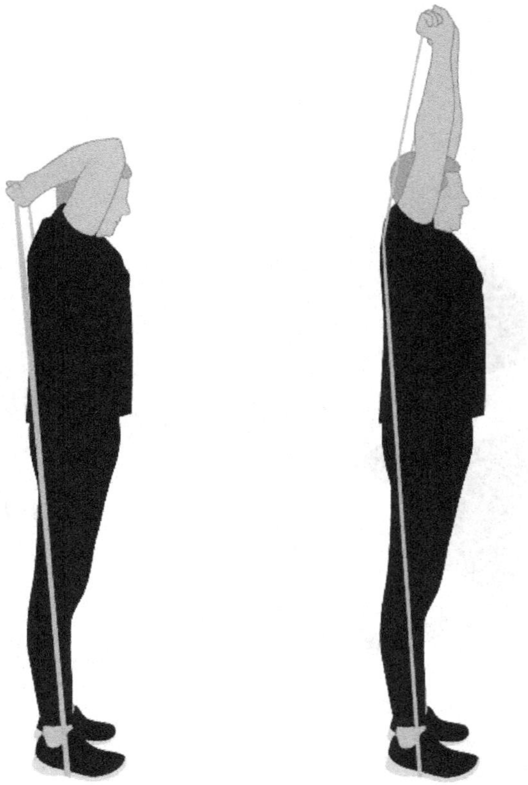

SCAN FOR VIDEO

Banded Deceleration Lunges #48

These lunges are intensified by the band to further challenge your quadriceps, glutes, and hips.

- Loop a larger band around your waist and attach the other end to a door handle or post, making sure the connection will hold under tension.
- From a standing position, step backward with your right leg, and bend your right knee until it just touches the floor. Keeping your upper body as upright as you can, step back far enough that your left thigh is parallel to the floor. Pause, then rise back up to the starting position for your first rep.
- Do 8 to 10 reps, then switch legs and repeat the same number of reps with your left leg rearward to complete the first set.

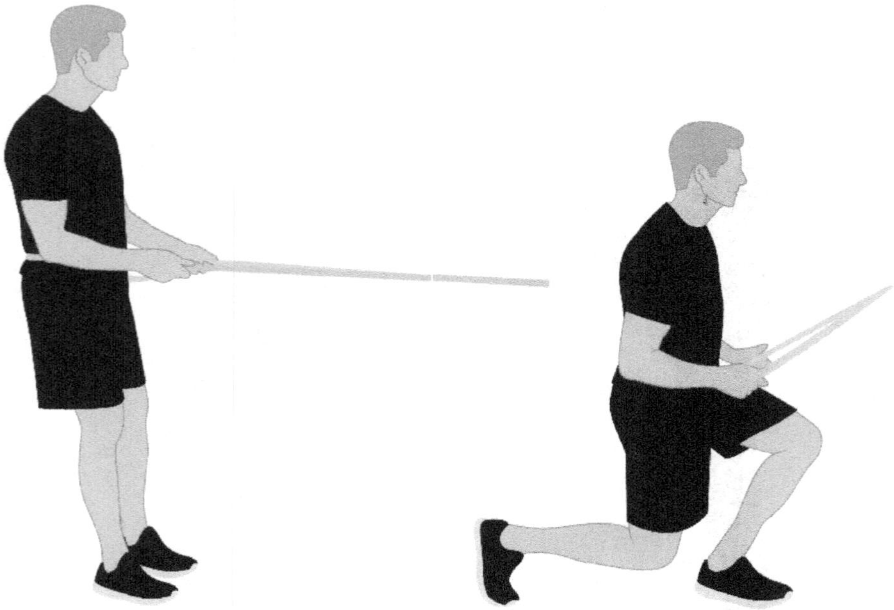

SCAN FOR VIDEO

Shoulder Press #49

This is almost the same as the Triceps Press, standing on a long loop or two flat bands or tubes, but with your hands held *in front of your shoulders*. You'll be pressing your hands and arms directly upward.

- Tighten your core and glutes and be sure there is sufficient resistance so that you have considerable tension when your arms are fully extended upward. Your hands should remain just forward of your head as you press upward, and your elbows should be pointing downward as you begin.
- Pause at the top of the movement, then slowly lower your hands to your shoulders to complete the first rep.

SCAN FOR VIDEO

X-Band Squat #50

This is a good intensifier of the thigh-building squat exercise. You'll need both a short and a long loop band for this exercise.

- Step both feet into the short loop band and place it just above your knees. Step on the lower section of the large loop band with your feet shoulder-width apart. Twist the loop to form an X shape, and insert your head into the upper loop, and slide the band behind your neck. Press your hands together and push them forward to help your balance.
- Press your bum back and keep your body upright as you lower into a squat. Your knees should be above your toes, pointing forward, not inward. Tighten your core and glutes and be sure to press your knees outward to further engage the glutes and hips. Pause, then rise back up to standing posture to complete one rep.

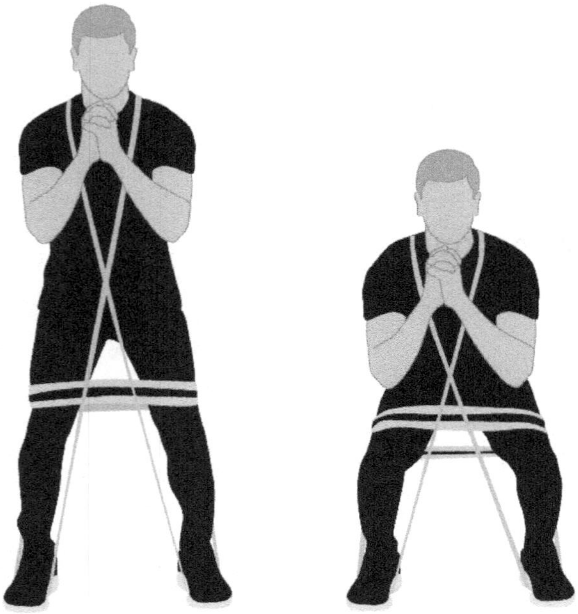

Wrapping up: The next and last chapters will keep you on the path of safety, good exercise practices, and how to follow a healthy, enjoyable dietary lifestyle practice.

CHAPTER 10

Safety Tips, Good Practices, a Healthy Diet

SCAN FOR AUDIO CHAPTER

Our greatest ability as humans is not to change the world; but to change ourselves.

Mahatma Gandhi

Putting More Life in Your Years; More Years in Your Life

It's time to wrap up your resistance band training by ensuring you'll be able to perform your workouts safely and beneficially, and avoid the common injuries that anyone, but especially seniors, can experience when stressing joints and muscles.

In the spirit of the Hippocratic Oath's "First, do no harm," we begin with the basic ways to protect and strengthen your joints, and reduce the risks of injury. We then follow this with a summary of the good practices that will keep you from hurting yourself and enable you to make your fitness program a part of your daily routine, putting more years in your life, and more life in your years.

This chapter will conclude with a straightforward presentation of a healthy diet that you can adopt with ease and without sacrifice; a diet you'll love, and that will optimize your health and ability to stay fit.

Protect Your Joints: Safety Tips for Exercising as a Senior

It is not a sign of weakness to acknowledge that your age will affect how you exercise. As a senior, the expression, "You're not a kid anymore" is of particular relevance when you put your joints, connective tissues, bones, and muscles through resistance training. No matter the exercise and dietary disciplines you have practiced, the years must be taken into account.

This means you are not as flexible as you once were and won't be able to bend or reach as deeply or as far as before. The flexibility of your muscles, ligaments, tendons, and joints gradually reduces as these connective tissues stiffen and become more resistant to stretching, as well as to the hard resistance work you're trying to impose. As a result:

Your joints are susceptible to injury as a result of reduced flexibility, strength and resilience, and longer recovery times. Virtually every movement we make involves flexing joints, from our fingers, hands, and wrists to our elbows, shoulders, neck, spine, hips, knees and ankles. We even have joints in our toes.

Your recovery times following a work out or any good amount of physical exertion will be longer. If you recall the concept of hypertrophy covered earlier, your muscle fibers and cells need time to repair and rebuild the damage to your muscles from these types of exertions. What used to take a day for recovery may take two or three days.

You are not as strong or resilient as you once were. If you could do bicep curls with a 25 lb or 30 lb dumbbell or resistance band equivalent when you were 35 years old, it is probably no longer possible if you are now 55 or 65; these days you may peak at 15 lb, or at most 20 lb.

Your aerobic capacity is also not what it once was, even if you've hit the trail or the treadmill faithfully for many years. As the data shows in the previous chapter, your optimal heart rate for sustaining a comfortable cardiovascular conditioning pace slows a little bit every year; adding up to six or seven *fewer beats per minute* every 10 years.

Furthermore, certain aerobic exercises can *damage your joints*, potentially permanently. Running, and other repetitive, sustained high impact activities can wear down the cartilage in your joints, especially knees and ankles; tennis can lead to tennis elbow, of course, and that abraded cartilage won't grow back!

Your back is at risk. We all experience back pain at certain times in our lives; it's as if the back is just waiting to inform us of its presence. There are many risks your upper and lower back can be exposed to, including dislocating spinal disks and pinching spinal nerves, causing sciatica. See the warning in the next section about lifting heavy objects with improper posture.

Okay, given those realities, what can you do to avoid injuries while getting into shape?

Good Practices for Seniors

Let's extend the timeless maxim, "Know thyself, with Know thyself and thy physical limits." Be aware of your true capabilities, and don't push beyond them. Take care not to try to keep up with others, whose strength and conditioning may give them advantages; just be yourself and respect your limits.

- **Form and posture:** Learn how to do each movement correctly, and maintain good form, especially good posture. Be attentive to the instructions for each movement, and don't try shortcuts or fast movements to get through the exercise quickly. Slower is better by being safer, and also more productive in creating resistance to make you stronger.
- **Lift responsibly:** This includes *all lifting* you may do, whether it's during your resistance bands workout, or when moving a dresser or hauling a heavy box. Bend your knees, keep your back straight without arching or bending your spine, and use your thighs to push yourself up. (This is why it's important to practice squats, and to do so correctly!)
- **Don't powerlift:** Avoid trying to lift or pull heavier resistance than you can handle, and don't try powerlifting, which involves resistance that is so intense that only 1 or 2 reps can be performed in a set. This may build bigger muscles when the person is young, but for seniors, it's a recipe for pulls, strains, and tears. You should be able to do at least 8 reps for the resistance level to be safe for you.
- **Safety first:** Be attentive to safety concerns when using your resistance bands and tubes. Take an extra few moments when attaching one end of the band to a stationary object, and ensure the band, or its handle, will not come loose and snap back and hit you in the face. If you are hooking the handle at the end of a tube, secure it with another band or strap.
- **Protect your equipment:** Make sure you are not exposing the bands and tubes to sharp or rough, abrasive surfaces, such as when placing the band over the top of a door, or a tree branch. Be careful when tying bands together to extend them or create a loop; use a slipknot so the knot can be untied, but make sure it will hold during use. Read the safety instructions that come with the equipment.
- **Get help:** If you have any doubts about how to use resistance bands and tubes, consult a trainer who is familiar with them (but not a trainer who will steer you away from bands and

over to weightlifting!). Be attentive to the instructions you receive, especially when the trainer shows you how to stand and maintain good posture, and how to do each movement.

- **See your doctor:** Finally, as you've been advised throughout the book, if you are new to exercise, or if it's been quite a while since you were in shape, get checked out medically before starting resistance and aerobic exercises. In the same spirit, get medical help if you experience serious pain during a workout; it may just be fatigue or a slight strain, but it's best to rule out anything serious, and attend to it immediately if necessary.

What About Diet?

Yes, what you eat (and how much) is essential to health and fitness, and we'll give you the lowdown on a diet endorsed by the medical professionals at the Mayo Clinic, Harvard Medical School, Johns Hopkins, and the Cleveland Clinic, especially for protecting heart health. "In January, US News and World Report named it the 'best diet overall' for the second year running" (Harvard Health, 2019). It's based on healthy, delicious foods, so you can ignore all those fad diets and go with the diet recognized by medical authorities to help you live your longest and best.

The Mediterranean Diet

The residents of the Mediterranean Basin live longer and healthier lives than worldwide average expectancies, and the consensus among cardiologists, and other medical professionals, is that these advantages trace to the quality and nature of their diets, along with being physically active and socially interactive.

You can learn about this diet, and find many good recipes online; Here is a brief summary of the components and benefits of the Mediterranean diet, profiled by WebMD (2022):

- **Heart healthy:** "Almost everything in this diet is good for your heart. Olive oil and nuts help lower 'bad' LDL cholesterol. Fruits, veggies, and beans help keep arteries clear." Fish from coldwater sources like salmon, tuna, and sardines help lower triglycerides and blood pressure. "Even a daily glass of wine may be good for your heart!" (More on this below).
- **No calorie counting:** Instead, trade heart-healthy fats like olive oil for unhealthy fats like butter, margarine, and shortening. Fish and lean poultry are healthier than saturated fats in red meat and full-fat dairy products. Have sweet-tasting, vitamin and fiber-rich fresh

fruit, and avoid the empty calories in sugar-laden desserts. You can have dark chocolate, but in moderate amounts.

- **Veggies unlimited:** Enjoy as much as you want of flavorful vegetables and salad greens, and you can also enjoy whole grains and beans. Nuts of every type, and seeds, like chia, flax, pumpkin, and sunflower, are great for you, but stick to a handful a day, since they're oil rich.
- **Avoid salty prepared foods:** like bacon and sausages, and canned, preserved meats that are low in nutrients, and focus on "Seasonal food that's made in simple, mouth-watering ways. Build a yummy salad from spinach, cucumbers, and tomatoes." Choose a diversity of colors for your salad for optimal minerals and vitamins.
- **Bread is back:** It's now recognized as good for you. But only if you choose breads made with whole grains, which have more protein, fiber, and minerals and are healthier than breads made with white flour. "Try whole-grain pita bread dipped in olive oil, hummus, or tahini, a protein-rich paste made from ground sesame seeds."
- **Eggs are back too:** and are recommended in moderation, given their quality protein and low saturated fats. One a day, or no more than about eight per week is okay with the cardiologists! Use little or no butter when cooking to keep saturated fat intake low.
- **Go easy on the salt:** and add spices for safer, better flavors. Drop in some bay leaves, sauteed onion, rosemary, coriander, cilantro, pepper, and cinnamon to add lots of flavor, so you can cut back on hypertension-causing salt. Many spices and herbs "Have health benefits, too; coriander and rosemary, for example, have disease-fighting antioxidants and nutrients."
- **More about wine:** A glass or two taken with meals is "Common in many Mediterranean countries, where dining is often leisurely and social." There's evidence that "One glass a day for women and two for men may be good for your heart. Talk to your doctor to see if it's a good idea for you." Other sources of alcohol—beer and distilled spirits—may also be beneficial if similarly consumed in moderation.
- **You won't be hungry:** because you'll be eating rich-tasting foods like "Roasted sweet potatoes, hummus, and even lima bean spread." These and other complex carbohydrates tend to digest slowly, letting you feel full for a longer time. In addition, "Hunger's not a

problem when you can munch on nuts, olives, or bites of low-fat cheese when a craving strikes." Just don't overeat!

- **Get smarter:** The nutrition that's good for your heart is also beneficial for your brain. By consuming antioxidant-rich foods and avoiding "bad fats and processed foods which can cause inflammation," you are making "this eating style a brain-friendly choice."

The DASH Diet

You may have heard of this medically endorsed diet; DASH stands for *Dietary Approaches to Stop Hypertension*, and its primary target group are those at risk for high blood pressure, and strokes this condition can lead to.

- DASH is very similar to the Mediterranean diet, with one important exception: it limits salt intake, since the sodium in salt directly affects blood pressure.
- Apart from this one distinction, DASH diets emphasize vegetables and fruits, whole grains, nuts and seeds, beans, low fat dairy, eggs, coldwater fish, less red meat, and no processed meats, like Spam, bacon, and sausages, all of which are commonly high in sodium.
- "DASH diet and Mediterranean diet are the most popular diet plans in the US. As per World Health Report and US News, both have been declared the top 2 best eating plans consistently over the years," reports Sarika Moghe in *Health Unplugged* (2022).
- If hypertension is a concern, be sure to read labels and check the sodium content. Many canned foods are high in salt, but some offer low-salt versions.

You've Made It!

You have now mastered the exercises within Resistance Bands For Seniors 50, 60 and Beyond – **Congratulations!**

This completes your resistance band training. Now on to Chapter 11: **Workout Programs**

To provide further encouragement we have designed 4 week workout routines specifically for you. They are intended to help you build a habit of regular exercise.

Initially, the workouts are to be performed twice a week. As your fitness and strength increase, consider working out more frequently, increasing the number of repetitions performed or using stronger Bands and when you feel ready and confident move to the next level workouts.

These whole body workouts are suggestions only. You can modify each workout to suit your particular interest.

The most important thing to achieve your goal is consistency.

Exercise regularly and you will see your strength and fitness improve!

CHAPTER 11

Workout Programs

SCAN FOR AUDIO CHAPTER

"what seems impossible today will one day become your warm-up."

Exercise Videos

It is often beneficial and easier to see an exercise being performed rather than following written instructions. Which is why, each exercise in this book has a QR code that links to it's video clip.

While all the exercises included in each workout routine below can be accessed individually by scanning their respective QR codes, **if you wish to see all the exercises included in a workout in a single video**, avoiding the necessity of scanning each exercise's QR code one at a time, become part of our community by scanning this QR code.

4 Week Workouts

Here we'll cover four different types of workouts you can do to keep things mixed up, so your body will end up constantly adapting, avoiding plateaus in your progress:

- Beginner's Workouts
- Intermediate Workouts
- Advanced Workouts
- Seated Workouts

See the next page for the programs ...

Beginner Workout (4 weeks)

Beginner - Week 1 (a)

Exercise	**#**	**Sets**	**Reps**	**Rest**
Chest Pull Apart	**#1**	3	10	30 seconds
Lat Pulldown	**#2**	3	10	30 seconds
Band Side Step	**#5**	3	30 seconds	30 seconds
Clamshell	**#6**	2 (each side)	10	30 seconds
Pallof Press	**#4**	2	5 (each side)	30 seconds

Beginner - Week 1 (b)

Exercise	**#**	**Sets**	**Reps**	**Rest**
Chest Press	**#8**	3	10	30 seconds
Seated Row	**#3**	3	10	30 seconds
Band Side Step	**#5**	3	30 seconds	30 seconds
Side Leg Lift	**#7**	2 (each side)	10	30 seconds
Pallof Press	**#4**	2	5 (each side)	30 seconds

Beginner - Week 2 (a)

Exercise	**#**	**Sets**	**Reps**	**Rest**
Chest Pull Apart	**#1**	3	10-12	30 seconds
Lat Pulldown	**#2**	3	10-12	30 seconds
Band Side Step	**#5**	3	35 seconds	30 seconds
Clamshell	**#6**	2 (each side)	10-12	30 seconds
Pallof Press	**#4**	2	6 (each side)	30 seconds

Beginner - Week 2 (b)

Exercise	#	Sets	Reps	Rest
Chest Press	**#1**	3	10-12	30 seconds
Seated Row	**#3**	3	10-12	30 seconds
Band Side Step	**#5**	3	35 seconds	30 seconds
Side Leg Lift	**#7**	2 (each side)	10-12	30 seconds
Pallof Press	**#4**	2	6 (each side)	30 seconds

Beginner - Week 3 (a)

Exercise	#	Sets	Reps	Rest
Chest Pull Apart	**#1**	3	12-15	30 seconds
Lat Pulldown	**#2**	3	12-15	30 seconds
Band Side Step	**#5**	3	40 seconds	30 seconds
Clamshell	**#6**	2 (each side)	12-15	30 seconds
Pallof Press	**#4**	2	7 (each side)	30 seconds

Beginner - Week 3 (b)

Exercise	#	Sets	Reps	Rest
Chest Press	**#8**	3	12-15	30 seconds
Seated Row	**#3**	3	12-15	30 seconds
Band Side Step	**#5**	3	40 seconds	30 seconds
Side Leg Lift	**#7**	2 (each side)	12-15	30 seconds
Pallof Press	**#4**	2	7 (each side)	30 seconds

Beginner - Week 4 (a)

Exercise	#	Sets	Reps	Rest
Chest Pull Apart	**#1**	3	12-20	30 seconds
Lat Pulldown	**#2**	3	12-20	30 seconds
Band Side Step	**#5**	3	45 seconds	30 seconds
Clamshell	**#6**	2 (each side)	12-20	30 seconds
Pallof Press	**#4**	2	8 (each side)	30 seconds

Beginner - Week 4 (b)

Exercise	#	Sets	Reps	Rest
Chest Press	**#8**	3	12-20	30 seconds
Seated Row	**#3**	3	12-20	30 seconds
Band Side Step	**#5**	3	45 seconds	30 seconds
Side Leg Lift	**#7**	2 (each side)	12-20	30 seconds
Pallof Press	**#4**	2	8 (each side)	30 seconds

Intermediate Workout (4 weeks)

Intermediate - Week 1 (a)

Exercise	#	Sets	Reps	Rest
Hip Thrust	**#9**	3	10-15	30 seconds
Bulgarian Split Squat	**#10**	3 (each side)	10	30 seconds
Bend Over	**#15**	3	10-20	30 seconds
Banded Push Up	**#12**	3	8-12	30 seconds
One Arm Row	**#14**	3 (each side)	10	30 seconds
One Arm Shoulder Press	**#13**	3 (each arm)	10	30 seconds

Intermediate - Week 1 (b)

Exercise	#	Sets	Reps	Rest
Hip Thrust	**#9**	3	10-20	30 seconds
Bulgarian Split Squat	**#10**	3 (each side)	10	30 seconds
Pull Down	**#11**	3	10	30 seconds
Banded Push Up	**#12**	3	8-12	30 seconds
Banded Dead Bug	**#16**	2 (each side)	12	30 seconds
Banded Plank Walk	**#17**	3	10	30 seconds

Intermediate - Week 2 (a)

Exercise	#	Sets	Reps	Rest
Hip Thrust	**#9**	3	12-15	30 seconds
Bulgarian Split Squat	**#10**	3 (each side)	12	30 seconds
Bend Over	**#15**	3	15-20	30 seconds
Banded Push Up	**#12**	3	10-12	30 seconds
One Arm Row	**#14**	3 (each side)	12	30 seconds
One Arm Shoulder Press	**#13**	3 (each arm)	12	30 seconds

Intermediate - Week 2 (b)

Exercise	#	Sets	Reps	Rest
Hip Thrust	**#9**	3	12-20	30 seconds
Bulgarian Split Squat	**#10**	3 (each side)	12	30 seconds
Pull Down	**#11**	3	12-15	30 seconds
Banded Push Up	**#12**	3	10-12	30 seconds
Banded Dead Bug	**#16**	2 (each side)	15	30 seconds
Banded Plank Walk	**#17**	3	12	30 seconds

Intermediate - Week 3 (a)

Exercise	#	Sets	Reps	Rest
Hip Thrust	**#9**	3	15	30 seconds
Bulgarian Split Squat	**#10**	3 (each side)	15	30 seconds
Bend Over	**#15**	3	20	30 seconds
Banded Push Up	**#12**	3	12	30 seconds
One Arm Row	**#14**	3 (each side)	12-15	30 seconds
One Arm Shoulder Press	**#13**	3 (each arm)	12-15	30 seconds

Intermediate - Week 3 (b)

Exercise	#	Sets	Reps	Rest
Hip Thrust	**#9**	3	20	30 seconds
Bulgarian Split Squat	**#10**	3 (each side)	15	30 seconds
Pull Down	**#11**	3	15	30 seconds
Banded Push Up	**#12**	3	12	30 seconds
Banded Dead Bug	**#16**	2 (each side)	15-20	30 seconds
Banded Plank Walk	**#17**	3	12	30 seconds

ntermediate - Week 4 (a)

Exercise	#	Sets	Reps	Rest
Hip Thrust	**#9**	3	15-20	30 seconds
Bulgarian Split Squat	**#10**	3 (each side)	15	30 seconds
Bend Over	**#15**	3	20	30 seconds
Banded Push Up	**#12**	3	12-15	30 seconds
One Arm Row	**#14**	3 (each side)	15	30 seconds
One Arm Shoulder Press	**#13**	3 (each arm)	15	30 seconds

Intermediate - Week 4 (b)

Exercise	#	Sets	Reps	Rest
Hip Thrust	**#9**	3	20	30 seconds
Bulgarian Split Squat	**#10**	3 (each side)	15	30 seconds
Pull Down	**#11**	3	15-20	30 seconds
Banded Push Up	**#12**	3	12-15	30 seconds
Banded Dead Bug	**#16**	2 (each side)	20	30 seconds
Banded Plank Walk	**#17**	3	15	30 seconds

Advanced Workout (4 weeks)

Advanced Workout - Week 1 (a)

Exercise	#	Sets	Reps	Rest
Pull to Face	**#30**	3	12-20	30 seconds
Front Squat	**#31**	3	8-12	60 seconds
Single Leg Deadlift	**#32**	3 (each side)	10	60 seconds
Bulgarian Split Squat	**#10**	3 (each side)	10	40 seconds
Hip Thrust	**#9**	3	10-15	30 seconds
Chest Crossover	**#35**	3	10-15	30 seconds
Lateral Raise	**#37**	3	10-12	30 seconds
One Arm Row	**#14**	3 (each side)	10	30 seconds
Resistance Crunch	**#36**	3	8	30 seconds

Advanced Workout - Week 1 (b)

Exercise	#	Sets	Reps	Rest
Pull to Face	**#30**	3	12-20	30 seconds
Clean and Press	**#33**	4	6-10	60 seconds
Hip Thrust	**#9**	3	10-20	30 seconds
Bulgarian Split Squat	**#10**	3 (each side)	10	60 seconds
Chest Press	**#8**	3	10	30 seconds
Lat Pulldown	**#2**	3	8-12	30 seconds
Bear Crawl	**#34**	3	10	60 seconds
Pallof Press	**#4**	2	10 (each side)	40 seconds
Banded Plank Walk	**#17**	3	10	30 seconds

Advanced Workout - Week 2 (a)

Exercise	#	Sets	Reps	Rest
Pull to Face	**#30**	3	15-20	30 seconds
Front Squat	**#31**	3	10-12	60 seconds
Single Leg Deadlift	**#32**	3 (each side)	10-12	60 seconds
Bulgarian Split Squat	**#10**	3 (each side)	10-15	40 seconds
Hip Thrust	**#9**	3	10-20	30 seconds
Chest Crossover	**#35**	3	15	30 seconds
Lateral Raise	**#37**	3	12	30 seconds
One Arm Row	**#14**	3 (each side)	10-15	30 seconds
Resistance Crunch	**#36**	3	8-10	30 seconds

Advanced Workout - Week 2 (b)

Exercise	#	Sets	Reps	Rest
Pull to Face	**#30**	3	15-20	30 seconds
Clean and Press	**#33**	4	8-10	60 seconds
Hip Thrust	**#9**	3	15-20	30 seconds
Bulgarian Split Squat	**#10**	3 (each side)	10-12	60 seconds
Chest Press	**#8**	3	10-15	30 seconds
Lat Pulldown	**#2**	3	10-12	30 seconds

Exercise	#	Sets	Reps	Rest
Bear Crawl	**#34**	3	10-12	60 seconds
Pallof Press	**#4**	2	12 (each side)	40 seconds
Banded Plank Walk	**#17**	3	15	30 seconds

Advanced Workout - Week 3 (a)

Exercise	#	Sets	Reps	Rest
Pull to Your Face	**#30**	3	20	30 seconds
Front Squat	**#31**	3	12-15	60 seconds
Single Leg Deadlift	**#32**	3 (each side)	12-15	60 seconds
Bulgarian Split Squat	**#10**	3 (each side)	15	40 seconds
Hip Thrust	**#9**	3	15-20	30 seconds
Chest Crossover	**#35**	3	15-20	30 seconds
Lateral Leg Raise	**#37**	3	12-15	30 seconds
One Arm Row	**#14**	3 (each side)	12-15	30 seconds
Resistance Crunch	**#36**	3	10-15	30 seconds

Advanced Workout - Week 3 (b)

Exercise	#	Sets	Reps	Rest
Pull to Face	**#30**	3	20	30 seconds
Clean and Press	**#33**	4	10-12	60 seconds
Hip Thrust	**#9**	3	20	30 seconds
Bulgarian Split Squat	**#10**	3 (each side)	12-15	60 seconds
Chest Press	**#8**	3	15-20	30 seconds
Lat Pulldown	**#2**	3	10-15	30 seconds
Bear Crawl	**#34**	3	10-15	60 seconds
Pallof Press	**#4**	2	15 (each side)	40 seconds
Banded Plank Walk	**#17**	3	15-20	30 seconds

Advanced Workout - Week 4 (a)

Exercise	#	Sets	Reps	Rest
Pull to Face	**#30**	3	20	30 seconds
Front Squat	**#31**	3	15-20	60 seconds
Single Leg Deadlift	**#32**	3 (each side)	15	60 seconds
Bulgarian Split Squat	**#10**	3 (each side)	15	40 seconds
Hip Thrust	**#9**	3	20	30 seconds
Chest Crossover	**#35**	3	20	30 seconds
Lateral Leg Raise	**#37**	3	15	30 seconds
One Arm Row	**#14**	3 (each side)	15-20	30 seconds
Resistance Crunch	**#36**	3	10-20	30 seconds

Advanced Workout - Week 4 (b)

Exercise	#	Sets	Reps	Rest
Pull to Face	**#30**	3	20	30 seconds
Clean and Press	**#33**	4	12	60 seconds
Hip Thrust	**#9**	3	20	30 seconds
Bulgarian Split Squat	**#10**	3 (each side)	15	60 seconds
Chest Press	**#8**	3	20	30 seconds
Lat Pulldown	**#2**	3	15-20	30 seconds
Bear Crawl	**#34**	3	15	60 seconds
Pallof Press	**#4**	2	20 (each side)	40 seconds
Banded Plank Walk	**#17**	3	20	30 seconds

Seated Workouts (4 weeks)

Seated Workouts - Week 1 (a)

Exercise	#	Sets	Reps	Rest
Chest Press	**#23**	3	10-12	30 seconds
Shoulder Press	**#24**	3	10-12	30 seconds
Tricep Extension 1	**#25**	2-3 (each side)	8-10	30 seconds

Exercise	#	Sets	Reps	Rest
Bicep Curl 1	**#27**	3 (each side)	8-10	30 seconds
Leg Press	**#20**	3 (each leg)	5-10	30 seconds
Leg Lift	**#19**	3 (each leg)	5	30 seconds
Pointed Foot Flex	**#18**	3 (each leg)	5	30 seconds
Abdominal Lean	**#22**	3	10	30 seconds

Seated Workouts – Week 1 (b)

Exercise	#	Sets	Reps	Rest
Chest Stretch	**#29**	2-3	10	30 seconds
Shoulder Press	**#24**	3	10-12	30 seconds
Tricep Extension 2	**#26**	2-3 (each side)	8-10	30 seconds
Bicep Curl 2	**#28**	3 (each side)	8-10	30 seconds
Hip Opener	**#21**	3 (each leg)	5-8	30 seconds
Leg Lift	**#19**	3 (each leg)	5	30 seconds
Pointed Toes	**#18**	3 (each leg)	5	30 seconds
Abdominal Lean	**#22**	3	10	30 seconds

Seated Workouts - Week 2 (a)

Exercise	#	Sets	Reps	Rest
Chest Press	**#23**	3	12	30 seconds
Shoulder Press	**#24**	3	12	30 seconds
Tricep Extension 1	**#25**	2-3 (each side)	10	30 seconds
Bicep Curl 1	**#27**	3 (each side)	10	30 seconds
Leg Press	**#20**	3 (each leg)	8-10	30 seconds
Leg Lift	**#19**	3 (each leg)	6	30 seconds
Pointed Toes	**#18**	3 (each leg)	6	30 seconds
Abdominal Lean	**#22**	3	15	30 seconds

Seated Workouts – Week 2 (b)

Exercise	#	Sets	Reps	Rest
Chest Stretch	**#29**	2-3	10-15	30 seconds
Shoulder Press	**#24**	3	12	30 seconds
Tricep Extension 2	**#26**	2-3 (each side)	10	30 seconds

Exercise	#	Sets	Reps	Rest
Bicep Curl 2	**#28**	3 (each side)	10	30 seconds
Hip Opener	**#21**	3 (each leg)	8-10	30 seconds
Leg Lift	**#19**	3 (each leg)	6	30 seconds
Pointed Toes	**#18**	3 (each leg)	6	30 seconds
Abdominal Lean	**#22**	3	15	30 seconds

Seated Workouts – Week 3 (a)

Exercise	#	Sets	Reps	Rest
Chest Press	**#23**	3	12-15	30 seconds
Shoulder Press	**#24**	3	12-15	30 seconds
Tricep Extension 1	**#25**	2-3 (each side)	10-12	30 seconds
Bicep Curl 1	**#27**	3 (each side)	10-12	30 seconds
Leg Press	**#20**	3 (each leg)	10	30 seconds
Leg Lift	**#19**	3 (each leg)	6-8	30 seconds
Pointed Toes	**#18**	3 (each leg)	6-8	30 seconds
Abdominal Lean	**#22**	3	15-20	30 seconds

Seated Workouts – Week 3 (b)

Exercise	#	Sets	Reps	Rest
Chest Stretch	**#29**	2-3	15-20	30 seconds
Shoulder Press	**#24**	3	12-15	30 seconds
Tricep Extension 2	**#26**	2-3 (each side)	10-12	30 seconds
Bicep Curl 2	**#28**	3 (each side)	10-12	30 seconds
Hip Opener	**#21**	3 (each leg)	10	30 seconds
Leg Lift	**#19**	3 (each leg)	6-8	30 seconds
Pointed Toes	**#18**	3 (each leg)	6-8	30 seconds
Abdominal Lean	**#22**	3	15-20	30 seconds

Seated Workouts – Week 4 (a)

Exercise	#	Sets	Reps	Rest
Chest Press	**#23**	3	15	30 seconds
Shoulder Press	**#24**	3	15	30 seconds
Tricep Extension 1	**#25**	2-3 (each side)	12	30 seconds

Exercise	#	Sets	Reps	Rest
Bicep Curl 1	**#27**	3 (each side)	12	30 seconds
Leg Press	**#20**	3 (each leg)	10-15	30 seconds
Leg Lift	**#19**	3 (each leg)	8	30 seconds
Pointed Toes	**#18**	3 (each leg)	8	30 seconds
Abdominal Lean	**#22**	3	20	30 seconds

Seated Workouts – Week 4 (b)

Exercise	#	Sets	Reps	Rest
Chest Stretch	**#29**	2-3	20	30 seconds
Shoulder Press	**#24**	3	15	30 seconds
Tricep Extension 2	**#26**	2-3 (each side)	12	30 seconds
Bicep Curl 2	**#28**	3 (each side)	12	30 seconds
Hip Opener	**#21**	3 (each leg)	10-12	30 seconds
Leg Lift	**#19**	3 (each leg)	8	30 seconds
Pointed Toes	**#18**	3 (each leg)	8	30 seconds
Abdominal Lean	**#22**	3	20	30 seconds

CHAPTER 12

Conclusion

SCAN FOR AUDIO CHAPTER

The Great Equalizer

Resistance bands represent what you could call 'The Great Equalizer' among the muscle and strength building alternatives. Resistance bands are accessible to virtually everyone, and are far less expensive than owning weightlifting equipment, or joining a fitness center. They are portable, easy to store, and can be used at home, or just about anywhere.

Yet resistance bands are equal to the weights and cable machines in building muscle mass, strength, and endurance:

- Performing 10 to 12 tricep presses, bicep curls, chest presses, or any other muscle-building movements with resistance bands and tubes will give the same results as the same movements with dumbbells and barbells, assuming equivalent resistance levels.
- You can replicate what you could do in a well-equipped gym with the many resistance band exercises we've covered in this book, and actually go farther and do more than most gym workouts entail.
- Resistance bands may be actually more effective than weights, because the intensity of the resistance increases as you lift or pull; weights tend to 'weigh less' when you get to the top of the lift. Your bands, conversely, intensify the challenge.
- Bodyweight calisthenics are a good supplement to resistance band training, because they too can be performed anywhere, without the costs and inconveniences of equipment.

Even better, in combination, resistance bands and calisthenics can optimize the results of your workouts.

Consider your safety: As a senior, you will appreciate that resistance bands are credited with being safer than weights. You won't injure yourself by dropping a weight or losing control of it so it pulls or tears a muscle or tendon, or yanks a joint out of place. You will be less likely to lift or pull too heavy a resistance level, and over-exhaust your muscles.

Mind your form: Effectiveness in getting stronger and doing it safely means being attentive to the instructions for each individual move. Make sure your form is correct and you're always maintaining good posture in order to reinforce it, rather than compromising the exercises and reinforcing bad posture!

Protect your back: Be especially attentive to your back, which you depend on continuously, and which is easily injured if you are careless when working out with resistance bands, or when lifting anything heavy. Remember that your flexibility is not what it once was, so respect your years with caution.

Respect rest: You need a brief rest between each set of reps, to give your muscles a chance to reoxygenate, and enable you to do the next set effectively. Of even greater importance is the need for you to rest for at least a full day between resistance workouts involving each muscle group, to allow hypertrophy to repair, rebuild, and make you a little bit stronger. If you are injured make rest your priority, to get you back to your regular routine sooner.

Include aerobics: in your weekly routine to increase your resistance to diseases, and potentially keep you alive longer, and able to enjoy a higher quality of life. Try to get at least 75 minutes of vigorous cardiovascular training into your weekly schedule, or 150 minutes at a moderate pace.

You are what you eat: so eat well, and in moderation. Read up on the Mediterranean and DASH diets for knowledge and recipe ideas, and don't be seduced by the risky fad diets that keep emerging online and in bookstores.

Spread the Word

If you enjoyed this book as much as I have enjoyed writing it, and if you feel (as I surely hope) that the resistance bands training you've received here will positively improve your lifestyle and your life, please tell others.

Spread the word by referrals to friends, family, and other seniors (and soon-to-be seniors) whom you know, and who you think can benefit.

Our Community:

To be one of the first people to receive notification of future books in the series "For Seniors 50, 60 and Beyond" when they are released join our community. I'll personally notify you as soon the next book in the series is available. Our monthly newsletter also contains tip, tricks and advice to help you on your fitness journey.

As a member you have access to the exercise videos directly from our website ***www.iaa.pub***, without the need to scan individual QR codes within the book. Plus **Exclusive Members Access** to workout videos showing the exercises contained in each of the 32 workouts (not available from within the book), a great reference and time saver!

Finally, I wish to thank you so much for reading *Resistance Bands for Seniors 50, 60 and Beyond*. It was written to provide helpful information to seniors, and I hope that you'll use what you've learned in this book to build strength, improve balance as well as to look and feel years younger, boosting your confidence!

I have a favor to ask:

Would you please take a couple of minutes to write a review of this book on Amazon? I'll be checking the reviews personally and your honest feedback will help me better help others on their fitness journey.

To leave a review:

You can either:

- Scan the QR Code on your mobile

- visit Amazon's website, search for *Resistance Bands for Seniors 50, 60 and Beyond*. Click the link for this book, scroll down, and click on "Write a Customer Review."

Thank you very much, and I look forward to reading your comments!

David O'Connor

For Seniors 50, 60 and Beyond

BOOK SERIES

Book 1: **Fitness For Seniors 50, 60 and Beyond**

It's never too early to improve your fitness and definitely never to late to start. Consider this a fitness guide book, dip into to its sections as and when required.

Book 2: **Resistance Bands For Seniors 50, 60 and Beyond**

Strength and flexibility training without the need to purchase expensive weights and with less risk of injury, or a gym membership.

Book 3: **Balance Exercise For Seniors 50, 60 and Beyond**

Improve your balance to significantly reduce the risk and overcome the fear of falling. Live an active life in your golden years with increased self-confidence.

Book 4: **Chair Yoga For Seniors 50, 60 and Beyond**

All the benefits of yoga achievable while sitting or using a chair for additional support. Chair yoga offers variations that are perfect for seniors, even for those with limited mobility.

Book 5: **Stretching For Seniors 50, 60 and Beyond**

Stretches to improve flexibility, balance, mobility and reduce muscle pain for beginner through to advanced practitioners. Stretching helps release muscle tension, soreness and reduces the risk of injury.

Book 6: **Core Training For Seniors 50, 60 and Beyond**

A strong core stabilizes your entire body, providing better balance and posture. Core strength is essential at any age but especially as you get older and your risk of falling increases.

An overview of the For Seniors 50, 60 and Beyond book series is available at www.iaa.pub or scan the QR code.

SCAN FOR BOOK INFORMATION

Glossary

Advanced Training. Resistance exercises for experienced individuals who have mastered the less complex and challenging groups of exercises; in addition to complexity, advanced training depends on higher levels of resistance.

Aerobic Exercise. Also called cardiovascular conditioning; aerobics are performed at a pace for a sustained period, with the objective of elevating the heart rate, and pumping more oxygen-rich blood through the heart to the muscles to help prevent heart disease, obesity, type 2 diabetes, and other diseases. Examples: Running, ellipticals cycling.

Beginner Training. A series of relatively simple and easy resistance exercises that are used to start a training program, and familiarize the user with usage of the various bands and tubes.

Calisthenics. A form of resistance exercises that use minimal or no equipment; relying instead on a person's body weight to provide the resistance force. Push ups, crunches, squats, and planks are examples.

Cardiovascular Conditioning. See Aerobic Exercise.

Free Weights. Dumbbells, barbells, and kettle weights used in the resistance training called weightlifting, and distinguished from weight cable machines generally found in gyms and fitness centers, which provide guided movements.

Hypertrophy. The intramuscular process of breaking down muscle cells and fibers as a result of resistance training, followed by rebuilding and overbuilding with added protein; it occurs during a rest of 48 hours following a hard resistance workout.

Intermediate Resistance. A series of resistance exercises that are more complex and challenging than beginner movements, and require a higher level of strength and a better sense of balance.

Managed breathing. Conscious inhalation with the abdomen and diaphragm extended outward to increase lung capacity, and exhalation with the abdomen and diaphragm tightly contracted to fully empty the lungs; used in yoga and other exercises.

Mediterranean Diet. A widely recommended dietary and lifestyle practice based on populations, whose health and longevity are above average; includes a wide range of unprocessed whole grains, vegetables and fruits, nuts and seeds, beans, fish, low fat dairy, eggs, and olive oil.

Monounsaturated Fats. A form of fat, generally an oil at room temperature, which is credited with lowering LDL ("bad") cholesterol and raising HDL ("good") cholesterol, and therefore recommended for heart health. Abundant in extra virgin olive oil, canola oil and avocados.

Polyunsaturated Fats. Usually an oil at room temperature, also credited with lowering LDL (bad) cholesterol and raising HDL (good) cholesterol, and therefore recommended for heart health. Found in corn oil, sunflower oil, soybean oil, safflower oil, and peanut oil.

Note: Both mono and polyunsaturated oils are considered heart healthy; but recently monounsaturated oil has gained a reputation of being the more effective. New studies indicate that both types are equally beneficial, per *VeryWell Health* (2022).

Reps and Sets. 1 cycle of a resistance exercise is a repetition, or rep, such as raising and lowering a weight one time; a series of continued reps, such as 10 bicep curls or 12 push ups, is a set. A typical routine is three sets of 8 to 12 reps.

Resistance Bands. Stretchable flat and tubular lengths of a rubber or latex-based material that provide varying levels of resistance during exercise; some (tubes, primarily) have handles, and most bands are color-coded to designate resistance levels.

Resistance Training. These are exercises that use free weights, cable machines, or resistance bands and tubes to exhaust muscles to make them stronger, build endurance and make connective tendons, joints and ligaments more flexible and resilient.

RICE Method. A widely recommended procedure for treating injuries to muscles and joints: Rest, Ice, Compression, Elevation.

Saturated Fats. Typically solid at room temperature, and associated with elevated levels of LDL (bad) cholesterol and triglycerides, and resultant buildup of plaque in the coronary arteries; a serious form of heart disease. Found in meats and full fat dairy products, and in coconut and palm oils.

Stretching. A form of exercise that is distinguished from resistance and aerobic training; its objective is to lengthen and flex muscles, and connective tissues and joints to increase ranges of motion, and prevent injuries and improve performance. (See Yoga).

VO2 Max. The highest level your pulse can achieve under extreme stress; it is used to calculate your ideal heartbeat during aerobic exercise, which is generally 65% of 220 minus your age.

Warmups. Any exercise or stretching that is performed before resistance or aerobic training, to increase flexibility, and begin to oxygenate the heart and skeletal muscles.

Yoga. An ancient practice of stretches and poses (called *asanas*) originating in India and Asia, and very popular worldwide today. The focus is on managed breathing, concentration, balance, and flexibility. Yoga is a good supplement to resistance training.

References

AZ Quotes. (2022). *Motivational inspirational sports quotes.*

https://www.azquotes.com/quotes/topics/motivational-inspirational-sports.html

Ali, M. (2011, February 3). *Top 25 quotes by Muhammad Ali (of 544).* AZ Quotes.

https://www.azquotes.com/author/242-Muhammad_Ali

Bodybuilding.com (2021, January 20). *Bodybuilding.com's highest rated resistance band workouts.*

https://www.bodybuilding.com/content/best-resistance-band-workouts.html

BodyGym. (2022). *Before and after results of using resistance bands.*

https://moveyourself.bodygym.com/post/before-and-after-results-using-resistance-bands

Cleveland Clinic. (2022, May 4). *How effective are resistance bands for strength training?* Health Essentials from Cleveland Clinic.

https://health.clevelandclinic.org/should-you-try-resistance-bands-for-strength-training/

Article adapted from Cleveland Clinic Men's Health Advisor

Clifton. T. (2021, June 25). *Resistance band workouts for abs: 11 Exercises to try.* Healthline.

https://www.healthline.com/health/fitness/resistance-band-workouts-abs

Fetters, K. A. (2022, March 29). *The total-body resistance band workout.* Silver Sneakers.

https://www.silversneakers.com/blog/total-body-resistance-band-workout-older-adults/

Fetters, K. A. (2021, October 17). *7 Quick moves to do before every strength workout.* Silver Sneakers.

https://www.silversneakers.com/blog/7-quick-moves-to-do-before-every-strength-workout/

Lerner, A. (2018, April 24). *The beginner's guide to exercise bands.* Silver Sneakers.

https://www.silversneakers.com/blog/pick-right-resistance-band/

Lopes, J. S. S., Machado, A. F., Micheletti, J. K., de Almeida, A. C., Cavina, A. P., & Pastre, C. M. (2019, February 19). *Effects of training with elastic resistance versus conventional resistance on muscular strength: A systematic review and meta-analysis*. SAGE Open Medicine, 7(PMC6383082), 205031211983111. National Institute of Health (NIH).

https://doi.org/10.1177/2050312119831116

Lyon, R. A. (2022, August 18). *Do resistance bands build bone density?* Senior Fitness.

https://www.seniorfitness.org/do-resistance-bands-build-bone-density/

Machowsky, J. (2022, March 29). *The total-body resistance band workout*. Silver Sneakers.

https://www.silversneakers.com/blog/total-body-resistance-band-workout-older-adults/

Migala, J. (2022, April 13). *How to get started with resistance band workouts: An absolute beginner's guide*. Everyday Health.

https://www.everydayhealth.com/fitness/how-to-get-started-with-resistance-band-workouts-an-absolute-beginners-guide/

Moghe, S. (2022, August 28). *DASH diet vs. Mediterranean diet*. Health Plugged.

https://healthplugged.com/dash-diet-mediterranean-diet/

Moll, J. (2022, August 24). *Saturated vs. unsaturated fats*. VeryWell Health.

https://www.verywellhealth.com/difference-between-saturated-fats-and-unsaturated-fats-697517

Porter, E. (2020, September 8). *9 Types of resistance bands and when to use each of them*. Trusty Spotter.

https://trustyspotter.com/blog/types-of-resistance-bands/

Samuel, E., et al. (2022, August 17). *56 Resistance bands moves you can do at home*. Men's Health.

https://www.menshealth.com/fitness/a32093962/resistance-band-workouts/

Samuels, M. (2013, October 19). *Exercises for ancillary muscles*. SportsRec.

https://www.sportsrec.com/exercises-ancillary-muscles-12320280.html

Stephens, D'A. (2022, March 12). *This 20-minute resistance band workout actually feels harder than weights*. Livestrong.

https://www.livestrong.com/article/13770019-20-minute-advanced-resistance-band-workout/

Stivey, G. (2022, April 20). *How to use resistance bands for injury recovery*. GND Fitness.

https://gndfit.com/blogs/gnd-fitness/how-to-use-resistance-bands-for-injury-recovery?shpxid=ab450fa2-f3d3-4df5-bfec-90020a13bf08

TB12 Team. (2021, February 10). *Tom Brady workout: His 9-exercise high-intensity favorite.*

https://tb12sports.com/blogs/tb12/tom-brady-workout

Waehner, J. (2022, June 22). *Beginner's total body resistance band workout*. Very Well Fit.

https://www.verywellfit.com/beginner-total-body-resistance-band-workout-1231110

WebMD. (2022). *Best resistance band exercises for beginners.*

https://www.webmd.com/fitness-exercise/resistance-bands-exercises-beginners#1

WebMD. (2021, April 24). *What is the RICE method for injuries?*

https://www.webmd.com/first-aid/rice-method-injuries

Yes2Next. (2022, August 4). *10 Chair resistance band exercises.*

https://yes2next.com/fitness-joy/resistance-bands

CORE TRAINING FOR SENIORS

50, 60 and Beyond

Home Exercises to improve Core Strength, Posture, Balance and Relieve Back Pain. Fully illustrated + Free videos

DAVID O'CONNOR

CORE TRAINING FOR SENIORS 50, 60 AND BEYOND

Core Training For Seniors 50, 60 and Beyond offers 60+ practical and easy-to-follow exercises to strengthen your core muscles and improve your overall health. This book provides three complete 24 week training programs tailored to differing levels and abilities, plus free videos of exercises to ensure good form and maximum benefit. You will discover how to reduce your risk of health complications and improve your quality of life.

Core training is more important with every passing year!

Benefits of reading this book:

- Strengthen your core and improve your quality of life
- Reduce your risk of health complications caused by inactivity
- Everyday tasks become easier
- Feel empowered to take control of your core strength and health

FOREWORD

This book is designed to provide exercises for people who are over 50 years old. As you can imagine, this encompasses a wide range of mobility levels. The exercises that a fit and healthy 50-year-old can perform are not going to be the same as the exercises that a 94-year-old can perform.

While a lot of effort has been put into creating training programs that are accessible to everyone, there may well be some people over 50 who are not able to properly follow the workouts in this book. Seated chair exercises are included however, there are floor exercises too. If you have very low mobility, disability, or health conditions that may affect your ability to perform very simple exercises, then this book may not be right for you.

Your best option would be to consult with your doctor and perhaps schedule some sessions with a physiotherapist. Not only will they be able to give you specific exercises that suit your capabilities, but they can also help you to improve your strength, fitness, and mobility, allowing you the opportunity to follow the exercises in this book at a later date.

It would be irresponsible to pretend that this book is for everyone. This is a shame, but it would be impossible to create a book that caters to every single person over 50. Some people need face-to-face coaching, which a book is not capable of recreating.

Equally, the advanced exercises require good mobility and previous fitness training. If you are unsure, my advice is start with the intermediate exercises and only when you feel comfortable performing them, and if you wish to increase the intensity of your workouts consider incorporation the advanced exercises into your program. You should not feel that you have to strive towards performing the advanced exercises, you do not!

A one size fits all approach to core exercise is simply impossible, this book however caters for the widest range of abilities as possible.

I did my best to make this book as comprehensive as possible so those new to core exercise or returning after a gap and looking for a detailed refresher would find the fullest information available within the book. Given the wide range of abilities this book caters for you may already be familiar with the contents of a chapter, in which case, feel free to skip ahead.

If you are new to exercise however, I would encourage you to read the book in its entirety to obtain a thorough understanding of core exercise.

FREE BONUS
FITNESS MATERIAL TO HELP YOU ACHIEVE YOUR GOAL

To ensure you gain as much value as possible from Core Training For Seniors 50, 60 and Beyond, I've put together some additional free bonus materials to help you achieve your goals, including:

1. ***24 Week Beginner's Workout Plan*** provided as printable PDF document.
2. **Exercise List:** all the exercises in this workout plan together with their video QR codes for easy reference. *Keep this handy as you train to locate videos without opening the book.*
3. **4 Fitness Word Puzzles**. As a bit of fun to help maintain brain fitness too.
4. **Direct access to the exercise videos** from our members area (without scanning QR Codes)
5. **Members Only Access** to videos showing the exercises contained in each of the workout plans (not available via QR codes from within the book)
6. **Monthly Newsletter** on topics to help you succeed on your fitness journey.

GET YOUR FREE BONUS MATERIAL

INTRODUCTION

SCAN FOR AUDIO CHAPTER

The world is becoming more and more sedentary with each passing year. This is due to many factors. We are more affluent, more jobs require you to sit down than at any point in history, and many adults tend to have weight-related health problems as they age.

It has never been easier to live a comfortable, sedentary lifestyle than at this moment in time. A study in 2018 found that over 80% of US jobs are sedentary, and that has increased by 83% since 1950 [1]. This increased sedentary during our younger years can have a knock-on effect in our retirement.

This is borne out in the data, with seniors reporting significantly more time per day spent pursuing sedentary activities. A 2015 study found that older adults in care facilities spent 79% of the hours they were awake sedentary and only spent 1% of their time performing moderate-to-vigorous physical activity [2].

Leading a sedentary lifestyle can have many health implications. It can increase your risk of heart disease, cancer, diabetes, and hypertension.

But it can also affect your musculature. A study in 2019 looked at the core strength and stability of bank employees, people who had highly sedentary jobs (75% of their day was spent sitting down) [3]. The study found that 72.73% of participants suffered from a weak core. Even participants who had healthy Body Mass Indexes (BMIs) had weak cores.

This study was in people who were 40-50 years old, and your core muscles will often weaken as you age. This means that if you are over 40 and you lead a sedentary lifestyle, then your core muscles are highly likely to be weak.

There are many downsides to having a weak core, and as you can imagine, there are many advantages to strengthening your core. In this book, we will take a look at what your core is made up of, how to train it, and the benefits of doing so.

You will have access to a huge range of core exercises, as well as exercises that strengthen the entire body (including your core). You will also receive a complete training program that can help you to strengthen your core, improve your cardiovascular fitness, and reduce your risk of health complications that can be exacerbated by inactivity.

Core training is often misrepresented as a way to build a six-pack. As such, the general public often overlooks it. "Oh, I don't want a six-pack. I just want to improve my health and be more active." Is a phrase that most personal trainers and fitness professionals hear thirty times per day in a gym setting. And it is usually seniors who say this.

Core training is seen as vain or something for the young and fit. Not something that regular people need to concern themselves with. As such, it is avoided, and many health-related complications may occur as a consequence.

One of the biggest goals of this book is to change the conversation surrounding core training for the seniors. It should no longer be seen as vain or unnecessary. Instead, it should be seen as a crucial component of overall fitness.

Core training is surprisingly accessible, and there are hundreds of variations that make it possible for people with all different levels of mobility to participate. The truth is that the less mobile you are, the less you need to do to see improvements in your core muscles.

While a fit and healthy person may need to perform several complicated and intense exercises, someone who hasn't exercised in decades could see significant improvements from a very simple, low-intensity movement.

This is why we have separated our core exercises into three groups (adjusted for the elderly): Beginner, medium, and advanced. You will easily find out what level you are, and then you will be able to follow a specific workout for your capabilities.

Don't worry if you find yourself in the beginner category. This means that you will get the most out of the book. You can follow the beginner training program, then step-up to the medium training program when you are ready, and finally, the advanced training program. As mentioned early, do not feel you must conquer the advanced exercises. Many fit seniors

I teach maintain their strong core without ever tackling the advanced exercises. There are however others who simply love the challenge and sense of achievement they receive from performing advanced exercises.

You may be worried that you've left it too late to strengthen your core. Isn't exercise just for the young and middle-aged? Well, science does not back this opinion up. Provided you are performing exercises that match your physical capabilities, then you can see huge benefits in the quality of your life and your health within a few weeks of regular exercise.

A 2018 study in the Journal of BioMed Research International found that exercise can protect against cardiovascular disease, strokes, diabetes, and cancer [4]. It can also improve mental health, help delay the onset of dementia, and it can improve your quality of life.

Regular, safe exercise is also much less likely to cause an injury than many elderly people suspect. In fact, it can reduce your risk of falling over and help you to respond better when you do. Injuries are not completely avoidable, but they are more likely the *less* you exercise.

Finally, before embarking on your core fitness journey, you should consider consulting your doctor. They can give you specific advice about what your limitations are and whether you are able to perform certain exercises.

Core training involves exercises that range from the very easy to the very difficult. However, almost all involve you creating a "block". This is where you breathe in and hold your abdominal muscles tight. Doing this makes the exercises safer and protects your lower back, but some people are not able to do this due to specific injuries and medical conditions.

The risks are very low, but it is still useful to schedule an appointment before following any new exercise regime. Your doctor will almost certainly advise you to follow a training program, but they may caution you against certain movements.

This information is not here to put you off exercising. It is to give you the context necessary to make an informed decision. No doctor will advise you *not* to exercise at all, but they can give you helpful specific tips that are beyond the scope of a book to offer.

Fully illustrated instructions plus exercise videos

What sets this book and the other books in the For Seniors 50, 60 and Beyond series apart is that I use my expertise and experience to describe each exercise in detail, so you can easily understand and follow along at your own pace. I keep the descriptions simple, but I still carefully explain the movements and positions with sufficient detail so you can perform each exercise correctly and avoid injury.

Often, no matter how precise a book's exercise instructions or detailed the accompanying illustrations are, they may still leave you unsure how to perform it. Incorrectly performed exercises reduce their effectiveness and can lead to injury, a possibility that increases with age. That is why I want you to be able to see how to perform each exercise to remove all ambiguity. Therefore, each exercise in this book is not only illustrated but accompanied by a QR Code, scan it on your mobile to watch a video clip of the exercise being performed.

Meet the Author

Who am I? Well, I'm a Personal Trainer and proud to say I've been studying and practicing physical training for most of my life and can appreciate the benefits this conditioning has done for my own health, not to mention many others whom I have trained so they were able to benefit from this same training and health information. Following are a few notes and quotes to give you a quick overview of my background and experiences.

- A fitness nut since my days at UCLA, cross-fit, trail running, and skiing are still my passions. During the last 25 years as a Ski Instructor and Personal Trainer, I've trained people of all ages and abilities to achieve their fitness goals. A couple of years ago my father required assistance to improve his health, having become increasingly sedentary with each passing year. It took a sustained effort to get him to accept that it's never too late to get fit, certainly not at just 65 years of age!
- I guided my father through a simple yet progressively challenging home exercise program, and introduced him to healthier eating habits appropriate for his stage of life and individual body type, also taking into account his specific needs due to a medical condition. Today, he lives a fulfilling, active Californian lifestyle, regularly beating me on the golf course.
- Another source of inspiration for me is George Jedenoff. He was still skiing Snowbird at the age of 103. George attributed a daily exercise program and a positive mindset for this vitality. He celebrated his 105th birthday in July 2022 and after a wonderful life sadly passed in October of that year.

The QR code below links to George's video where he shows his daily workout routine. Please take a look, I'm sure you will find it inspirational!

Leave a Review:

If you enjoy this book and it helps you achieve your goals, as I most definitely trust it will, please take a minute to leave a short Amazon review. Your feedback will help others considering starting their fitness journey and are the lifeblood of indie authors competing with established publishing houses and their large advertising budgets.

Every review is therefore greatly appreciate!

CHAPTER 1

What is the Core?

SCAN FOR AUDIO CHAPTER

The public's understanding of what muscles make up the core is, at best, mixed. Most people point vaguely to their abdominal muscles when asked where their core is located. This is understandable because what muscles make up the core is rarely communicated properly by the fitness industry. In fact, many fitness instructors and personal trainers may not be able to mention which muscles make up the core.

So, what is the core?

It might interest you to know that the term "core muscles" isn't actually an anatomical term. Students who study anatomy at University are not taught this specific grouping. Some people claim that there are 29 muscles that make up the core, while others are much more conservative with their number. This variance is due to the core being quite a vague concept.

The core muscles help:

- Support posture – particularly as resistance to forces
- Connects upper and lower body, allowing them to move together
- Assist continence
- Assist labour (giving birth)

While all of these functions are important, the ones that are focused on when exercising are the connection between the upper and lower body and the ability to support the spine, which impacts posture.

As an example, a boxer's punch is dependent on power from the legs not his arms! To properly connect, you need to generate power from your legs and transfer it into your arms, chest, and shoulders. Your core muscles do that.

But that's not all. The muscles of your core also provide stability. Imagine trying to throw a punch while off balance. It would be a lot weaker, as you wouldn't be able to generate force. A weak core will not provide stability, and it won't allow you to transfer power from your legs, and you will throw a weak punch.

This is not just a boxing thing. Stability and the transfer of power from upper to lower (and vice versa) affect every movement we make.

To give a more specific example, imagine you slip on some ice whilst out walking. Your lower body will be travelling in one direction while your upper body travels in another. Your core muscles will work hard to keep your spine stable.

A strong core could potentially help you to maintain your balance or to lessen the damage. A controlled fall is far better than an uncontrolled fall. The core as a stabilizer could make a huge difference to the amount of damage that your fall causes.

The following section describes in detail the core muscles and the benefits that accrue from having a strong core. If this level of detail is more than you require skip ahead to chapter two.

What Muscles Make Up the Core?

In this section, we will go over all of the muscles that make up the core, and then we will divide them into the main core muscles and the lesser core muscles. This is not meant to say that one set of muscles is better than another, just that some muscles are larger contributors to the functions of the core in an exercise setting.

The Core Muscles

- Pelvic Floor Muscles
- Rectus Abdominus (six-pack muscles)
- Transverse Abdominus

- Internal Obliques
- External Obliques
- Erector Spinae
- Multifidus
- Diaphragm
- Lumbar Muscles (several muscles make up this group)
- Longus Coli (neck muscle)
- Latissimus Dorsi (upper back muscle)
- Trapezius (upper back muscle)
- Gluteus Maximus

Don't worry if you don't recognise these muscles, it is not crucial to learn most of them and we will be going into more detail about each of the important core muscles for this book. But first, we shall separate the core muscles into major core muscles (for exercise and stability) and lesser core muscles (equally important, but for different reasons).

Major Core Muscles

- Rectus Abdominus
- Transverse Abdominus
- Internal & External Obliques
- Lower Back Muscles (Erector Spinae, Multifidus, Lumbar Muscles)

These are the main muscles that we will be focusing on in this book. You have the muscles around your abdomen (where most people point when you say "abs"), which includes the rectus abdominus, transverse abdominus and the internal and external obliques. Then there are the erector spinae and spinal muscles, which are situated in your lower back.

Rectus Abdominus

The rectus abdominus is better known as the six-pack, and it is a collection of six portions that are separated by a band of tissue that travels down the middle. They are all connected but can be separated in women when they give birth (it is called diastasis recti).

The rectus abdominus plays a crucial role in good posture, and it is important for natural movements like sitting up in bed or raising your knees. It is also very important for breathing, particularly the form of breathing that is required for lifting weights.

The rectus abdominal muscles are best worked using the traditional abdominal crunch. Lying on your back with feet flat on the floor and curling your shoulders and head up off the floor and towards your knees requires the rectus abdominals to flex; returning to the starting position causes them to stretch out, also placing a lot of stress on the muscles.

Transverse Abdominus

The transverse abdominus is directly behind (or underneath) the rectus abdominus. It is a deep-lying muscle and wraps around your lower torso a little like a cummerbund or very wide belt. The role of the transverse abdominus is to provide stability, and works a little like a corset (it is often referred to as the corset muscle) to hold in the abdomen, preventing your organs from pushing outwards.

A strong transverse abdominus can help you to perform many compound lifts (squats etc.) without risking your lower back or spine. You train the transverse abdominus with exercises such as the plank, bird dog, dead bug, and leg raises (all exercises described in the following chapters).

Internal & External Obliques

The oblique muscles are situated on the sides of your torso, starting at the bottom of your ribs and travelling down to your hips. They create our abdominal walls alongside the transverse abdominus.

The deepest layer of the abdominal wall is the transverse abdominus, which, as mentioned above, travels all the way around your lower torso like a belt.

Your internal obliques then form a second layer, one on each side of your rectus abdominus muscles.

Your external obliques then form a third layer, and the one closest to the skin.

Like the rectus abdominus and transverse abdominus, these muscles provide stability to the torso. They also allow you to twist and lean side to side. They benefit from twisting variations of the exercises that work the rectus abdominus.

For example, instead of a regular crunch that targets the six-pack muscles, you could perform a crunch where you twist your torso from side to side (touching your right elbow to your left knee and vice versa) to also target the obliques.

Lower Back Muscles

There are many lower back muscles that make up the major muscles of the core, but they mostly provide the same function and are worked in the same way, so it makes sense to group them together. These muscles are all located in the lower back, but many of them travel all the way up the spine.

It's a little too complicated to go into details, which is why we're going to refer to them as lower back muscles. These muscles allow you to straighten and rotate the spine. They also provide stability. Bowing forwards and returning is all down to the lower back muscles. Swaying from side to side is also a function of your lower back muscles.

You can work the lower back muscles with a huge variety of exercises.

Minor Core Muscles

- Pelvic Floor Muscles
- Diaphragm
- Longus Coli
- Latissimus Dorsi
- Trapezius
- Gluteus Maximus

As mentioned above, these muscles are all important and have crucial roles to play in how you move. But they aren't as important to your core when it comes to movement as the others. The lats and traps are ideal for pulling movements and upper back stability.

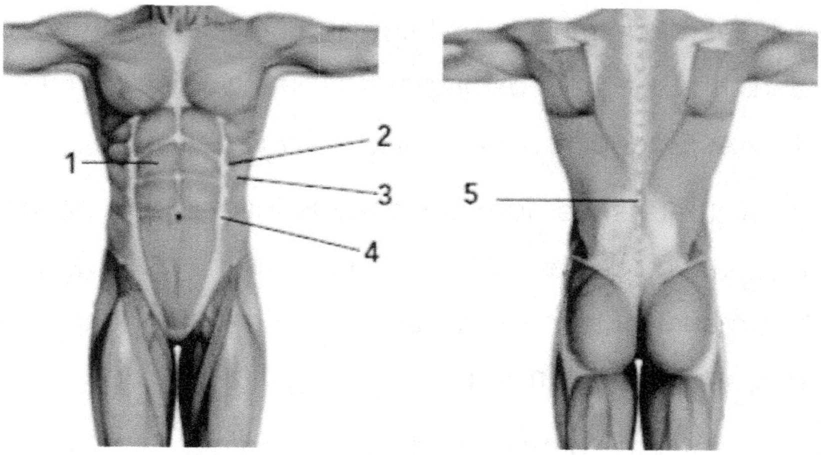

Major abdominal muscle group:

(1) Rectus abdominis

(2) External oblique

(3) Internal oblique

(4) Transverse abdominis

Main stabilizer muscles of the spine

(5) Iliocostalis

(5) Longissimus

(5) Spinalis

Why Our Core Muscles Weaken As We Age

There are few people who would argue that a 90-year-old will have weaker core muscles than a 20-year-old. But why is that? Well, there are two main reasons:

1. Biological changes
2. Lifestyle changes

The first reason is just a natural part of ageing. As we age, our muscles become weaker and smaller. This is called sarcopenia. There are many theories as to what causes sarcopenia, but one of the biggest causes is that the body becomes less efficient at absorbing an amino acid called leucine.

Protein plays a crucial role in muscle building and muscle maintenance. Protein is made up of amino acids, and three of the most important amino acids for muscles are branched-chain amino acids (BCAAs) – leucine, isoleucine, and valine.

Studies have shown that as we age, our body is less able to absorb the BCAA called leucine [5]. This means that you can eat the same amount of protein that you would at age 20 but not get the same amount of leucine. As leucine is crucial for muscle maintenance, your muscles will begin to lose size and strength.

This theory has been mostly proven, and there is evidence that supplementation with leucine can help to prevent sarcopenia or at least reduce its severity. If you feel you are eating sufficient protein daily and exercising yet are losing muscle mass seek advice from your doctor regarding leucine supplementation.

But this is only one cause of muscle loss. Reductions in hormones such as testosterone in men and estrogen in women can also have an effect, as can increases in inflammation and a reduction in motor neurons [6].

Anyway, the point is that your core muscles will always weaken as you age, but regular exercise can help to reverse age-related muscle loss. A 2018 study found that aerobic and resistance exercises can help to prevent muscle loss [7].

The second cause of weakened core muscles is lifestyle changes. The use-it-or-lose-it mentality is as true of exercise as anything. As we age, many of us become less independent, lead more isolated lives, and tend to spend more time sitting down and sedentary.

This can lead to a weakening of the core muscles, as they aren't required as often during the day. This creates a vicious cycle where your lack of movement weakens your core, and then your weakened core makes movement more difficult.

Luckily, it is never too late to reverse this process. A very simple core workout can help to improve core strength and capability in anyone, provided they are consistent, work hard, and use good form.

The point of this book is to prevent core weakness and increase core strength.

The Benefits of a Strong Core

Having a strong core has many benefits that can be noticed during exercise sessions, at home, or going out and socialising. Here are some of the best benefits:

Reduced Injury Risk

This is such a huge benefit and the number one reason why you should be training your core in later life. A strong core can protect you from injury in two ways:

1. It can help you to move better, which reduces your risk of injuries.
2. It improves stability which further reduces your risk of injuries.

Let's say that somebody knocks into you. A strong core can help you to stabilize yourself and find your balance, helping to reduce the likelihood that you will fall over and hurt yourself.

Posture

The muscles of the core are all able to improve stability, but many of them also help to keep the spine erect. Even muscles, such as the abdominals, can help you to perform movements with excellent posture.

Improving your posture brings many benefits. It can help to reduce your risk of certain injuries, it can make your movements more efficient, and it can help you to perform certain exercises safely. You will also look taller and more confident.

Increased Athleticism

By improving your core strength, you are making more activities accessible. A strong core can help you to generate more power as it helps to transfer energy from the lower body to the upper body (and vice versa).

Think about that golf swing of yours. As you swing the club, your back heel rises off the floor and rotates, driving power from your legs up through your core muscles and into your torso and shoulders. Helping to generate extra power.

You will also be more agile, able to change directions faster and with more efficient results. This is useful for almost any activity from avoiding people on the sidewalk to sport. You can react to forces better with a strong core. Your posture will also be much better, and you won't fatigue as fast. This can be very important in sports such as golf, pickleball, and even sports such as ten-pin bowling.

Better Balance

This is tied into the improved posture and athleticism that a strong core can provide you with, but balance is absolutely crucial as we age. A strong core allows you to twist, rotate, flex and extend the spine, all of which can help you to balance better.

Imagine you were pushed hard in the chest. How would you react? You would try to find your footing, your arms would wave around for balance, and you would stick your glutes out for balance. All of these movements require a strong core to transfer energy back and forth between your upper and lower body.

Increased Stability

Every muscle in your core's main function is to increase your stability, so it should be no surprise that a stronger core means increased stability. Stability allows you to react better to forces that would destabilize you and to generate more power (think golf swing).

Protects Your Organs

Our organs are vital to our survival, but they are incredibly vulnerable. Your stomach, intestines, liver, kidneys, and pancreas are all situated in your lower torso. All of which could be easily damaged if it were not for your core muscles. The stronger these muscles are, the better they can protect your organs from harm.

Reduces Lower Back Pain

A strong core can improve your posture, improve your balance, and reduce your risk of injury. They can also help to support the spine and therefore reduce lower back pain. Gentle beginners core exercises are therefore recommended for those suffering lower back pain.

Makes Tasks Around the Home Easier

By now, you should have an inkling of just how integral your core muscles are to daily life. Any household task you can think of will require your core muscles. Washing the car, wiping down the kitchen surfaces, scrubbing the bathroom floor, and walking the dog. The list goes on and on. Of course, you can do most of these things with a weak core, but it is so much harder and less efficient.

You will be pleasantly surprised to find that as your core muscles strengthen, tasks that used to leave you tired and aching are now easy to do.

The Downsides of a Weak Core

Now that you know the many benefits of having a strong core, here are a few downsides to having a weak core.

Increased Injury Risk

A weak core can increase your risk of getting seriously injured. You will have poor balance and poor posture, and you won't be able to react to accidents or sudden movements as well as you could. You are in danger of both acute injuries (falling over) and chronic injuries (lower back pain from prolonged posture issues).

Poor Posture

Without a strong core, it is very difficult to maintain good posture for long. Your spine won't have the same level of support, your abs won't be as strong, and you won't be as mobile. This can all lead to poor posture, which has several unwanted side effects of its own.

Reduced Metabolism

This is an interesting one, but it makes a lot of sense. Poor core strength means that you will find it harder to be active. Less walking, playing sports, exercising etc. This means that your daily calorie expenditure (calories burned) will be reduced. The number of calories you burn through exercise and non-exercise activities (walking etc.) contribute to your overall metabolism.

A reduced metabolism can often lead to weight gain, as it is much more likely that you will be in a daily calorie surplus. Weight gain can lead to obesity, which can then create a vicious cycle. It also increases the risk of high blood pressure, type2 diabetes and coronary heart disease. The 2023 prevalence of obesity in the US is 36.2% compared with 13% in 1960.

Loss of Independence

If you are less mobile, you are moving less, and you find it harder to perform everyday routine activities such as carrying your shopping bags then you are going to become less independent.

If you can't walk to the shops, can't lift your shopping bags out of the car, and can't unload the shopping when you're home, then you are going to need to ask for assistance. Once that begins to happen, you are no longer living to your own schedule, and your independence will be eroded.

Muscular Compensation

So, how do people with weak cores manage to perform any movement in the first place? Well, your body is a marvellous thing, and it is able to call on other, stronger muscles to carry the load. This is called muscular compensation. For example, the glutes and hamstrings may take on a lot of the work if your lower back is weak.

This can then lead to other injuries cropping up. If your hamstrings are doing more work because your lower back isn't strong enough, then a hamstring injury is more likely. People with tight hamstrings or pain in the upper back and shoulders may, despite the location of the pain, well have a core issue.

Strong Core vs Visible Abdominals

The final thing to discuss in this chapter is the common misconception about the core. Many people think of core training as a way to get a visible six-pack. The problem is that training for a visible six-pack and training for a strong core can actually be very different.

We all have a six-pack, absolutely everyone (except people who have had an injury or specific disability). Right now, reading this, you have a six-pack. Most people have no idea because their six-packs are hidden behind a layer of body fat.

To see visible abs, you need to reduce your body fat levels significantly. If you lost all the body fat from around your waist and abdomen, your six-pack would become visible. To do this, you would need to follow a calorie-deficit diet, where you consume fewer calories than you burn each day.

You wouldn't even *need* to work your abs, though it would help slightly. The point is that getting a visible six-pack is not really about strengthening your core. It's about changing your diet.

This book is focused on building core strength not stripping away fat to make your abs visible!

Unless you are particularly lean, you may not actually *see* much change. But training your core has so many benefits (see above), while getting a visible six-pack doesn't really have *any* benefits except that some people think it looks good.

Before those of you who want a visible six pack put this book down, that doesn't mean that you can't get visible abs while performing the exercises in this book. It's just not the main goal. If you combine the workouts in this book with a calorie-deficit diet, you can simultaneously strengthen your core and burn body fat. Eventually, this will lead to a six-pack. But ask yourself whether you really need a six-pack. It's up to you, but it will make the next few months a lot more challenging if you do!

CHAPTER 2

What Does the Science Say?

SCAN FOR AUDIO CHAPTER

In this chapter, we will be looking at how to train your core muscles according to the latest scientific research. We will look at the differences between isolation exercises and compound exercises (don't worry if you don't know what these are yet), the best way to incorporate core training into your regular workout program, and an explanation of what works and what doesn't when it comes to core training.

How to Train the Core Muscles?

To understand how best to train the core muscles, you need to know a little bit about muscle fibres. Your muscle fibres are what make up each muscle, and there are three main types:

- Type 1 = Slow-twitch
- Type 2 = Fast-twitch
- Type 2B = Fast-twitch

Every muscle in your body will be made up of a combination of slow-twitch and fast-twitch fibres. Some will be almost all slow-twitch, some will be almost all fast-twitch, and many will be around 50/50 or 60/40.

The muscles in your abdominals are 58% Type 1, slow-twitch [8]. Without going into too much detail, muscles that are predominantly slow-twitch tend to respond better to high-rep sets. So, you would perform 10-20 reps instead of 4-6 reps in each set.

But not all of the muscles in your core are predominantly Type 1. Some can be more fast-twitch and therefore suit lower reps.

In this workout program, we will be changing the rep ranges as the weeks go on, but most of them will be higher-rep sets, as this will suit your core muscles slightly better.

Isolation vs Compound Lifting

There are two main forms of resistance exercise. Isolation exercises and compound exercises. An isolation exercise is one that targets one muscle in particular, with very little input from other muscles.

For example, a bicep curl will almost exclusively target the biceps muscle. There are other muscles involved such as the muscles in your forearm, the muscles that help you grip, and even your core muscles, but for all intents and purposes, it is a single muscle exercise.

Compound exercises are ones that work multiple muscles at the same time. For example, the bench press works the pectoral muscles, the deltoid muscles, and the tricep muscles. While the pectorals are the main focus of the bench press, unlike the bicep curl, it requires a lot of input from other muscles. Your deltoids and triceps will be fatigued after you finish.

Core exercises are mostly isolation exercises. An abdominal crunch works the abdominals and little else. So, many people tend to only use isolation exercises when training the core.

But compound lifts such as the barbell deadlift actually work the core to an even greater extent than an abdominal crunch. Some trainers believe therefore that isolation exercises aren't worth performing. They believe, if you have enough big compound lifts, such as deadlifts, squats, pull-ups, and presses, in your program, you don't need isolation exercises.

I believe both arguments are wrong. You want a combination of the two.

You can build a lot of strength in your abdominal and core muscles through compound lifts, but adding in exercises that directly target the core muscles can help to boost your strength much further. If you are looking to get yourself a six-pack (very hard but not impossible once you pass 50) then isolation abdominal exercises are vital to your progress.

One thing that it is very important though is to ensure that you have a number of compound lifts in your routine. While it is possible to build a strong core without isolation exercises, it would be foolish to try and build a strong core without including compound lifts in your workout routine.

Why? Because compound lifts work the core in the way that it should be worked. The purpose of the core is to tie all of your muscles together and help them to work as one. This is exactly what compound lifts require.

My experience has shown a good core training program should be 75% compound lifts and 25% core-specific movements. You can change the ratios slightly, but the majority of your training plan should work the whole body rather than just the core.

How to Incorporate Core Training into a Regular Workout

Your core-specific exercises are very important to your training program, but you need to add them in sensibly. There is no point performing a plank at the beginning of the workout, as it will make all other exercises too difficult (due to fatigued muscles).

While core exercises are obviously important, they are also isolation movements and will therefore require less strength and power to perform.

There are two options for adding core exercises into your regular workouts. You can either train them on a separate day entirely, or you can add them in to the end of your session. There are positives and negatives to each approach.

The positives of training your core separately is that you have more energy and more time available to train them. Core exercises are the easiest to neglect during a hard workout, partly because they are at the end of the session, when you are feeling tired and fatigued, and partly because you can justify skipping them (those deadlifts really worked my core, no need for any planks today).

Having more time to perform them also allows you to have more rest between sets, which allows for greater recovery. You can also add in more exercises and therefore more variety.

The negatives of training your core separately is that you will have one less recovery day between workouts, and your body may not have enough time to recover before your next session. Again, there is also the issue that you may want to skip the core workout entirely, as it feels like a bonus session.

So, what are the positives of training your core at the end of your session? Well, you get more rest days, and you are already in the gym (or your specified exercise area if you are training at home or in a park), making it easier to train.

The downside is that you are more likely to skip them (as mentioned previously), and you may be too fatigued to perform them properly.

The truth is, both options are fine, but some people will suit one better than the other. This program includes core exercises as part of each session, but if you find that you can't manage them at the end of your session, then training them separately is fine.

What Will a Core Training Session Look Like?

By now, you are probably wondering what your core training sessions are going to look like, so this section will deal with that and give you an idea as to why it is designed this way.

The structure will look like this:

- Warm-Up
- Full Body Workout
- Core-Specific Exercises
- Cool-Down/Stretching (optional)

You may be wondering where cardio is in this training session, but for the vast majority of people reading this the workout itself will be highly cardiovascular. Any additional cardio you want to add in should be done on rest days.

Warm-Up

A solid 5-10 minute cardiovascular warm-up. How intense it is will be based on your mobility and fitness levels. Gentle cardio on an exercise bike for some, a bodyweight workout for others. The importance of a warm-up is often overstated, training without one is not necessarily a bad thing for many people, but as we age the importance of warming up your muscles increases.

Full Body Workout

This is the main part of the workout, and it will involve exercises that work multiple muscle groups at the same time (compound). What specific exercises you perform will depend on your mobility and fitness. But whatever group you are in, the exercises will work the upper and lower body.

Examples of exercises include squats, chair sits, push-ups, leg swings, seated shoulder press, and for the more mobile among you there can be more challenging exercises.

Core Specific Exercises

This is where the majority of your direct core work will happen. Crunches, planks, leg raises, side planks, and all of the other core exercises that you need. As with the full body workout, these exercises will be split into groups based on mobility and fitness, that way you won't risk injury by attempting anything too ambitious!

Cool-Down/Stretching

Whether you perform a cool-down or not is really up to you. Unlike warm-ups research suggests, cool-downs don't appear to reduce your injury risk or provide many health benefits. Some people find that a structured cool-down helps them to relax after a session, but feel free to skip it if you don't enjoy it. The core workout should help you cool down in any case, as it is low in intensity.

CHAPTER 3

What to Know Before Your First Workout

SCAN FOR AUDIO CHAPTER

No matter where you are planning on performing your first workout, whether it be in the park, your house, or your local gym, there are certain things you should consider. In this chapter, we will be looking at what you need to know before embarking on your core fitness journey.

If in Doubt: Ask

This first consideration is important no matter what age you are, but the older you get, the more crucial it is to ensure that you know what you are doing. This book will give you detailed descriptions of each exercise, but if you aren't certain about something, it is very important that you check with a professional beforehand.

Whether it be a doctor, a personal trainer, a physiotherapist, or even a fitness instructor at your local gym, just ask them to clarify. There really aren't any bad questions when it comes to exercise.

But it's not just technical help you should seek. Consult your doctor before embarking on any fitness program is very sound advice. Particularly if you have any medical issues.

Prepare Your Exercise Area

When you exercise, the last thing you want is a loss of balance or stability. This can be caused by an improperly prepared exercise area. Before you start any workout, clear your exercise space and make sure that there is nothing to bump into.

If you are training in the gym, then remember that you are in a public space. This means that people may be walking past or through your exercise area. If this is likely to happen, then you may want to train in a different, less busy part of the gym.

If you are outside, then check the ground beforehand. Is there any broken glass? What about uneven ground? You also want to check the weather beforehand, as well as the light. You don't want the last half of your workout performed in darkness!

Warming Up

This is not something that you want to skip, no matter your mobility level, these workouts are designed to test your physical limits. A properly structured warm-up is a fantastic way to prepare yourself for intense exercise and reduce your risk of injury.

This book is packed full of top quality warm up exercises and routines to help you complete your workouts in complete safety. Please don't just skip past them, they form an integral part of your workout!

Equipment Check

This is great advice for any workout program. Whether you are using a dumbbell, an exercise bench, a fully stacked barbell, or just a sturdy chair, you want to check that it is in a good condition before you use it.

If you are using a dumbbell, is it stable? Are there any loose parts? Is it the right weight for your needs? If you are using a sturdy chair then you should check if it is placed on a level surface, if it can handle your weight, and whether it is stable or wobbly. You get the idea.

If you are using equipment in your gym then you should check that it is working properly, that it is set to the correct weight, and that you know how to use it correctly. If in doubt, ask.

Exercise has many benefits, but if you don't treat your equipment with respect, it can easily lead to accidents.

Rest Between Sets and Exercises

Exercise is designed to be tiring, and this means that you will be breathing heavily between sets and after each exercise. If you aren't, then you might not be working hard enough. But to keep yourself safe and efficient, you need to recover properly before starting a new set.

There has actually been a lot of research into the optimal rest time between sets. A 2009 study in the Journal of Sports Medicine found that the ideal rest period between sets is 3-5 minutes for strength training, 30-60 seconds for hypertrophy (muscle size), and 20-60 seconds for muscular endurance [9].

While this information is interesting, it doesn't necessarily apply in this instance. The study in question was based on a review of 35 similar studies, almost all of which would have been performed on people in their 20s and 30s.

People in their 50s, 60s, and beyond will have different goals, but also different capabilities. This may not apply to everyone over 50, but the majority of people over 50 will be less fit than 20 and 30 year olds.

You might think that this means that you will require longer rest periods, and for many this is sensible advice. But the truth is a little more complicated.

One of the reasons why you need to rest is to allow your nervous system to recover. Interestingly, the heavier the weight you are lifting, the harder your nervous system is worked.

At 75 years of age, you are unlikely to be lifting anywhere near as much as a 20-year-old, so your nervous system may not need as long to recover. This is part of the reason why women require shorter rest periods between sets than men.

As there is no clear consensus on the ideal rest period for people over 50 years of age, and there is so much variation in this age group, the best advice is to find a time that suits your unique fitness level and goals.

When choosing your rest time, you want to have enough time to catch your breath, but you don't want it to be overly long. Having a 5-minute conversation with your gym friend between sets is not going to help you to build your fitness level or core strength.

Somewhere between 45 seconds and 90 seconds should be enough for most people over 50, but if you need a little longer then take it. When starting out, your fitness may not be very good, so longer rests may be required, which can be reduced as your fitness improves.

There is a difference between the time you take in between sets and the time that you take in between exercises. For example, if you are performing 3 sets of 10 reps of bodyweight squats, you would be resting twice. After the first set, and after the second set.

In this time, you have nothing to do except rest and relax, and perhaps analyse your performance. After the third set of ten reps, you will then have to move on to a different exercise.

Not only do you have to recover from the third set, but you also have to prepare for the next exercise. For example, you may need to grab a sturdy chair to perform a chair-assisted box squat.

All this means is that the length of time you spend between exercises needs to be a little longer than the time you spend in between sets of the same exercise.

A rest period of 2-3 minutes between exercises is about right, provided you are setting up for the next exercise. If you feel fresh and there isn't much to set up then cut that rest time down to 45-90 seconds.

Heart Rate, Breathing, and Signs of Fatigue

One of the most useful things that you can do when starting an exercise program is to purchase a heart rate monitor, one that can be used while you exercise. Wearable technology such as FitBits are great, but there are less expensive options around.

You can use your heart rate to measure how hard you are exercising and to give you an indication of when to adjust your intensity.

Your maximal heart rate is measured using this simple equation:

$$220 - \text{Your Age} = \text{Max Heart Rate}$$

So, the maximal heart rate of a 50-year-old is around 170 beats per minute, and 145 beats per minute for a 75-year-old. You can use this to set yourself a target.

But how do you do this?

With something called the **Rate of Perceived Exertion** (RPE) scale. This is a scale from 1 to 10, with 1 representing no exertion whatsoever (sitting down) and 10 representing the absolute peak of exertion (imagine running from an angry bear). Here is a quick breakdown of the scale:

- 1 = sitting down, very light activity, regular heart rate
- 2-3 = light activity, slightly raised heart rate

- 4-6 = moderate activity, you can still talk fluently while performing it, heart rate is elevated
- 7-8 = high activity, running, you struggle to talk fluently, heart rate is high
- 9 = near maximal activity. You cannot talk as it is too hard, and your heart rate is nearing its max
- 10 = Maximal intensity. You can only keep this up for a couple of seconds

It's very useful to use the RPE scale, even without checking your heart rate, because you can just estimate. But, if you have a heart rate monitor, then you can combine the two. A 10 on the scale represents 100% of your max heart rate.

You can go down the scale just like that, a 9 would be around 90%, 7-8 would be around 70-80%, and so on.

Let's take a look at what that would look like for a 50-year-old, 60-year-old, and a 70-year-old:

Age	RPE 1	RPE 2	RPE 3	RPE 4	RPE 5	RPE 6		RPE 7	RPE 8	RPE 9	RPE 10
50	Normal heart rate				85	102	119		136	153	170
60		80	96	112		128	144	160			
70		75	90	105		120	135	150			

As you can see, the heart rate/RPE scale doesn't really work for the first few levels, asking someone to have a heart rate of 17 while sitting down is a little extreme! But the RPE scale from 1-4 is all about relaxing and gentle exercise, so you don't really need to keep track of your heart rate for that.

Another good thing to keep track of, though in a much less organised way than heart rate, is your breathing. As you will be aware, the harder we exercise, the harder it is to breathe normally. We can use this to our advantage when training.

If you are sitting down on a chair, your RPE score is a 1, and you should find breathing to be very easy. You should be able to have a conversation normally. This should stay the same if you get up and go for a gentle stroll.

Once your exercise becomes sufficiently challenging (a score of 5+) you will notice that your ability to have a conversation will be affected. Try talking normally while jogging at a fast pace and you'll see the problem immediately.

You can use this as a way to gauge how hard you are working, and how long you need to recover.

Important: If you are supposed to be following a gentle exercise routine, but you are breathing so hard that you can't talk, then you are training too hard and should reduce your intensity.

If you are supposed to be really challenging yourself and yet you are able to talk normally to the person next to you, then you may want to increase your intensity slightly.

You get the idea. Breathing and the ability to talk are a great way to work out how hard you are training, how much time you need to rest between sets and exercises, and whether you are over or underperforming in terms of exercise intensity.

There are of course other signs of fatigue. Feeling nauseated, muscles aching (more than they should be), a loss of control/ability (think about playing tennis when exhausted and not being able to serve properly), sweating, and an inability to focus/concentrate.

All of these are signs that you are very fatigued. Now, that's not necessarily a bad thing, the point of exercising is to get out of your comfort zone, but it is vital that you know the signs so that you can adjust your sessions before something bad happens.

If you are sweating profusely, feel sick, and can't think straight, then that final set of squats is better left unperformed. The maxim is listen to your body.

Finding Your Fitness Level

It is very difficult to definitively assign someone a fitness level, as there are so many variables that can affect your fitness. Often, mobility and strength are included when talking about fitness. For example, someone not being able to perform a full push-up may be classified as less fit than someone who can.

Though this is not actually a measure of cardiovascular fitness. Perhaps they cannot perform a push-up, but they can run a half marathon?

There are many forms of fitness tests out there, but many of these are unsuitable for the majority of people who are over the age of 50 (though there will also be many people over 50 who are fit enough to perform them).

Luckily, there are many fitness tests that are specific for seniors. One of these is called the Groningen Walking Test, which was developed in the 90s and re-examined in 2001 by Lemmink *et al* [10].

As accurate as this test is, it does require quite a lot of organisation. A simpler procedure is the 2-minute step-in-place test developed by Rikli & Jones in 2002 [11].

For this test, all you need is a wall or chair (for support if required), and a stopwatch (you can use your mobile), and ideally, you would want someone who can make sure that you are performing each step correctly.

Stand next to a wall or chair

March in place for 2-minutes, ensuring that your knees are raised as high as your hip each time

You can stop and rest as many times as you need to within these 2-minutes

Record the number of times that your right knee is raised to hip height throughout the 2-minutes

One downside of the test is that it does not provide results guidance for those aged 50-60, so we will have to improvise (see table below):

Male

Age	Below Average	Average	Above Average
50-60	< 115	120	120
60-64	< 87	87-118	118
65-69	< 87	86-116	116
70-74	< 80	80-110	110
75-79	< 73	73-109	109
80-84	< 71	71-103	103
85-89	< 59	59-91	91
90-94	< 52	52-86	86

Female

Age	Below Average	Average	Above Average
50-60	< 107	107	107
60-64	< 75	75-107	107
65-69	< 73	73-107	107
70-74	< 68	68-101	101
75-79	< 68	68-100	100
80-84	< 60	60-91	91
85-89	< 55	55-85	85
90-94	< 44	44-72	72

The test is not perfect. For example, you may be very fit while having bad knees, but it is the best test available for the majority of people over 50.

Once you have completed the test, you will have a rough idea of what your current fitness level is based on your age and gender. You can use this to decide how long to rest in between sets (people with poor fitness will need longer), and you can use this to gauge progress over time.

This is not a measure of mobility or core strength, though there is going to be a correlation for a lot of people. If you have very good mobility, then raising your knee high is a lot easier and you can therefore score higher on this test.

Finding Your Mobility Level

While establishing your fitness level is very important before embarking on an exercise program, your mobility level is even more so. Particularly as you age. It is beyond the scope of this, or any, book to accurately measure your individual mobility and tailor a program for you.

That's why, if you have a specific mobility issue, you should consult with your doctor and/or a physio. But it is possible to get a general idea of what your mobility level is. The workouts in this book have been separated based on mobility level, so this section is very important.

Low Mobility – This means that you have several minor/medium mobility issues or one very big one. The number of exercises that are available to you will be limited, and you should definitely consult a physio before embarking on the program.

Medium Mobility – This means that you have one or two minor/medium mobility issues, but there will be some areas where you have no mobility issues. For example, you may have a problem with your shoulder, but your knees are fine.

High Mobility – You have no minor or medium mobility issues, and you can perform most exercises without noticing any pain or an inability to perform the exercise unhindered.

Finding Your Core Strength Level

This test is quite difficult to perform, but even if you can't perform it, you can use it to inform you about your core strength level. Quite simply, if you cannot perform the test, then your core strength level is low! Not a bad thing, and many may struggle to perform the test. Particularly if you have low mobility.

After reading how to perform the test, decide whether it sounds possible. If you don't think you can do it, then score yourself a low, and you can work towards it over time. If you can perform it, you can then use the results to give yourself a more specific rating.

Before starting, try to perform a plank for 30 seconds (see step #1 below)**. If you can manage this, then you can manage to perform the full test. If you cannot manage 30 seconds, then score yourself low and skip the test entirely. If you manage 30 seconds (or very close to 30 seconds) then you may attempt the test safely.**

For this test you will need a stopwatch, an exercise mat, and the ability to get into the plank position. This is a standard core exercise, that will feature in the medium and advanced workout programs. The test was designed by Brian Mac (a Sport Scientist) in 2002 [12].

Warm-up beforehand, a 10-minute walk or some time on an exercise bike (for example) would be ideal.

Step #1 Get into the plank position.

Lie on the floor in a straight line, then place your forearms flat with your elbows directly below your shoulders. Raise your hips off the floor so that there is a straight line from your shoulders down to your ankles. This is your starting position.

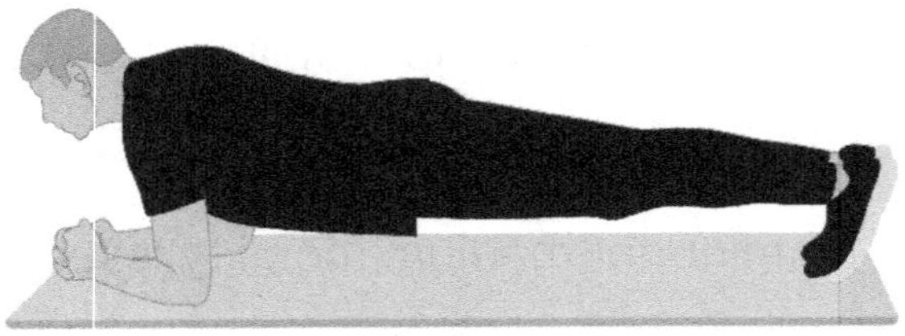

Step #2 Raise your right arm off the ground and push it out in front of you. Hold for 15 seconds.

Step #3 Return to the starting position, and then repeat with your left arm.

Step #4 Return to the starting position, and then raise your right leg off the floor and hold for 15 seconds.

Step #5 Return to the starting position and repeat with your left leg.

Step #6 Return to the starting position and then raise your right arm and your left leg off the floor at the same time. Hold for 15 seconds.

Step #7 Return to the starting position and repeat with the opposite arm and leg, holding for 15 seconds.

Step #8 Return to the starting position and hold for 30 seconds.

If you cannot complete any of the steps in this, then your core strength is currently low. If you don't even attempt the test, then your score is also low. If you can complete step #1-5 but no further, then your core strength is medium.

If you can complete the entire test, then your core strength is high. If you almost completed the test but fell at the final hurdle, then you can still group yourself into the high core strength group.

Don't take these groupings personally. There may not be a 90-year-old on the planet who could complete this test, so remember the context. This is not a core test that has been developed exclusively for seniors, it is one that has been designed for the general population.

Beginner, Medium, and Advanced

In this book, all of the exercises are grouped into beginner, intermediate (medium), and advanced. When choosing your group, please be as conservative as you can. It is better to embark on a program and then realise that it is too easy, then to realise that you've picked a program that is too hard.

There are three criteria that affect which group you should pick. And a fourth that is a little rougher, but probably effective for most people.

The three criteria are:

1. Fitness
2. Mobility
3. Core Strength

The fourth is age. This is a controversial choice, as there are many 68 year olds who are fitter and more mobile than some 50 year olds, etc. But if you are 90 years old, it is a fair guess that you should be in the beginner group.

Use your age if you think that is a sensible option, but you can also use the fitness, mobility, and core strength tests if you are not sure.

- **Beginners**: If you score low in any of the three tests, then you should be a beginner. Even if you score high in the other two.
- **Intermediate**: If you score medium in two of the three tests, then consider yourself an intermediate. If you score highly in two tests but medium in one, then you can decide for yourself whether you suit being an intermediate or an advanced lifter. However, the advice to be conservative is still valid.
- **Advanced**: If you score highly in all three tests, then you are advanced. If you score highly in two tests and medium in one, then you may qualify, but it may be safer to start at intermediate and work your way up.

If you score low in any of the three tests, then it is advisable to see a doctor and physio before embarking on this program. Just to ensure that the exercises are suitable for you. But the beginner program has been specifically designed with you in mind.

If you are basing the groups by age, then anyone over 75 should be in beginner, those aged 50-60 may be suited to intermediate or advanced (but it is a good idea to perform the tests before attempting advanced). 60-75 should be either beginner or intermediate, unless you feel that you are fitter/more mobile/have better core strength than the majority of your peers.

CHAPTER 4

Goal Setting

SCAN FOR AUDIO CHAPTER

In this chapter, we will be talking about creating realistic goals, what a good goal looks like, and the importance of measuring your progress, including finding your baseline statistics beforehand. This is a chapter that you may be tempted to skip, but having well-defined goals can make a huge difference to your chances of success.

A badly defined goal can lead to a drop in motivation while having no defined goal at all can be even worse. How do you know if you are progressing if you have no idea of where you started and no idea of what you want to achieve.

Yet this is the situation that so many adults find themselves when they begin a new fitness program. You will have had motivations for purchasing this book, but are they defined? Are they practical? Is there a timeframe involved?

Without any of these, it is of course still possible to succeed, but your odds of doing so are lower. So, let this chapter help you to create realistic, effective goals that prevent a loss of motivation, and boost your chances of success.

Creating Realistic Goals

The fitness world can be very misleading when it comes to creating realistic goals. Many of you will probably have seen magazines with "Lose 20 lbs in 2 weeks using THIS workout" on the front cover (or similar). But that is not at all realistic, some would say that it was actually impossible without some form of amputation!

This book is about core training, so we will avoid discussing fat loss where possible, but it is a good way to demonstrate realistic goals.

The recommended amount of fat loss per week is around 1 lb, possibly 2 lbs at a stretch. So 20 lbs in 2 weeks is not realistic, while 20 lbs in 20 weeks is. While many people are preoccupied with the idea of losing fat *fast*, they should instead be thinking of the simplest and easiest ways to achieve their goals.

In the previous chapter we discussed how to perform a core fitness test. We identified how to use it to measure your current core fitness level, as low, medium, or high.

The low core fitness group are those who cannot yet perform the test. Would it be realistic to expect someone who cannot perform the test in week one to master it within 2 weeks?

No. This would be very unlikely. Depending on how difficult the test was for you to even attempt, it may not be realistic to complete the test in 20 weeks.

Therefore for those currently at the lowest end of the scale for core fitness, the test should be disregarded in terms of setting realistic goals. Instead, you should look for a different type of goal. Working your way up from zero training sessions per week to three 15-30 minute sessions per week is a better (realistic) goal.

If you can complete the core fitness test, or you came quite close, then creating a realistic goal around this makes a lot of sense.

Whatever route you decide upon, find a goal that is realistic over a 24-week period.

SMART Goals

SMART is an acronym for goal setting. You want your goals to be:

- Specific – You are embarking on a core fitness training program, so your goal should be specific to that.
- Measurable – Avoid goals that cannot be measured, "I want to lose weight" is a bad example of a goal. How much weight? Within what timeframe? At what rate per week or month?
- Achievable – Can you actually complete this goal if you try very hard? Setting yourself a goal of a 9 second 100m sprint is an example of a goal that is unachievable, even if you're Usain Bolt.

- Realistic – As covered in the previous section, you want goals that are within your capabilities. This differs from achievable, in that you can create goals that are possible but not within the selected timeframe, or not specifically for you. A 10 second 100m sprint is achievable for someone who can run a 10.2 second 100m sprint, but it is not realistic for seniors approaching their ***70th birthday.***
- Time-Bound – While it is possible to have goals that do not have a deadline, creating time-bound goals is a fantastic motivator, and it makes it easier to pace yourself. Going back to weight loss example, if you want to lose 20 lbs, give yourself a deadline of 20 weeks and you have a very realistic, achievable goal of 1 lb per week.

This core fitness program has been designed to ensure that you all have at least one goal that is set up for you.

The program lasts 24 weeks, and it has a core fitness test that you can perform at the beginning, middle, and end of the program.

For example:

Week 1: Perform core fitness test, struggle to complete the final 30 seconds of the test. Create a goal that within 24 weeks you will be able to master the test.

The goal is specific, it is a core fitness-related improvement that you are seeking. It is realistic, you came quite close to completing the test in week 1, so 24 weeks of hard work should help you to improve your score. The test is measurable as each section is timed. You can see at what point you failed the test, and use that to measure progress.

The program is time-bound, you have 24 weeks to improve your score.

If you didn't attempt the test because you knew that you would not be able to achieve it safely. Then you have several options for goals. You could aim to attempt the test after 24 weeks, which is a very good goal.

But if you don't think that this is realistic, then you can go in a different direction. Perhaps you could set a goal to complete all sessions within the 24 weeks? That is a specific goal, it is measurable, achievable, realistic, and time-bound.

Setting Baseline Stats

For this program, setting baseline stats is very easy. All you have to do is take the tests for mobility, core fitness, and cardiovascular fitness. Write all of your results down, and you will have your baseline stats.

If you are using this program as a weight loss tool (perfectly possible when combined with a good diet), then you will want to measure your weight and possibly take measurements of the circumference of your waist, abdominals, chest, thighs, and arms (use tailor's tape for this).

If you want to go a step further, then you can get your doctor to measure your blood pressure, resting heart rate, body fat percentage, and other measurements that can be improved with exercise. Record them, and re-measure them at the end of the 24 weeks.

Measuring Progress

As with setting baseline stats, measuring your progress is simply a matter of retesting your scores. The trick is to do it regularly enough so that you can see how you are progressing but not so regularly that you waste time and effort.

This is a 24-week program, so retesting every 4-6 weeks makes sense. As the tests are not too strenuous, you can fit them into your week without having to sacrifice a session. Perform the test on a non-workout day during the week.

CHAPTER 5

Core Training Program Structure

SCAN FOR AUDIO CHAPTER

While this is a core training program, and obviously, training your core is of the utmost importance, your training sessions will not be made up exclusively of core exercises. This is partly because compound lifts will also work the core, but also to help you maintain a well-balanced physique. Yes, the core is important to focus on, but so are your legs, back, arms, and chest.

Think of this as a well-balanced full-body workout, with emphasis placed on the core. The structure is simple, and it is perfect for fat loss, building muscle, and improving your cardiovascular fitness.

Each session starts with a warm-up, and then it will have a few compound lifts which work multiple muscle groups. After that, you will perform some core training, and you can finish off the session with some cardio.

The following chapters will teach you warm-up exercises, compound lifts, core-specific exercises, and finally, cardio. After that, Chapter 12 will provide 24-week training programs for beginners, intermediates, and advanced group members.

Warm-Ups

The purpose of a warm-up is to prepare you for the workout ahead, reduce your risk of injuries, and gradually build up your workout intensity. If you are young and fit, then warm-ups are not essential but as we age, the importance of warm-ups increases significantly. A good warm-up will combine some gentle cardio and some bodyweight exercises that increase mobility and raise your heart rate. None of the exercises should be taxing, and you should be able to maintain a conversation while you perform your warm-up. Recall the **Rate of Perceived Exertion** (RPE) scale discussed earlier.

If you are out of breath and your muscles are aching, then you are working too hard during your warm-up. Consider reducing the number of reps, lowering the difficulty, or just giving yourself a little bit more rest between your sets.

Compound Lifts

Exercises that work multiple muscle groups at the same time are considered to be compound lifts.

The compound lifts in this book have been chosen to suit people of all abilities, but mostly they have been chosen for people with low mobility. You won't see any heavy barbell squats in this book, but you will see box squats and seated leg extensions.

Core Training

This section represents the most important part of the training program. There will be a large variety of core exercises that can suit most ages and mobility levels. The variety will help to work your core muscles in different ways and will keep you entertained throughout. Performing the same core exercises every session can get boring very quickly!

You train your core after your compound lifts, as a fatigued core can prevent you from performing compound lifts properly, but not vice versa.

Cardio (optional)

The final part of each program is made up of cardiovascular exercises such as walking, jogging, running, or even cardio machines (if you have access to them). Think of the cardio section as a chance to improve your health and fitness but also as a nice way to finish off your workouts. At the end of your cardio session, you will have fully cooled down from the workout. You will also have burned more calories and improved your fitness.

The cardio section is not compulsory in the same way that a warm-up, compound lift or core exercise is compulsory. If you are already fatigued, you can skip it. But it is a great bonus, and those that manage to fit it into their schedule will see better results in a shorter period of time.

Training Session Structure

Your warm-up should take 5-10 minutes, your compound lifts should take around 10-15 minutes, your core training should take around 10 minutes, and your cardio can take around 10-30 minutes (depending on your goals and abilities). Your cardio will also count as your cooldown, hence the lack of a specific cooldown in this training session structure. Yes, I'm aware of the many booking promising seniors fantastic results with only 5-10 minute workouts, but are they realistic? Probably not if you are seeking 'real' improvement within a realistic timeframe.

CHAPTER 6

Warm-Up Exercises for Core Training

SCAN FOR AUDIO CHAPTER

The warm-up exercises for this book have been split into three groups: Low-mobility, medium-mobility, and high-mobility. If you have performed your mobility examination (see chapter three), then you will know which group of warm-up exercises to follow.

These warm-ups have been designed to be performed at home, outside, or in the gym. They require no equipment unless you want to use it. The warm-ups should last around 10-15 minutes, depending on how much time you have available to spend on each section.

Low-Mobility Warm-Up

This low-mobility warm-up is very simple to learn and can be performed by pretty much anyone, regardless of their mobility score. The only people who should avoid this warm-up are those with known shoulder or neck injuries. If this is an issue for you, then ask your physiotherapist for an alternative warm-up.

Exercise #1 Gentle Cardio (5 minutes)

Gentle cardio can be anything from walking at a medium to fast pace to jogging on the spot or even climbing onto a cardio machine such as a treadmill or exercise bike. Find something that you enjoy and have easy access to. If you are at home, then walking up and down the stairs would qualify as gentle cardio.

Ideally perform it for 5 minutes, but you can do it for less if you feel that your heart is already racing. As your fitness improves, you will be able to perform the warm-up at a higher intensity (or for longer) without it becoming too burdensome.

Exercise #2 Neck & Shoulder Warm-Up (2 minutes)

This exercise routine will warm up your neck, your shoulders, your arms, and your back. It is very low-impact and simple to learn.

---

1. Stand upright with your chest pushed forward and your shoulders pulled back. Look straight forward.
2. Raise your chin upwards at a slow pace until you are looking at the ceiling (or sky) directly above you.
3. Pause, and then lower your chin to your chest, at a nice and slow pace.
4. Return to the starting position.
5. Bring your chin towards your right shoulder, and then slowly bring it over to your left shoulder. Keeping your body still throughout this movement.
6. Perform this entire movement five times.
7. Raise your shoulders up towards your ears then roll your shoulders forwards, and then slowly raise them up and backwards.
8. Repeat this five times.
9. Raise both arms into the air above your head, pause, and then lower them back down to the starting position.
10. Repeat this five times.

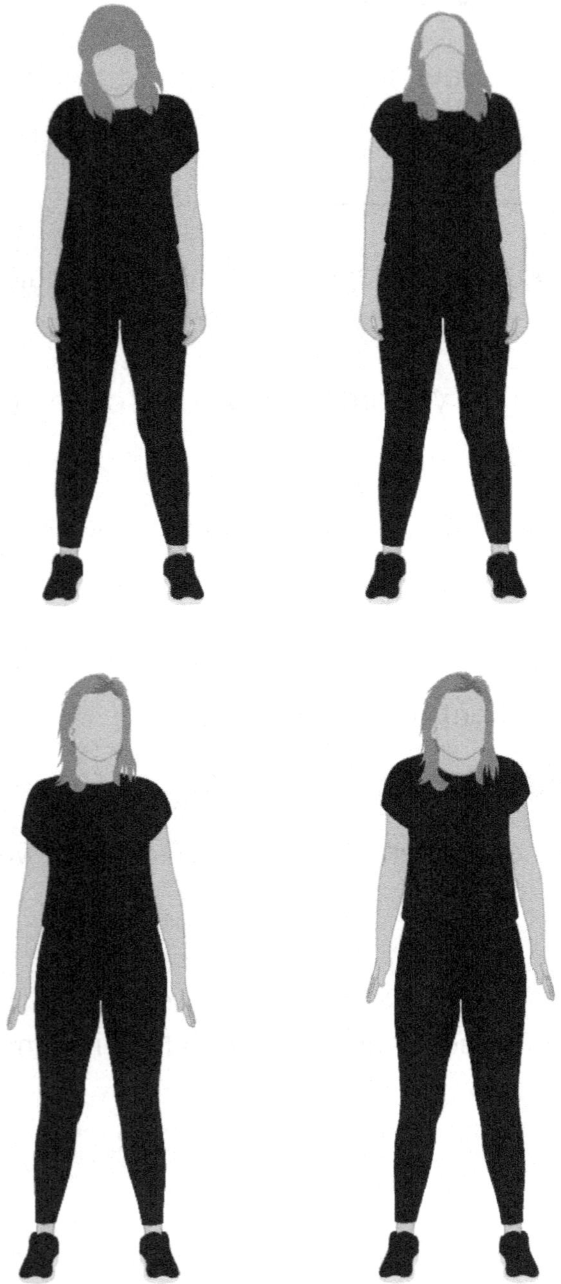

SCAN FOR VIDEO

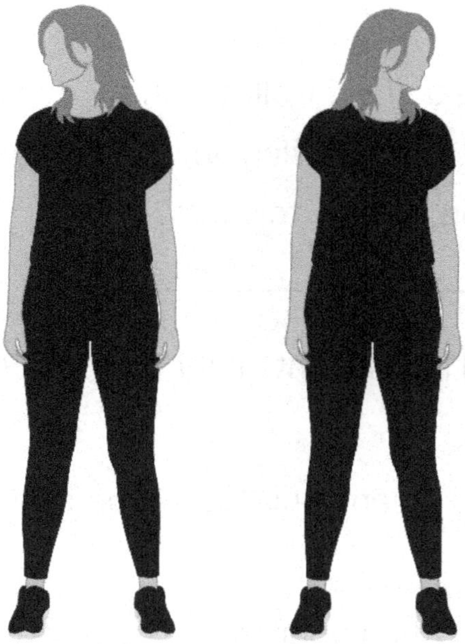

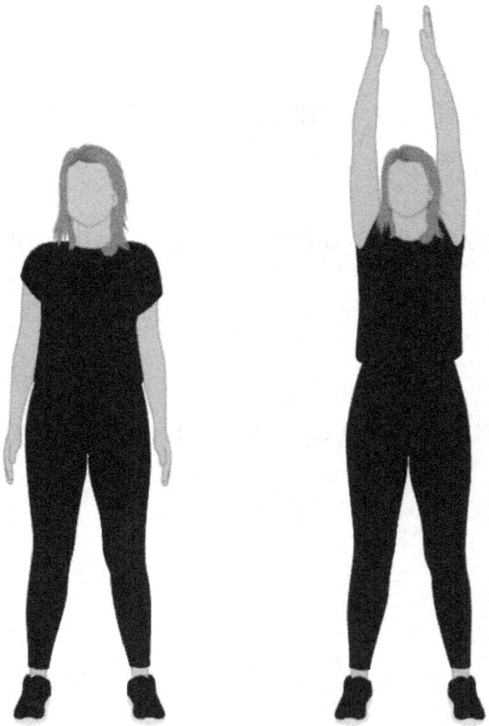

SCAN FOR VIDEO

As you can see, there are a lot of movements to remember, but they all flow into each other smoothly. If you forget one, then you can add it on to the end without any issue. Though the order above is optimal.

Exercise #3 Leg Warm-Up (2 minutes)

This exercise routine works best when you have a chair, wall, or sturdy object to hold onto for balance. Though, if you are able to perform it without using anything for balance, you will get a great core workout. Perhaps it is something to work towards?

---

1. Stand beside a chair or a wall, with your hand holding onto it for balance. Push your chest out and pull your shoulders back.
2. Raise your right foot off the ground, pausing when your thigh is parallel to the ground. Lower it back down.
3. Raise your left foot off the ground, pausing when your thigh is parallel to the ground. Lower it back down.
4. Perform this 5-10 times with each leg.
5. Then, you want to raise your right foot behind you, until your shin bone is parallel to the ground. Pause, and then lower it back down.
6. Raise your left foot behind you, until your shin bone is parallel to the ground. Pause, and then lower it back down.
7. Repeat this 5-10 times with each leg.
8. Raise both heels off the ground so that you are on your tiptoes. Pause, and then lower both heels back to the ground.
9. Repeat 10 times.

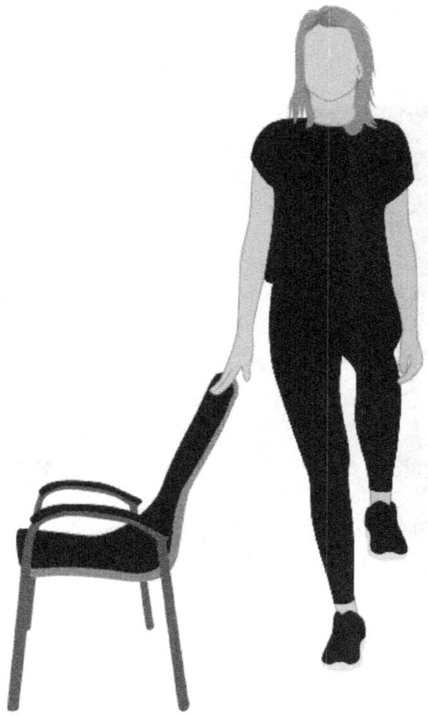

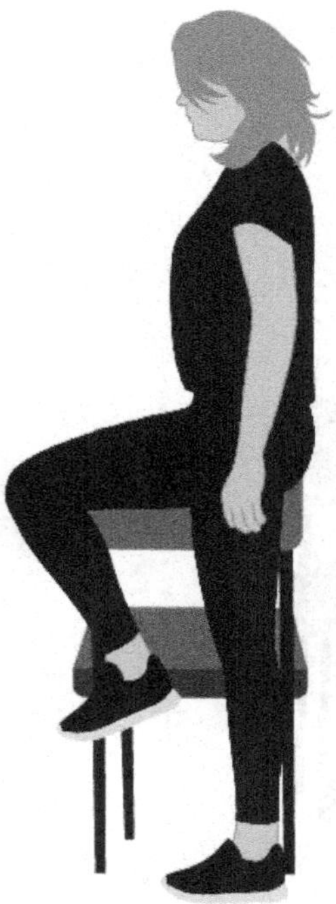

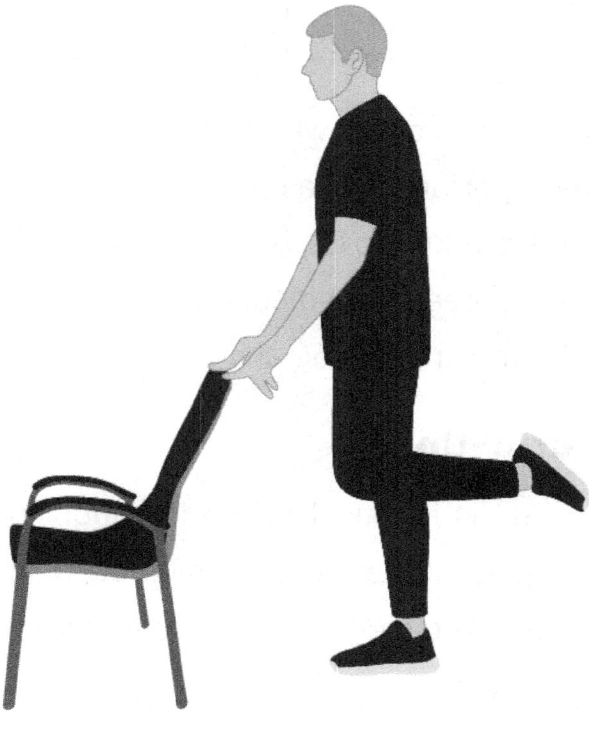

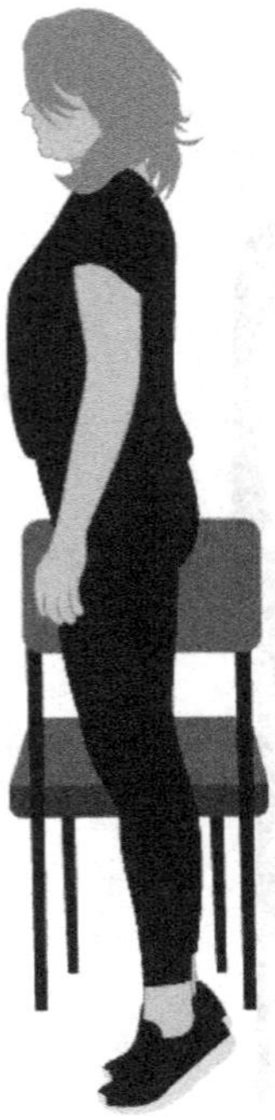

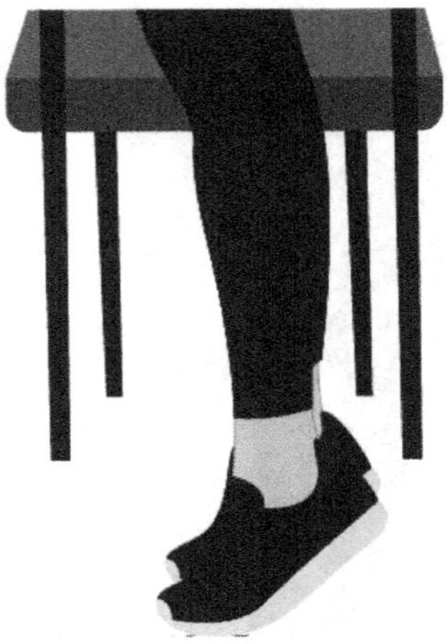

SCAN FOR VIDEO

Exercise	Sets	Reps	Rest Between Sets
Gentle Cardio	1	5 minutes	n/a
Neck & Shoulder WU	1	5	n/a
Leg Warm-Up	1	5-10	n/a

This warm-up may sound complicated when you first read it, but it really is a nice and simple routine. Once you have performed it a couple of times, you will know the routine off by heart. What's great about this warm-up is that it works your upper and lower body, as well as your core. The lack of rest between movements will also increase your heart rate, but not too much. Perfect for people who are over 50 and have low mobility.

Medium-Mobility Warm-Up

The medium-mobility warm-up is identical to the low-mobility warm-up. However, it is performed at a slightly faster pace, it therefore has more reps (as you can fit more reps into the same timeframe when training faster) and you are less likely to need to use a chair or wall for support during the leg warm-up.

Exercise	Sets	Reps	Rest Between Sets
Gentle Cardio	1	5-7 minutes	n/a
Neck & Shoulder WU	1	10	n/a
Leg Warm-Up	1	10-15	n/a

One thing should be made clear, though you are more likely to be able to perform these reps at a faster pace than someone in the low-mobility group. That doesn't mean that fast reps should be your goal. Perform each rep safely and smoothly, and you should naturally perform them faster, thanks to improved mobility. Don't rush them, as this could lead to poor form and injury.

High-Mobility Warm-Up

If you have high mobility, then you should be able to perform most bodyweight exercises with ease. That means that your warm-up can be a little more creative and varied than that of someone with medium or low mobility.

If at any point you find this warm-up to be too intense, then just drop down to the medium or even low-mobility warm-up instead. **Remember, you are looking to slowly increase your heart rate and prepare yourself for the upcoming workout.** The goal is not to exhaust yourself before the proper program begins!

You may find it useful to watch the High-Mobility Warm-Up video before reading on, it will help support the exercise instructions to ensure the movements involved are clear.

Exercise #4 Cardio (5 minutes)

Due to the more intense nature of the exercises in this warm-up, you may think that the cardio also has to be more intense. But not really. Just perform some gentle cardio for 5 minutes. If you are more mobile than most, your efforts will almost certainly be faster and more intense, but the point is not to exhaust yourself but gently warm the muscles and raise your heat rate to prepare the body for the training to come.

Use a treadmill, exercise bike, or even just go for a walk or run. If you are in your home, then climb up and down the stairs at a decent rate to get that heart pumping (though you can shorten the duration of the warm-up if you are using stairs as they are quite intense).

Exercise #5 Deep Squats

Deep squats are a fantastic mobility exercise for the legs, glutes, and lower back. They also serve as a heart rate raiser, making them one of the best warm-up exercises out there. Just remember that the focus is on form rather than hitting as many reps as you can.

1. Stand upright with your chest pushed out and your shoulders pulled backwards. Place your feet slightly wider than shoulder-width apart.
2. Turn your toes out slightly and clasp your hands together in front of your chest. Take a deep breath and hold it in your lungs.
3. Push your hips backwards and lower your glutes towards the floor. Try to ensure that your back stays straight throughout. Holding your hands close to your chest can help with this.
4. Go lower than you would with a normal squat, but only as low as you feel comfortable with. Once you have reached your personal stopping point, hold this position for 3-5 seconds.
5. Rise back up, pushing your hips forwards and squeezing your glutes as you do so. Breathe out while you rise upwards.

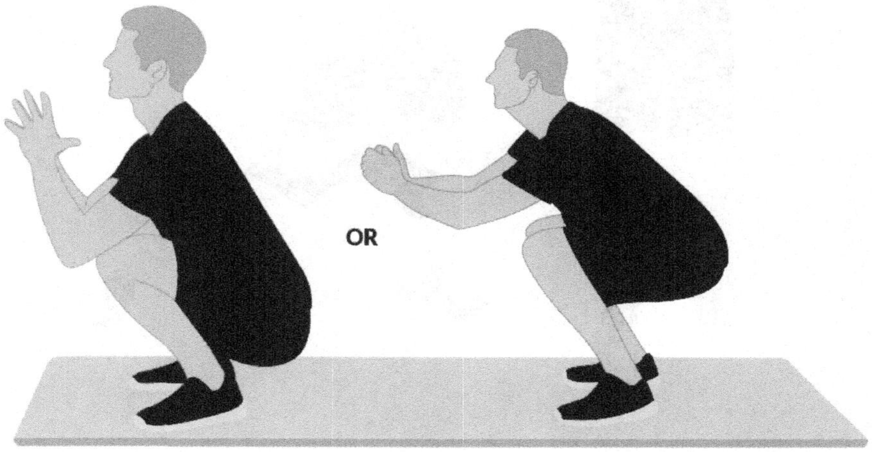

Exercise #6 Lateral Lunges

A lateral lunge is a great warm-up for the inner and outer thighs, and it can also help you to improve your squats over time. If you feel knee pain while performing them, then experiment with placing your foot forwards or backwards slightly. You can also take smaller or larger steps and experiment with how shallow or deep your lunge is.

1. Stand upright with both of your feet together, and your chest pushed out and shoulders back.
2. Take a large step to the right, straightening your left leg and bending your right knee slightly.
3. Pause, then return to the starting position. Repeat this with your other leg.

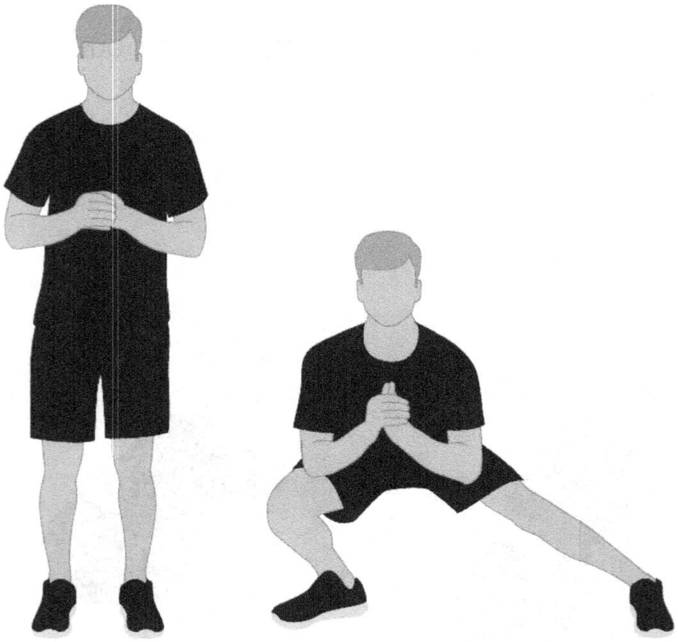

Exercise #7 Slow Burpees

Burpees are often talked about in hushed tones due to their extreme reputation, but the image of performing burpees at lightning speed while sweat pours down your face does not represent the many types of burpees out there.

Slow burpees are a fantastic full-body exercise that is great for warming up. The name explains it all, you are performing burpees at a deliberately slow pace. There is no jumping, and each movement is performed with care.

---

1. Start in the push-up position, with hands shoulder-width apart and feet close together.
2. Bring one knee forwards until it is directly below your chest and place your foot down, then repeat with the other leg until you are in a crouched position.
3. Carefully stand up until you are fully upright. This is one rep.
4. Reverse the movement and get back into the starting position.

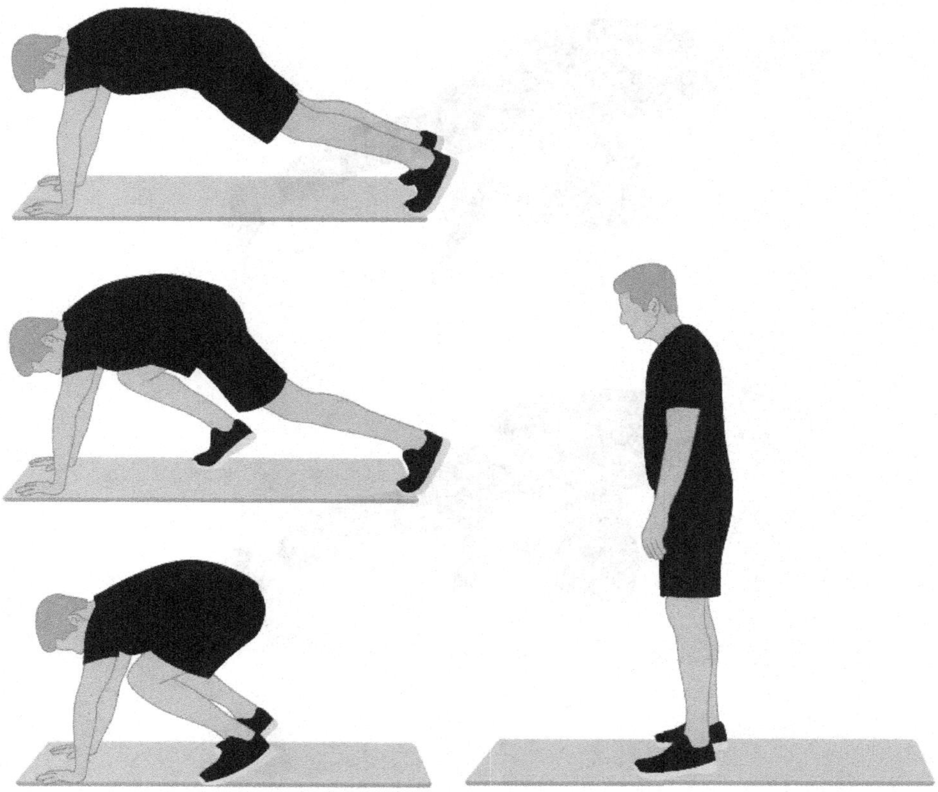

Exercise #8 Mountain Climbers

As with the gentle burpees, mountain climbers are exercises that are often performed at a fast pace during circuit-style workouts. But they are also able to be completely transformed into a useful warm-up exercise by slowing down the movement.

Not only can slow mountain climbers raise your heart rate sufficiently, they are also a great way to warm up your core muscles.

---

1. Place your hands on the floor and get into a push-up position or you can place them on a chair or bench.
2. Push your chest out, then slowly bring your left knee in towards your chest, pause and then return it.
3. As you are doing so, bring your right knee into your chest.
4. You can increase the pace slightly as you continue to move your knees back and forth.

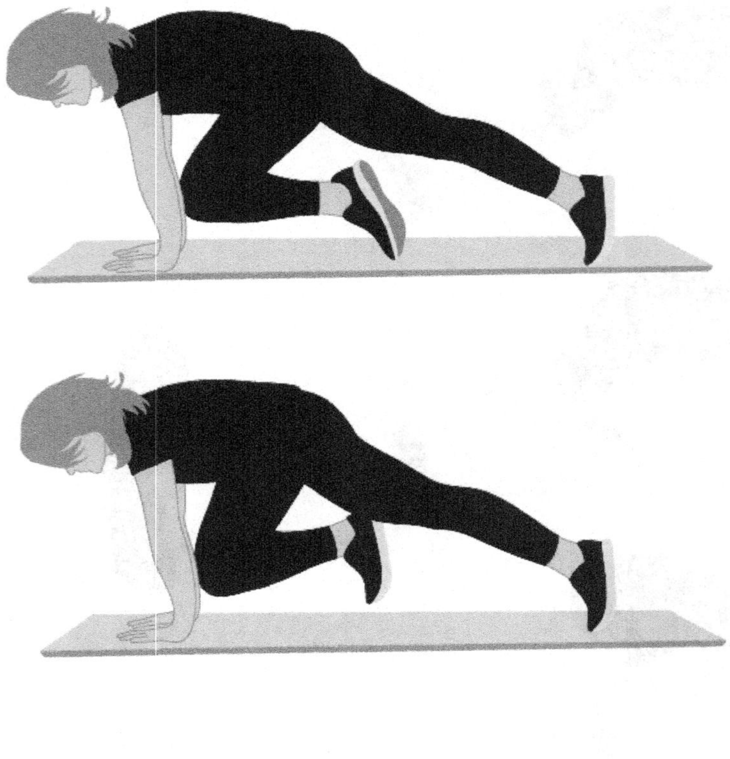

High Mobility Warm-Up Sequence

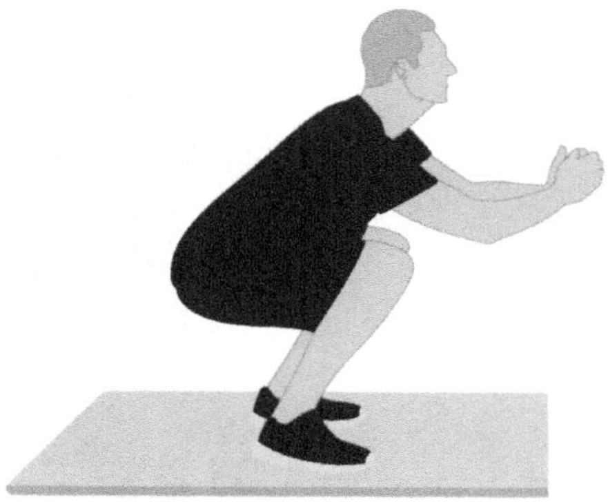

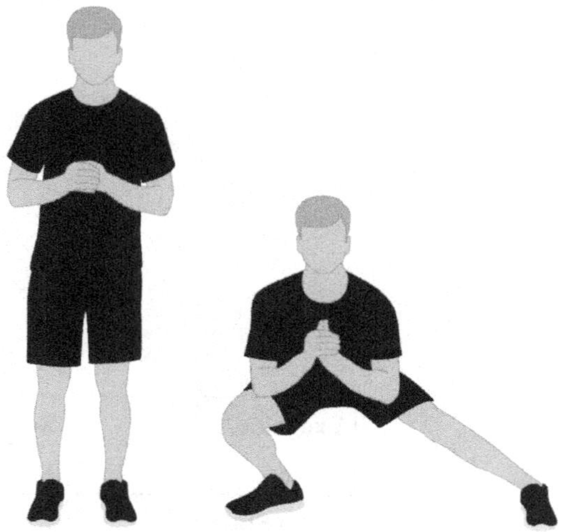

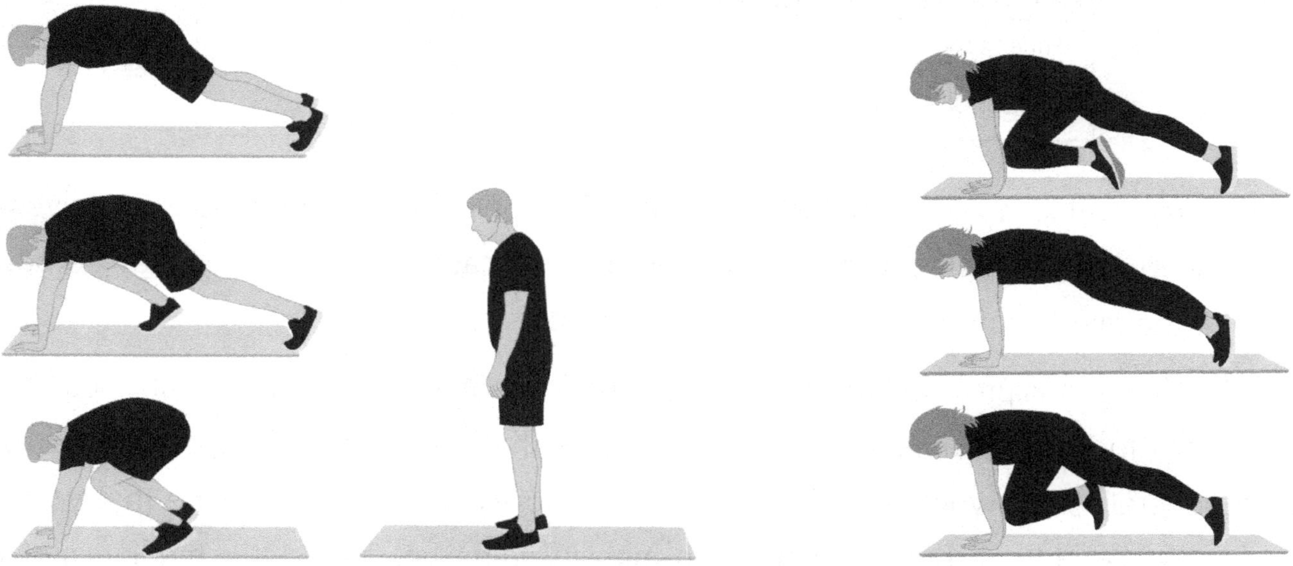

High Mobility Warm-up Video

Exercise	Sets	Reps	Rest Between Sets
Cardio	1	5 minutes	n/a
Deep Squats	1	8-10	n/a
Lateral Lunges	1 (each leg)	10	30 seconds
Gentle Burpees	1	10	n/a
Mountain Climbers	1	30-40 seconds	n/a

Remember, this is a high-mobility exercise for people who would class themselves as experienced exercisers. If you don't fit either of these categories, then you may be better suited to the medium or even low-mobility warm-up.

This chapter has provided three warm-up routines that are based on your abilities. When working out for the first time, you should make sure that the warm-up is appropriate. If you would generally class yourself as having a high mobility, but you aren't sure that you can manage several of the exercises on the high-mobility warm-up, then try the medium mobility warm-up and see how that suits you.

Whatever you do, don't avoid the warm-ups completely as they are crucial for any core training session.

CHAPTER 7

Compound Lifts for Core Training

SCAN FOR AUDIO CHAPTER

In this chapter, we will be taking a look at the compound lifts that you will be performing during your core workouts. Compound lifts work multiple muscle groups simultaneously, and they also target your core muscles in a different way to core-specific exercises.

A good core program should comprise several compound lifts that target the upper and lower body, as well as exercises that target the core muscles in isolation. While many compound lifts can sound intimidating (squats, deadlifts, presses, rows), they are actually the safest exercises to learn, with many variations that can suit seniors and people who are new this form of exercise.

As with the warm-up exercises, we are splitting the compound lifts into lifts for beginners, intermediate lifters, and experienced lifters. They can also be split into low, medium, and high-mobility if that is a better fit. For instance, you may be very experienced but have low mobility, in which case following a beginner's program makes more sense.

This chapter will provide exercise descriptions for each exercise, and the following chapters will deal with core exercises and cardio. Chapter 12 will place all of the exercises into a 24-week core training program.

Beginner Compound Lifts (Low-Mobility)

For these beginner compound lifts, you will need a sturdy chair that you can trust to take your weight. A set of light dumbbells is useful for one exercise, but you can substitute the dumbbells for two cans of food if you don't have any dumbbells. You may even find that not using any weights at all will be challenging enough!

Exercise #9 Box Squat

The box squat is an incredibly safe and yet effective exercise for the lower body. It works the glutes, the hamstrings, the quadriceps, and, yes, even the core muscles. It is also a fantastic exercise for beginners because it has so many variations that you can learn once you have mastered it.

How to Perform:

1. Stand directly in front of a chair with your feet shoulder-width apart and your toes turned out very slightly.
2. Take a deep breath, push your chest out, pull your shoulders back, and slowly lower your glutes until they touch the seat.
3. Pause, then rise back up again, breathing out as you go.

The trick with the box squat is to ensure that you don't slump down into the chair like you would if sitting recreationally. It's all about control. You lower yourself onto the seat carefully, keeping your chest out and your shoulders back. Once you touch the seat, you drive back up again.

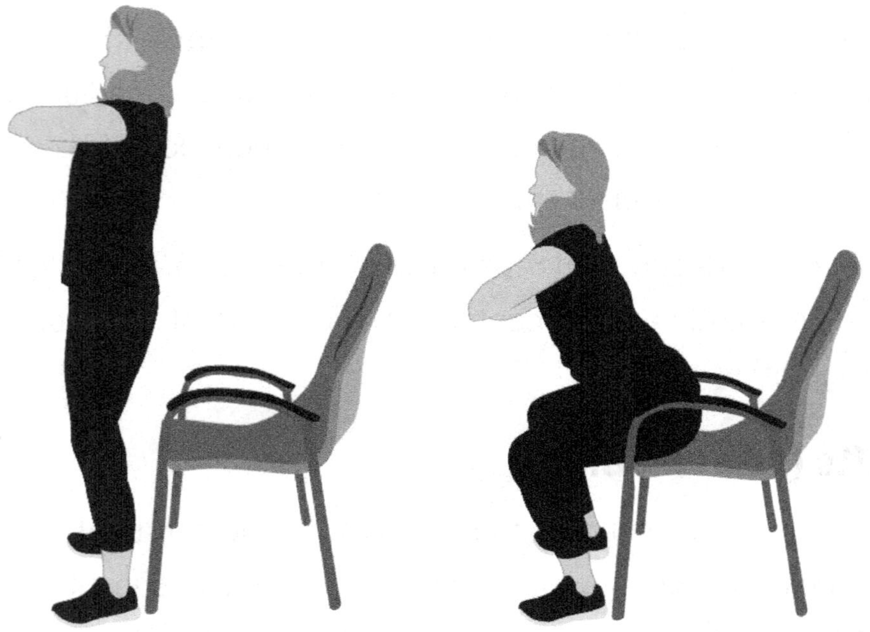

SCAN FOR VIDEO

Exercise #10 Squats while Holding Chair

This exercise sounds very similar to a box squat, which also involves a chair, but the two exercises are markedly different. Rather than sitting carefully on a chair, you are instead using the back of a chair for balance as you perform a squat.

Just make sure that the chair is both secure and balanced so that it does not topple when you use it for support. Place some heavy books on the seat if you find that the chair rises slightly when you place weight on it.

How to Perform:

1. Stand behind a chair with your hands holding onto the back. Place your feet shoulder-width apart and turn your toes out slightly.
2. Push your chest out and pull your shoulders back.
3. Slowly lower your glutes towards the floor, keeping your heels flat on the ground and your hands on the back of the chair.
4. Pause when your thighs are parallel to the floor, and then rise back up again.

You can go lower than parallel if you are finding the movement easy but don't try and force it. It is better to have a shorter range of motion while maintaining good form than to lose your form while trying to get too low.

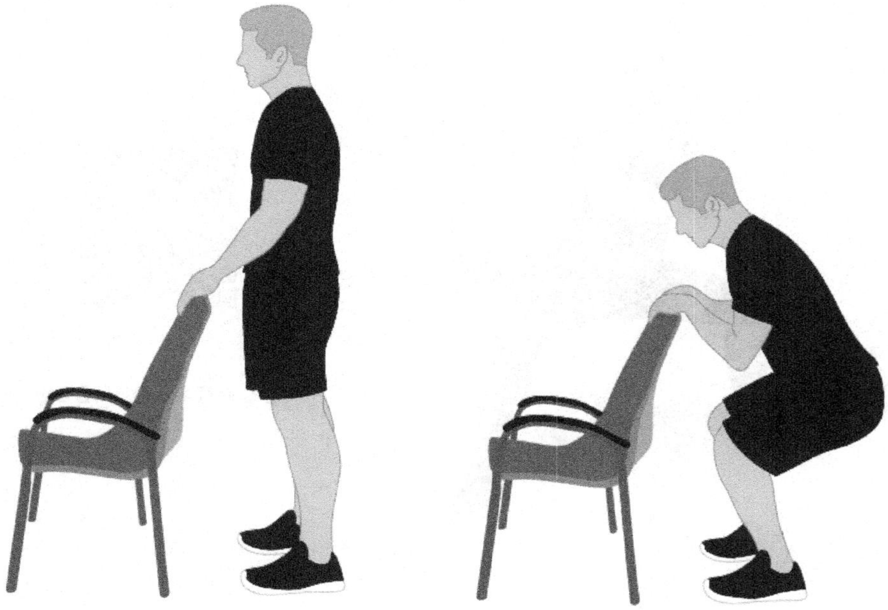

SCAN FOR VIDEO

Exercise #11 Sumo Box Squat

This exercise is very similar to a regular box squat (see exercise #9), but you use a much wider stance. This means that some chairs may be too high for you to perform this exercise comfortably. As the exercise has a shorter range of motion.

If the seat of your chair is too high, then you can bring your feet narrower until the seat becomes comfortable to sit on. Or just stick to regular box squats.

How to Perform:

1. Stand directly in front of a chair with your feet wider than shoulder-width apart and your toes turned out.
2. Take a deep breath, push your chest out, pull your shoulders back, and slowly lower your glutes until they touch the seat.
3. Pause, then rise back up again, breathing out as you go.

Because your legs are wider, your glutes won't travel as far backwards as usual, so start off a little closer to the chair than you would for a box squat.

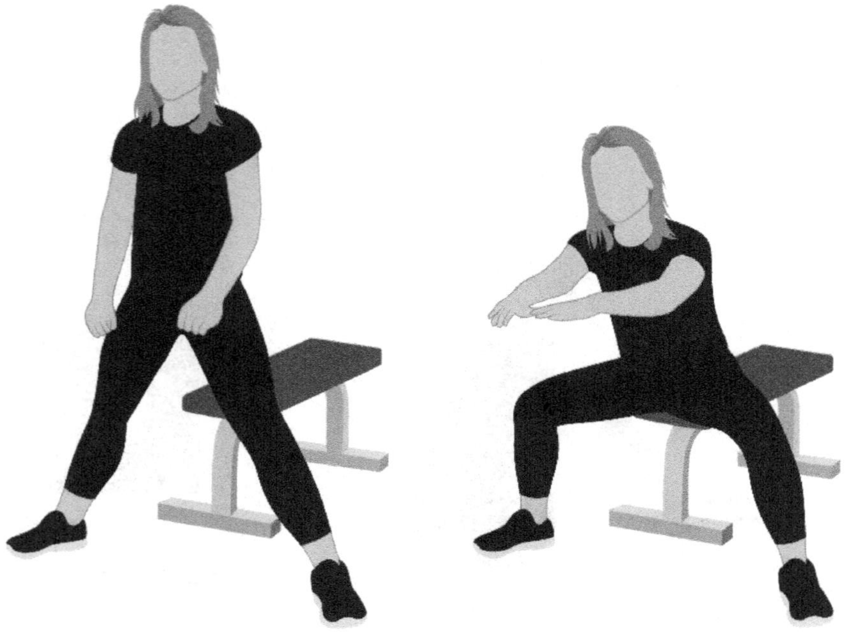

SCAN FOR VIDEO

Exercise #12 Box Push-Ups

The push-up is one of the best chest exercises out there, also targeting the triceps and the shoulders (deltoids). However, it can be very difficult for beginners as you are basically lifting 80% of your body weight.

Box push-ups are easier as you don't need to lift as much of your body weight, it is closer to 40%. It is the equivalent of replacing two heavy dumbbells with two very light dumbbells. The same muscles are worked, but the exercise is a lot more accessible.

How to Perform:

1. Place your hands on the floor, shoulder-width apart. Push your chest out and pull your shoulders back.
2. Place your knees on the floor, and rest your feet on the floor
3. Lower your chest down to the ground by bending your elbows
4. Pause when your chest is almost touching the ground, then rise back up

What's great about box push-ups is that as you begin to find them easier, you can increase the difficulty quite easily. Just raise your feet off the floor and slide your knees back. This causes you to lift more of your body weight, making the exercise harder.

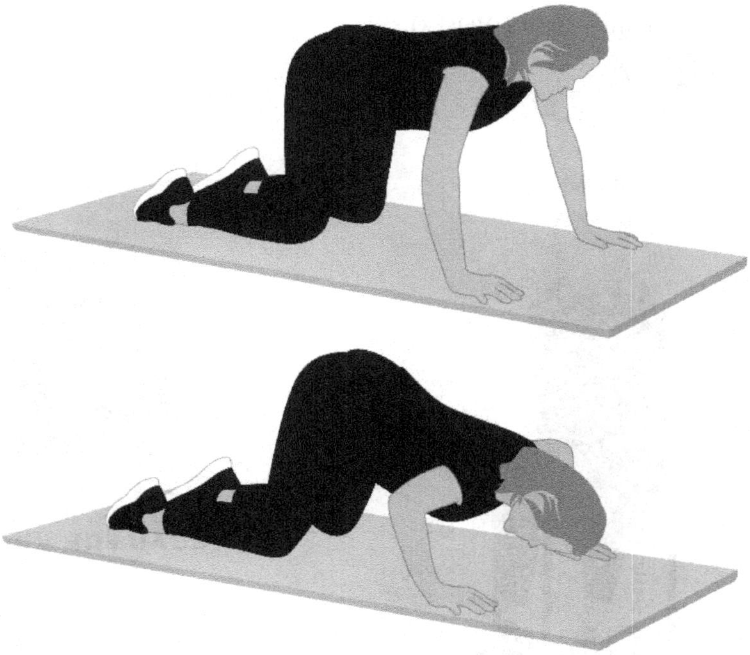

SCAN FOR VIDEO

Exercise #13 Seated Dumbbell Shoulder Press

For this exercise, you will want a set of light dumbbells. But if you don't have any dumbbells to hand, you can use two cans of food or similar items that have equal weight. Dumbbells are best because they are designed to be held safely, but not all households have dumbbells in them.

How to Perform:

1. Sit on a sturdy chair with a dumbbell held in each hand, resting on each of your knees.
2. Kick one knee up, using the momentum to raise the dumbbell up to shoulder height. Repeat with the other knee. You should now have both dumbbells at shoulder height.
3. Push your chest out and pull your shoulders back, and bring your elbows out in front of you with the dumbbells held in a neutral grip (both palms facing each other).
4. Take a deep breath, and then push the dumbbells up into the air above your head. Keep your feet flat on the ground while doing so. Breathe out as you raise the dumbbells.
5. Pause, and then lower the dumbbells back to shoulder height.

The most common way to perform a dumbbell shoulder press is with your arms out to the side rather than your elbows pushed out in front of you. But the option chosen in this book is safer and easier to perform. If you want, you can experiment with your elbows out to the side instead of in front of you to find out which suits you best.

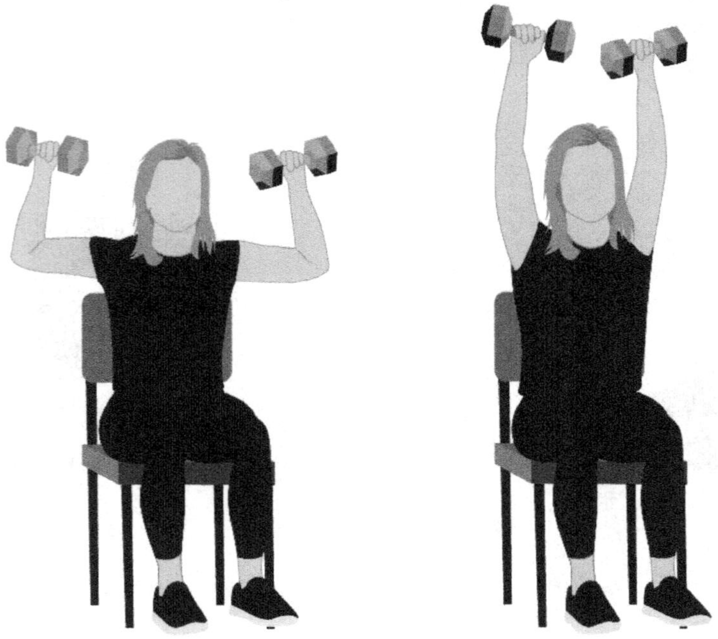

SCAN FOR VIDEO

Exercise #14 Wall Push-Ups

The wall push-up is a fantastic introduction to push-ups and a great alternative to box push-ups (which may be painful for people with knee injuries). All you need is a flat wall that you can push against.

How to Perform:

1. Stand in front of a wall with your chest pushed out and your shoulders pulled back. Place both hands on it, about shoulder-width apart. Your arms should be fully extended
2. Bend your elbows and lean forwards until your chest is almost touching the wall
3. Pause, and then drive your chest back to the starting position

You can make this exercise easier or harder by changing how close you are to the wall when you start. The closer you are to the wall, the easier the exercise. The further away you are, the harder.

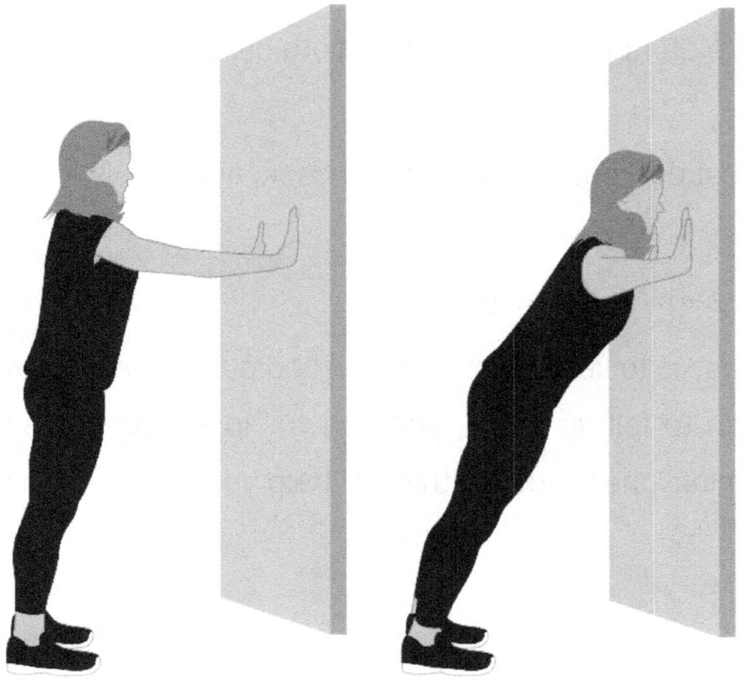

SCAN FOR VIDEO

Intermediate Compound Lifts (Medium-Mobility)

For these intermediate compound lifts, you will need a sturdy chair or bench that can support your weight. You also need a set of dumbbells. These dumbbells can be replaced with two cans of food if that is all you have available.

Exercise #15 Box Squat with Dumbbell

As with the dumbbell shoulder press (exercise #13), this exercise is best performed with a dumbbell, but if you don't have one to hand, then you can use alternatives. Because this exercise requires you to hold one weight with both hands, you have a lot more options (as you don't need two identical weights that can be held in each hand).

You can use a ball, a rucksack (which you can wear backwards across your chest), or even something like a heavy book. Just make sure that the weight isn't too big (as this can affect your movement and comfort while performing each rep).

How to Perform:

1. Stand directly in front of a chair or bench with your feet shoulder-width apart and your toes turned out very slightly. Hold a dumbbell (or weight) in both hands so that it is close to your chest.
2. Take a deep breath, push your chest out, pull your shoulders back, and slowly lower your glutes until they touch the seat.
3. Pause, then rise back up again, breathing out as you go.

The important thing with this exercise is to keep your chest pushed out and your shoulders back. Otherwise, the weight will begin to fall forwards, and you will lose your form. When performing the exercise, constantly think 'chest out', as this will help you to nail each rep.

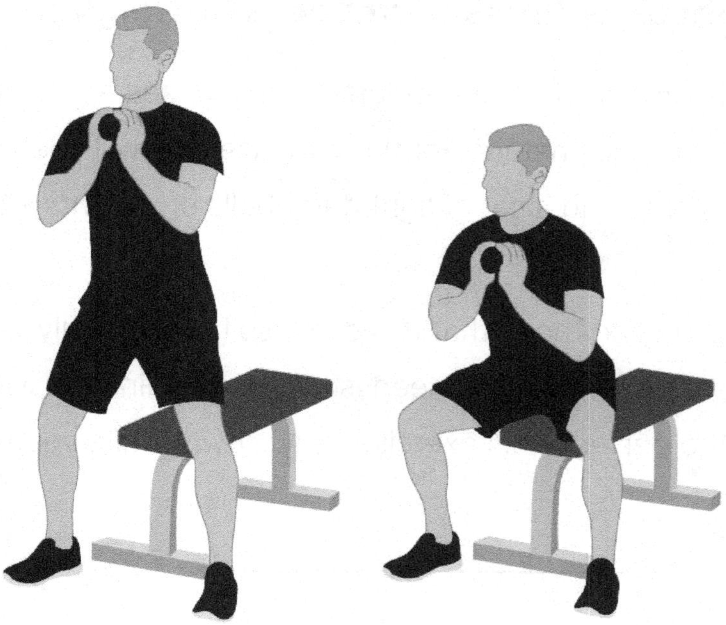

SCAN FOR VIDEO

Exercise #16 Box Squat into Shoulder Press (Dumbbells or Weights)

The box squat into shoulder press is one of the most underrated exercises for seniors, it is also very challenging due to its cardiovascular nature. For this exercise, you will need a sturdy chair or box that you can squat down onto and a set of light dumbbells or weights which you can use to press up in the air.

The transition from the lower to the upper body that this exercise has will really work your core muscles, as well as get your heart racing. All you need is a little coordination, which will come with practice. Don't be afraid to perform this exercise very slowly while you are learn the movement.

How to Perform:

1. Stand in front of a chair or box with your feet shoulder-width apart and toes turned out very slightly.
2. Hold a light dumbbell or weight in each hand, resting at shoulder height with your palms facing each other.
3. Take a deep breath, push your chest out, pull your shoulders back, and slowly lower your glutes until they touch the seat.
4. Pause, then rise back up again, breathing out as you go. As you do so, raise the dumbbells or weights up above your head until your arms are almost fully extended.
5. Lower them back down, and then sit back down to continue the exercise.

You can use heavier weights to turn this into a muscle-building exercise, one that really works the core. Or you can use lighter weights and turn this into a more cardiovascular and fat-burning exercise.

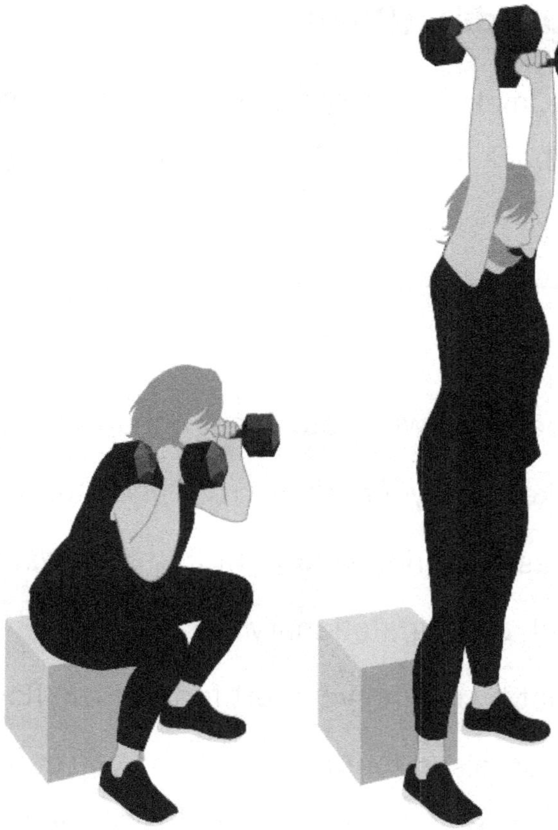

SCAN FOR VIDEO

Exercise #17 Single-Leg Romanian Deadlift (Chair)

This exercise requires quite a lot of balance, making it very taxing on the core muscles. But it is primarily a hamstring, glute, and lower-back exercise. All you need for it is a strong and sturdy chair that you can hold onto.

How to Perform:

1. Grip the back of a chair while standing behind it with your chest out and shoulders back.
2. Raise your right foot off the floor while keeping your left leg nice and straight.
3. Keeping left leg straight, lean forwards as you bring your right foot backwards
4. You should feel a nice stretch in the back of your stationary leg
5. Return to the starting position and repeat by raising your left foot off the floor.

The trick with this exercise is to keep your raised foot as straight as you can rather than having your toes pointing out and bringing your leg out wide. This will keep the focus on your hamstrings and glutes without bringing your hips into the exercise.

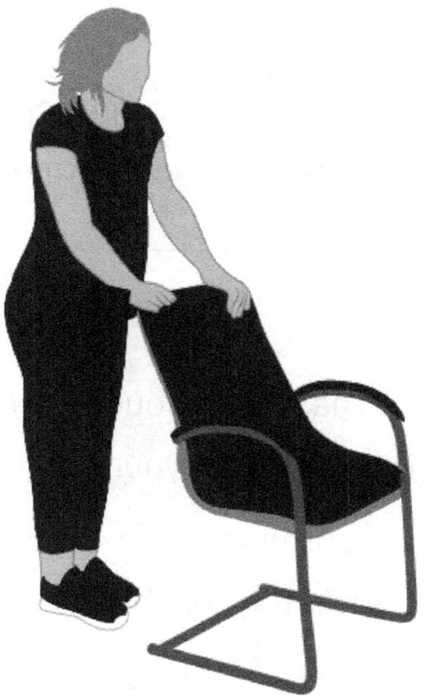

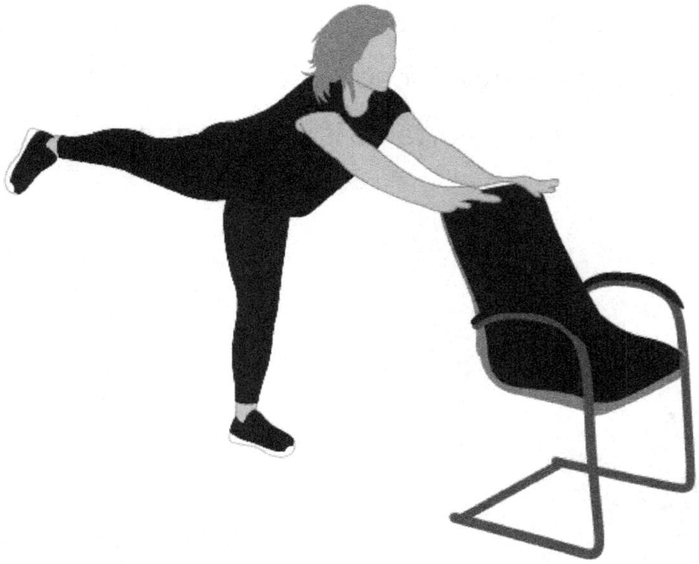

SCAN FOR VIDEO

Exercise #18 Glute Bridges

The glute bridge is a superb bodyweight exercise that can be performed without any equipment, though an exercise mat would make the exercise significantly more comfortable to perform.

How to Perform:

1. Lie on your back with your feet flat on the floor, shoulder-width apart, and your knees bent. Rest your arms on the floor on either side of your body.
2. Take a deep breath in and then raise your hips up as high as you can until there is a straight diagonal line from your knees down to your shoulders. Breathe out as you do so.
3. Squeeze your glutes tight and then lower your hips back down to the starting position.

You can make this exercise more difficult by resting a weight on your hips. This is usually okay for light weights, but once the weights get heavy, it can become uncomfortable. You can wrap the weight in a sweater to make it more comfortable if you need to.

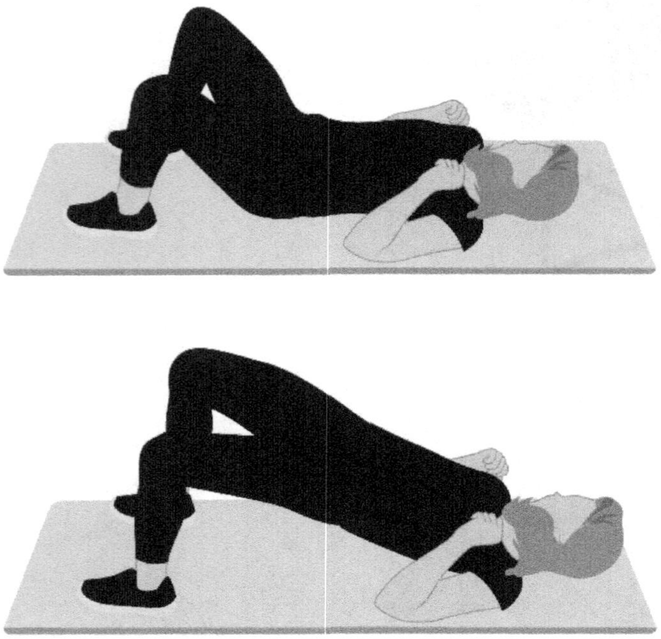

SCAN FOR VIDEO

Exercise #19 Lateral Lunges

The lateral lunge is a great exercise for your inner and outer thighs, as well as your quadriceps. It's simple to learn and can be easily adjusted to make it easier if you need it to be.

How to Perform:

1. Stand upright with your chest pushed out and your shoulders pulled back. Your feet should be next to each other.
2. Take a large step to the side with your left leg, keeping your right leg straight and bending your left knee.
3. You should feel a stretch on the inside of your right leg. If you don't, then you may not have taken a large enough step.
4. Pause, and then return your left leg to the starting position. Repeat this movement for the required number of reps, and then swap legs.

You can make this exercise harder by holding a weight in your hands so that it rests in front of your chest.

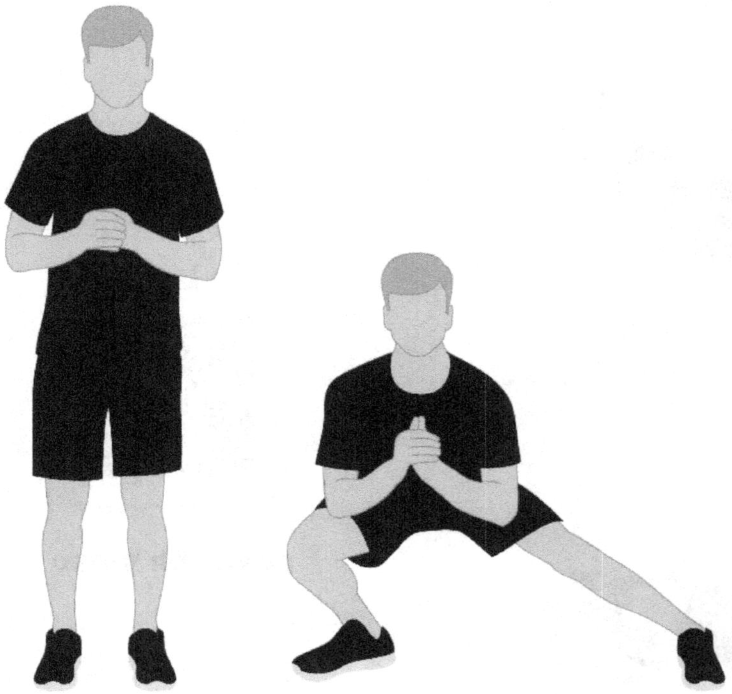

SCAN FOR VIDEO

Exercise #20 Knee Push-Ups

The knee push-up is a more difficult version of the box push-up, which we looked at earlier. As with box push-ups, you can easily adjust the difficulty by bringing your knees forwards or backwards. The closer your knees get to your torso, the easier the exercise is to perform.

How to Perform:

1. Place your hands on the floor, shoulder-width apart. Push your chest out and pull your shoulders back.
2. Place your knees on the floor, slide them backwards and raise your feet off the floor
3. Lower your chest down to the ground by bending your elbows
4. Pause when your chest is almost touching the ground, then rise back up

Another way in which you can adjust this exercise is by bringing your hands closer and wider apart. Bringing your hands closer together (and tucking your elbows in) will place more emphasis on your shoulders and triceps.

While bringing your hands out wide will place more emphasis on your chest. However, when bringing your hands wider, make sure that your elbows are at a 45-degree angle from your side as this will protect your shoulders.

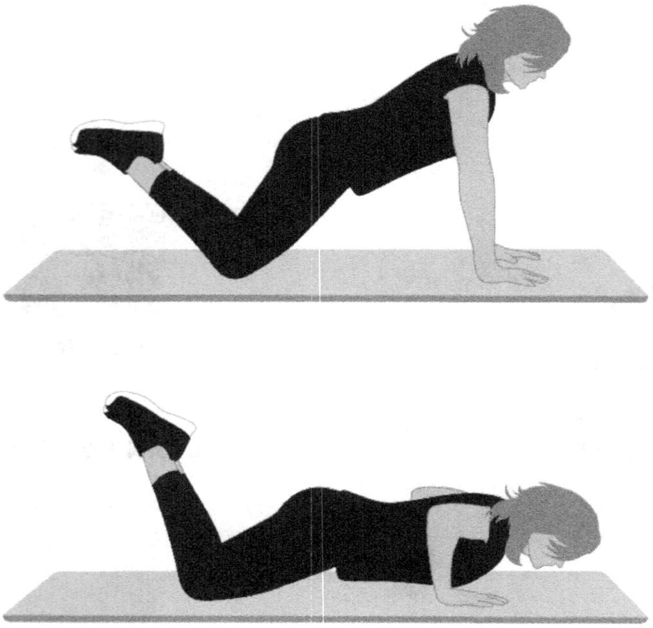

SCAN FOR VIDEO

Advanced Compound Lifts (High-Mobility)

The following exercises are for advanced lifters only, though if you are medium level and find that the exercises have become easier as the weeks go by, you may be able to start adding some of these exercises into your program but do so gradually and take notice how your body responds.

Exercise #21 Bodyweight Squats

The bodyweight squat is not particularly difficult to perform, but it requires balance and good form, which many people over 50 may struggle with. Hence its inclusion in the advanced compound lifts section. If you find this exercise easy, then you can hold a dumbbell, kettlebell, or even a barbell to increase the difficulty.

How to Perform:

1. Stand upright with your chest pushed out and your shoulders pulled back
2. Place your feet shoulder-width apart with toes turned out slightly, take a deep breath
3. Ensure that your heels stay in contact with the ground at all times
4. Push your glutes backwards and down as if you were about to sit on a small chair
5. Keep lowering your glutes until your thighs are around parallel to the ground
6. Pause, and then rise back upwards, breathing out as you do so.

Once you have mastered the bodyweight squat, you can begin to learn more complicated versions of this exercise. Goblet squats, barbell squats, bodyweight sumo squats, and even jumping squats. Just ensure that you are doing the basics right and that your body is responding well to the increased challenge.

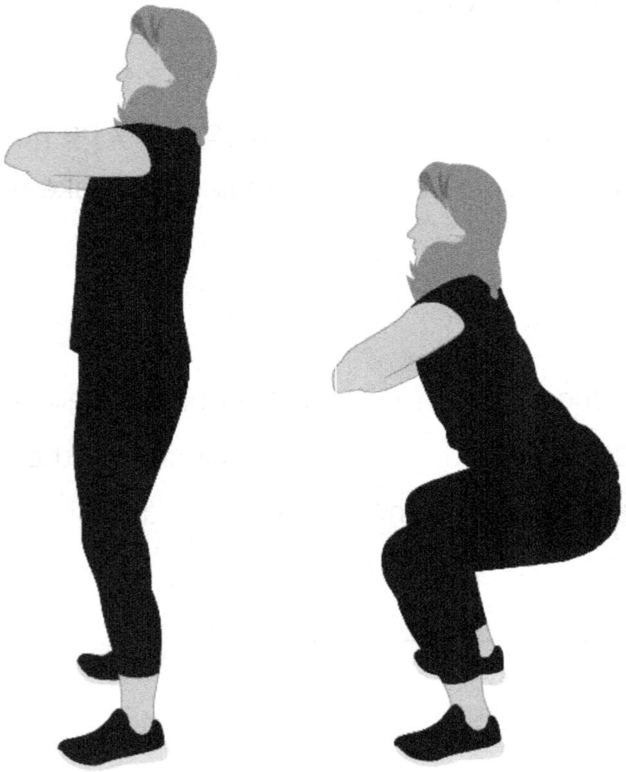

SCAN FOR VIDEO

Exercise #22 Walking Lunges

The walking lunge is an incredible exercise for the glutes and the quadriceps. It also works the core muscles really effectively. The only issue is that it can be hard from a balancing point of view. If you find that you struggle to keep your balance, then try static lunges instead.

How to Perform:

1. Stand upright with chest out and shoulder blades pulled together. Your feet should be together
2. Take a large step forward with your left foot, raise your right heel off the floor
3. Drop your right knee towards the floor, pausing just before it touches
4. Your left thigh should now be parallel to the floor
5. Keep your chest upright, and your shoulders pulled back throughout
6. Pause, and then rise back up and bring your right foot forwards.
7. Repeat the movement with the opposite legs to walk forward

Again, this is an exercise that, once you have mastered it you can upgrade it quite easily. Hold a dumbbell between your two hands (against your chest) or a dumbbell in each hand beside your body to increase the intensity.

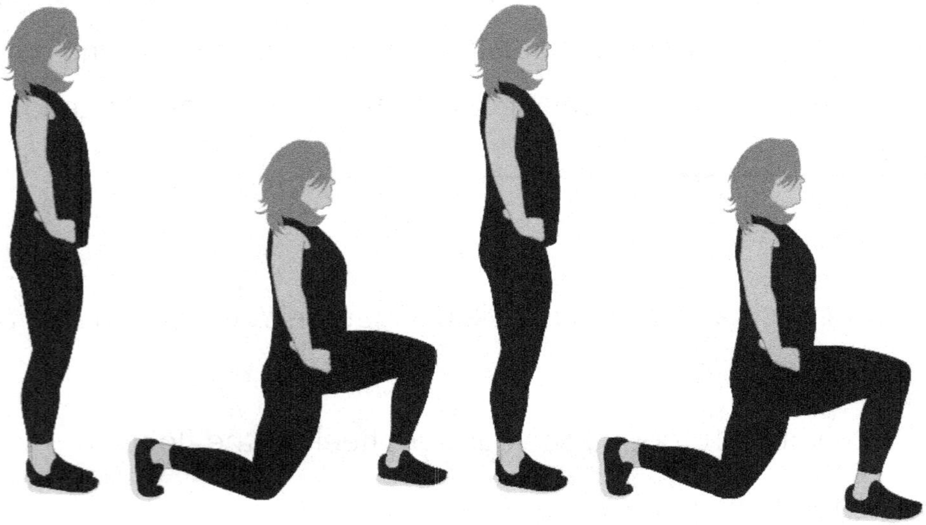

SCAN FOR VIDEO

Exercise #23 Bodyweight Sumo Squats

The sumo squat is very similar to the bodyweight squat, except that you use a much wider stance. This means that you won't push your glutes as far backwards as you would normally. Other than that, the difference is minimal.

How to Perform:

1. Stand upright with your chest pushed out and shoulders pulled back
2. Place your feet wider shoulder-width apart with toes turned out
3. Ensure that your heels stay in contact with the ground at all times
4. Push your glutes backwards and down as if you were about to sit on a small chair
5. Keep lowering your glutes until your thighs are around parallel to the ground
6. Pause, and then rise back upwards

If you find the bodyweight sumo squat is not challenging you enough, then you can attempt to perform it while holding a dumbbell to your chest with both of your hands.

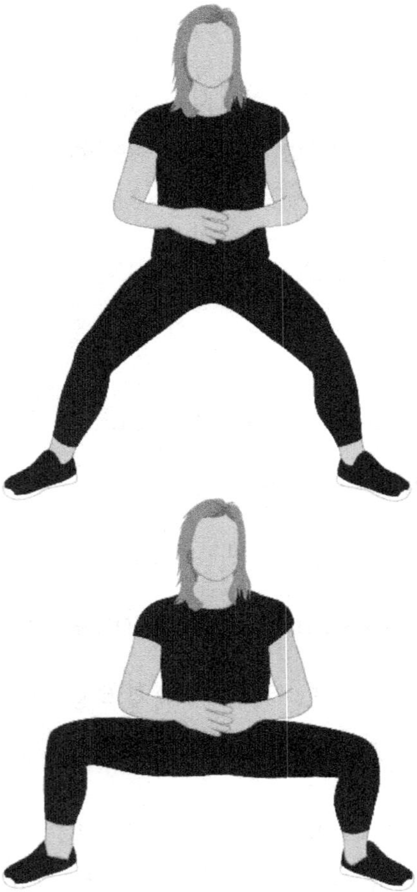

SCAN FOR VIDEO

Bodyweight Sumo Squats (Modified)

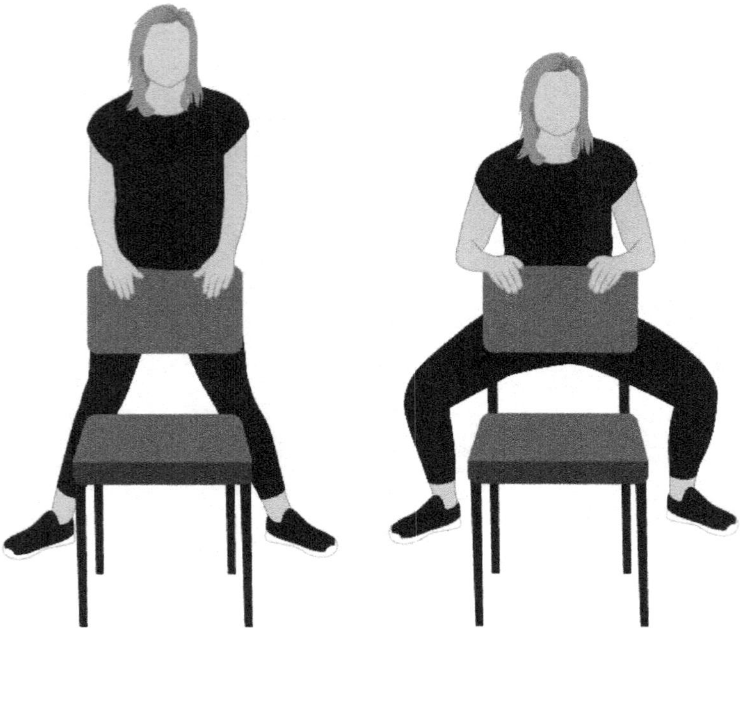

SCAN FOR VIDEO

Exercise #24 Squats into Shoulder Press (Dumbbells or Weights)

This exercise is a great compound lift as it works the upper and lower body simultaneously, burning a lot of calories and working the core very hard. It's also fun to learn and perform.

How to Perform:

1. Stand upright with your feet shoulder-width apart and toes turned out very slightly.
2. Hold a dumbbell in each hand, resting at shoulder height with your palms facing each other.
3. Take a deep breath, push your chest out, pull your shoulders back, and slowly lower your glutes until your thighs are at least parallel with the floor.
4. Pause, then rise back up again, breathing out as you go. As you do so, raise the dumbbells up above your head until your arms are almost fully extended.
5. Lower them back down, and then squat back down to continue the exercise.

If you find the exercise easy, then consider using heavier dumbbells or weights. If, however, you find the exercise very hard, then try to perform the box version of this exercise (sit on a chair rather than squatting in mid-air).

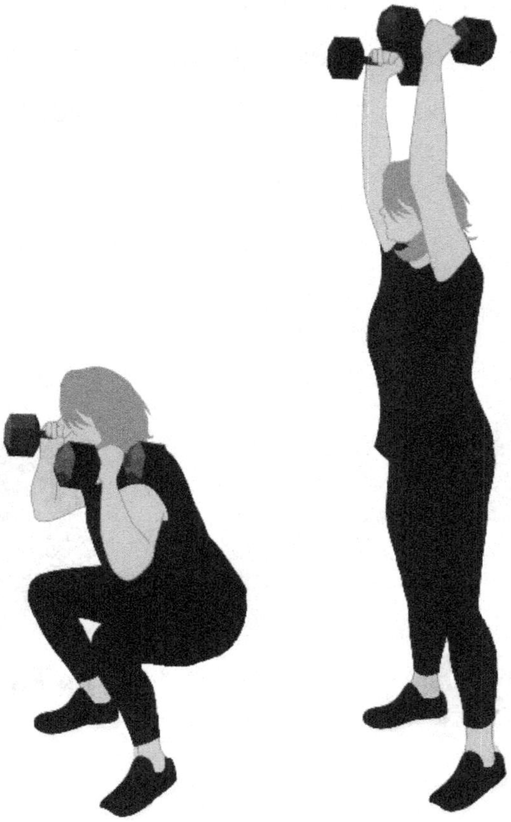

SCAN FOR VIDEO

Exercise #25 Push-Ups

The push-up is one of the best chest, shoulder, and tricep exercises out there. It is also one of the hardest bodyweight exercises there is! Many people will really struggle to perform a full set of 10 push-ups.

If this is the case, then perform as many full push-ups as you can before dropping to your knees and performing knee push-ups (exercise #20), and then performing box push-ups (exercise #12) when you can no longer perform knee push-ups.

How to Perform:

1. Place your hands on the floor, shoulder-width apart
2. Place your feet on the floor, and raise your hips up until there is a straight line from your shoulders down to your heels.
3. Keeping your elbows at a 45-degree angle from your body, lower your chest all the way down until it almost touches the ground.
4. Pause, and then rise back upwards to complete your push-up.

If your wrists start to hurt, then you may want to consider investing in a set of push-up stands, which take the strain off the wrists. Not everyone finds push-up stands more comfortable, but for those who do they can make a huge difference to your results. May be worth considering!

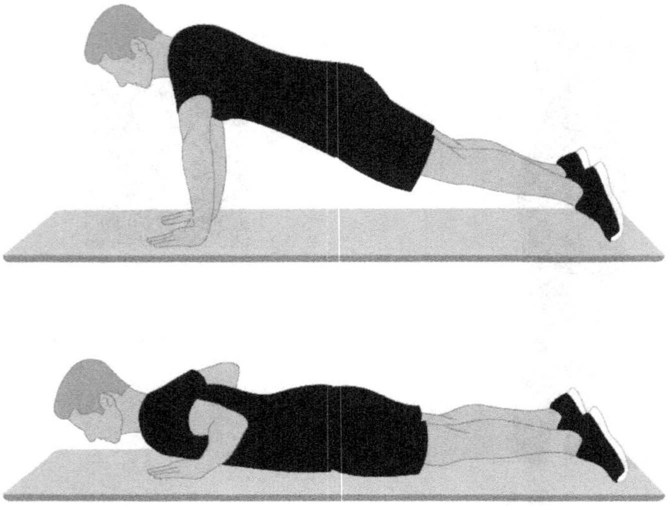

SCAN FOR VIDEO

Exercise #26 Dumbbell Shrugs

The dumbbell shrug is a great exercise for your upper back and shoulders, it is also very easy to learn and perform. The only thing to focus on is keeping your arms straight throughout.

---

1. Stand upright with your chest pushed out and your shoulders pulled back together. Place your feet shoulder-width apart, and hold a dumbbell in each hand resting by your side.
2. Keeping your arms straight, shrug your shoulders up as high as you can.
3. Pause, and then slowly lower them back down to the starting position.

The important thing to focus on when shrugging is tempo and range of motion. You really don't want to rush your shrugs. Raise your shoulders up nice and slowly until you can raise them no longer. Pause, and then slowly lower them back down again. Don't drop them.

So, there you have it, fifteen compound exercises that you can add to your training program. A beginner may find that they don't have much variety in the number of compound movements that they can perform, but as their strength grows, this variety will increase. Intermediate and advanced lifters will have very varied training programs, as the number of exercises that they can perform is significantly larger.

The important thing to focus on with all of these exercises is your safety. Before performing any exercise, check your workout area for hazards. Make sure that you have something to grab hold of if you lose your balance, and please make sure that you have a plan in case something goes wrong. Not that this is likely, of course, but it is better to be safe than sorry.

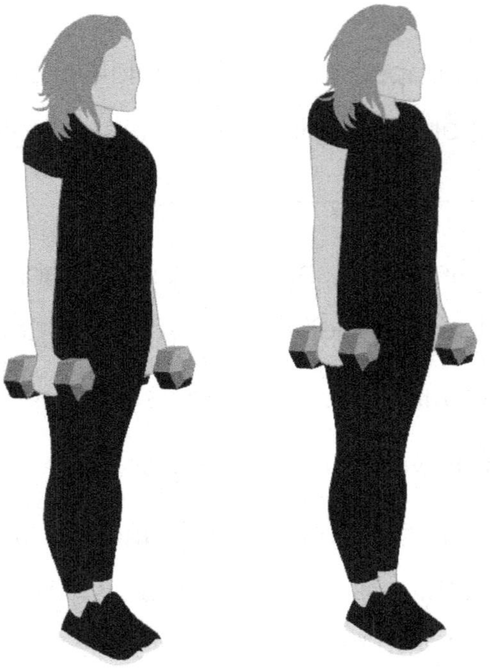

SCAN FOR VIDEO

CHAPTER 8

Core Exercises for Beginners

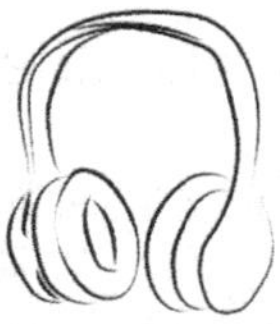

SCAN FOR AUDIO CHAPTER

In this chapter, we will be taking a look at basic core exercises that are suitable for beginners and those with limited mobility. As you may have already gathered, the core muscles are used in many exercises, and those with weak cores may find that they are getting a decent core workout from the compound lifts mentioned in the previous chapter.

However, it is always a good idea to perform some core-specific exercises, even as a beginner. This chapter will take you through some basic core exercises, giving you detailed instructions in how to perform them safely and effectively.

Exercise #27 Modified Plank

The modified plank is a really effective core exercise for people who are not yet capable of a full plank or a push-up position plank. It is ideal if you have mobility issues, and it can really help you strengthen your abdominal muscles in a safe position.

How to Perform:

1. Place your forearms on the floor, shoulder width apart.
2. Place your knees on the floor, and raise your feet off the ground. Keep your hips slightly raised.
3. Squeeze your abs tight, and squeeze your glutes
4. Hold this position for 30 seconds and then relax

If the exercise becomes a little too easy, particularly if you've been following the training program for a few weeks, then you may want to increase the difficulty. Bringing your knees further backwards will make the exercise harder. You can even attempt to raise your knees off the ground so that your legs are straight. Though this is quite an advanced movement, so don't rush into it.

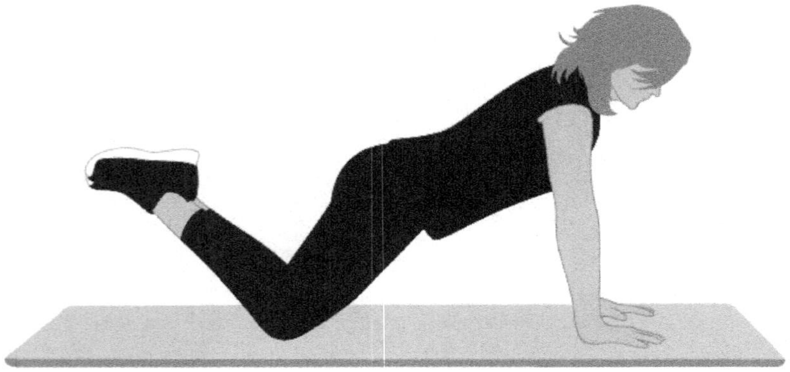

SCAN FOR VIDEO

Exercise #28 Seated Forward Roll-Ups

For this exercise, you will need a sturdy chair. It is an exercise that sounds almost too easy, but it is highly effective, particularly for older lifters. Don't try to push yourself too hard, and perform the exercise nice and slowly.

How to Perform:

1. Sit on a chair with your legs straight out in front of you and your feet together.
2. Push your chest out and pull your shoulders back so that you have a nice, straight back.
3. Bring your arms out in front of you, keeping them straight and pointing towards your toes.
4. Curl your chin towards your chest, slowly rolling forwards with your hands travelling towards your toes.
5. Pause when you cannot roll forwards any further and then slowly return to the starting position.

There is often a belief that the faster you perform a core exercise, the more powerful it is. This could not be more wrong! Core exercises are almost always best when performed as slowly as possible, and the seated forward roll-up is no exception. Move slowly and feel every second of the movement in your abdominal muscles.

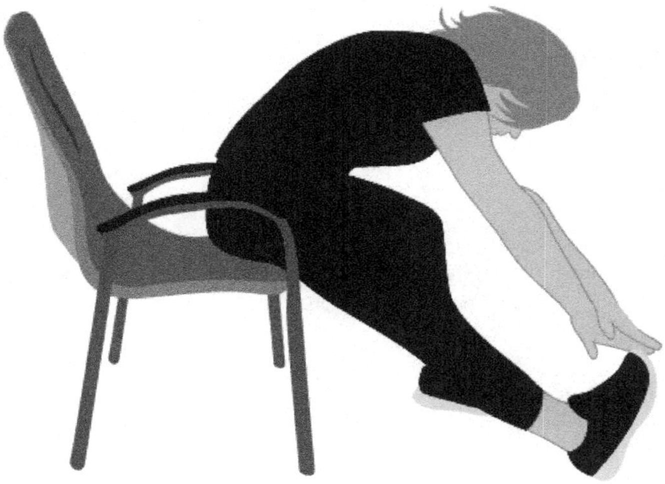

SCAN FOR VIDEO

Exercise #29 Seated Leg Extension

This exercise may sound similar to the quadricep-focused leg extension, but you are instead engaging your core muscles to bring your straightened leg upwards.

How to Perform:

1. Sit on a sturdy chair with your feet flat on the floor, your chest pushed out, and your shoulders pulled back. Place your hands on either side of the chair so that you can hold it for support.
2. Squeeze your abs (imagine you are about to get punched in the stomach) and then raise your legs off the floor, straightening them out as you do so.
3. Pause when your legs are fully straightened out, and then slowly return your legs to the starting position.

The longer you can hold your legs straight out in front of you, the harder the exercise will work your core muscles. If you are very new to exercising, then you may find it too difficult to even get your legs straight. This is perfectly normal, so just straighten your legs as much as you can, and don't force it.

Exercise #30 Seated Single-Leg Extension

This exercise is almost identical to the previous exercise, but instead of lifting both legs simultaneously, you lift one leg and then the other. The important thing to focus on is not leaning to one side while lifting only one leg, as this is a subconscious way in which your body tries to balance you.

How to Perform:

1. Sit on a sturdy chair with your feet flat on the floor, your chest pushed out, and your shoulders pulled back. Place your hands on either side of the chair so that you can hold it for support.
2. Squeeze your abs (imagine you are about to get punched in the stomach) and then raise one leg off the floor, straightening it out as you do so. Keep your other leg still.
3. Pause when your leg is fully straightened out, and then slowly return your leg to the starting position. Perform the required number of reps and then swap to the other leg.

You could increase the difficulty of this exercise by wearing ankle weights, but this will mostly place more emphasis on your quadriceps than your abs.

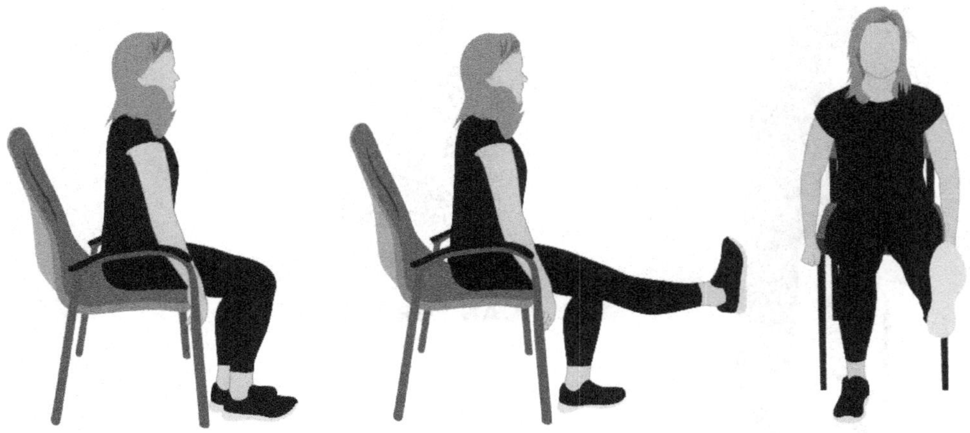

SCAN FOR VIDEO

Exercise #31 Seated Side Bends

This exercise works many of the core muscles, but it particularly works the obliques. It is a highly effective exercise and one that is easy to learn and perform.

How to Perform:

1. Sit on a sturdy chair with your feet flat on the floor. Place one hand by your side, and raise the other hand up in the air as if you were about to ask a question in class at school.
2. Keeping that arm up in the air, lean to your opposite side (if your left arm is raised, lean to your right) as if you are swaying to the music at a concert. Pause when you feel a stretch in your side, and then return to the starting position. This is one rep.
3. Perform the required number of reps and then swap arms.

Make sure that you are not leaning forwards or backwards when you perform this exercise. You are moving laterally only.

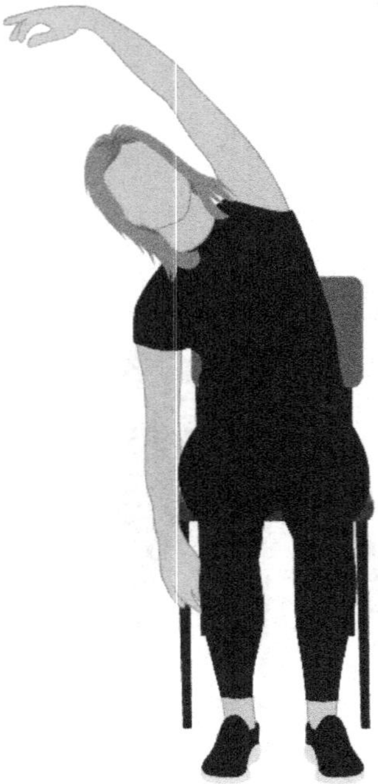

SCAN FOR VIDEO

Exercise #32 Bent Arm Seated Side Bends

This is very similar to the previous exercise, but instead of having your arm fully extended, you have your arm bent as if you are holding a phone or speaker to your ear.

How to Perform:

1. Sit on a sturdy chair with your feet flat on the floor. Place one hand by your side, and raise the other hand to your ear as if you are taking a call. Make sure that your elbow isn't forwards but out to the side.
2. Keeping that hand to your ear, lean to your opposite side (if your left arm is raised, lean to your right). Pause when you feel a stretch in your side, and then return to the starting position. This is one rep.
3. Perform the required number of reps and then swap arms.

Try this and the previous exercise and see which one you prefer, both have their benefits, and a good program will include each variation.

Exercise #33 Chair Planks

There are two things that you need to ensure before attempting this exercise. Firstly, you want a sturdy chair that isn't going to slide along the floor. Place it up against a wall if you have to. Secondly, you want to also ensure that your feet are not going to be sliding along the floor. Otherwise, you may end up falling and hurting yourself.

How to Perform:

1. Place your hands on either side of the seat of a chair, and place your toes on the ground so that your body is in a diagonal line from your shoulders to your heels.
2. Push your chest out and pull your shoulders back. Keep your head in a neutral position (don't raise it up in the air, or bring your chin down to your chest).
3. Once you are in position, squeeze your abdominal muscles (yet again, imagine you are about to get punched in the stomach and brace yourself).
4. Hold this position for the amount of time required, and then relax by bending your knees and getting out of the plank position.

Chair planks are a fantastic modification of the traditional plank, and they work well when rotated with exercise #27, the modified plank. Squeeze your glutes together while in this position for even better results.

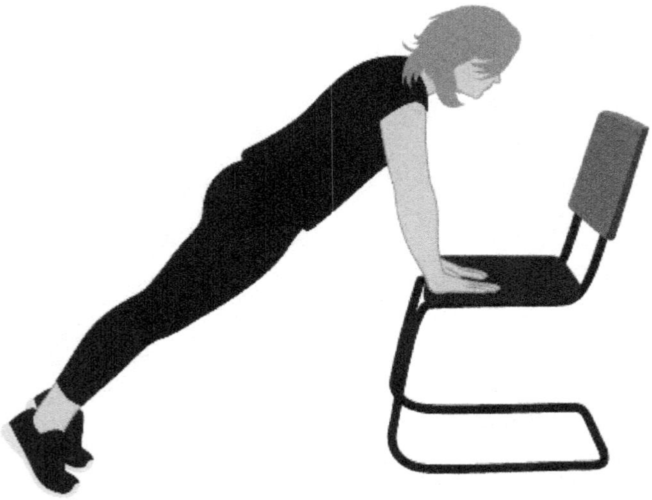

SCAN FOR VIDEO

Chair Plank (Modified)

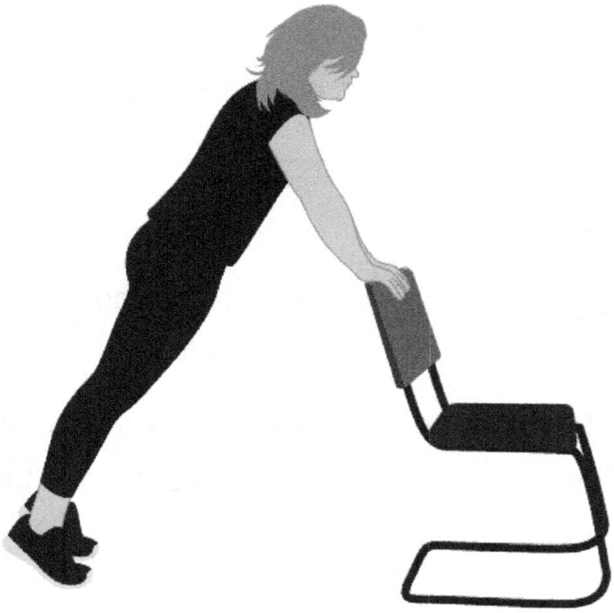

SCAN FOR VIDEO

Exercise #34 Seated Knee Lifts

This exercise sounds similar to exercises #29 and #30 which are leg extensions, but there are subtle differences. For this exercise, you are sitting on the edge of a chair and using your abs to raise both knees up into the air (keeping them bent). The leg extensions involve straightening your legs, which is easier, but also works the core in a different way.

How to Perform:

1. Grab a sturdy chair and sit on the edge of it, with your hands gripping the sides of the seat for support.
2. Brace your abs (yes, you know the drill. Imagine you are about to get punched in the stomach and you are tensing) and then raise both legs (knees bent) simultaneously as high as you can.
3. Pause, and then slowly lower both feet back to the ground.

The slower you lower your legs, the more your core will be worked. If it becomes too much, then place a small step for your feet to touch, which will reduce the range of motion, making the exercise easier.

If you don't have a strong grip, then you may find that this exercise is a little too hard, in which case you can switch to exercise #29. You can add ankle weights if you find the exercise too easy.

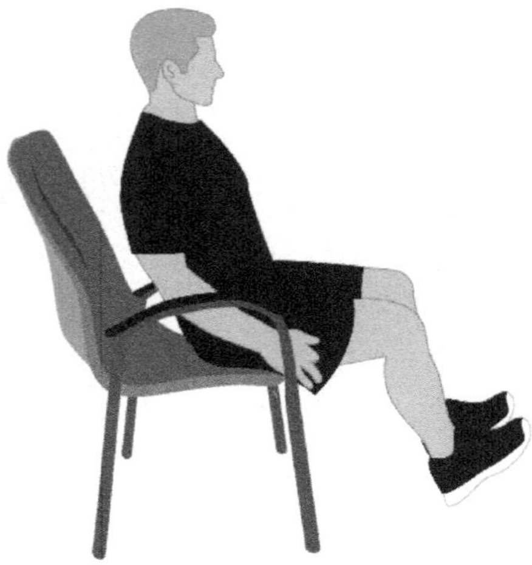

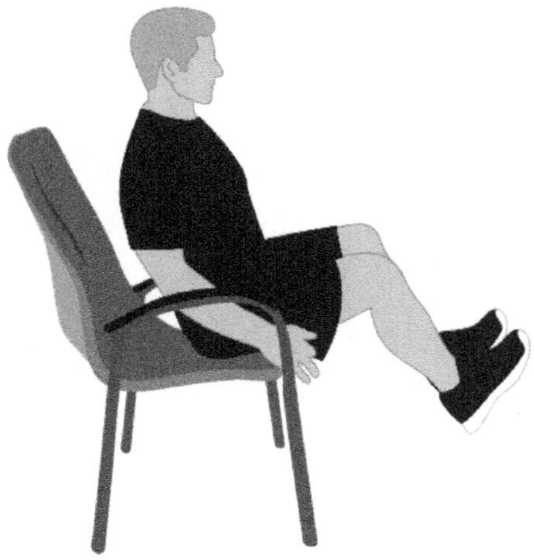

SCAN FOR VIDEO

Exercise #35 Marching in Place (Prone)

This exercise looks nothing like you would expect. You are not standing upright and marching in place. You are actually lying on your back and marching. This is a really good core exercise for people who have limited mobility.

How to Perform:

1. Lie on your back with your knees bent and your feet flat on the floor. Place your arms by your sides with your hands resting on the floor.
2. Keeping your leg bent, raise your right leg off the floor towards your chest.
3. Return your foot to the starting position, and then repeat with your left leg.

The trick with this exercise is for your lower back to stay flat on the floor. If it begins to rise, then stop moving your leg. There can be a little movement (the exercise would be impossible without it), but what you don't want is for your hips to be rising too far off the mat.

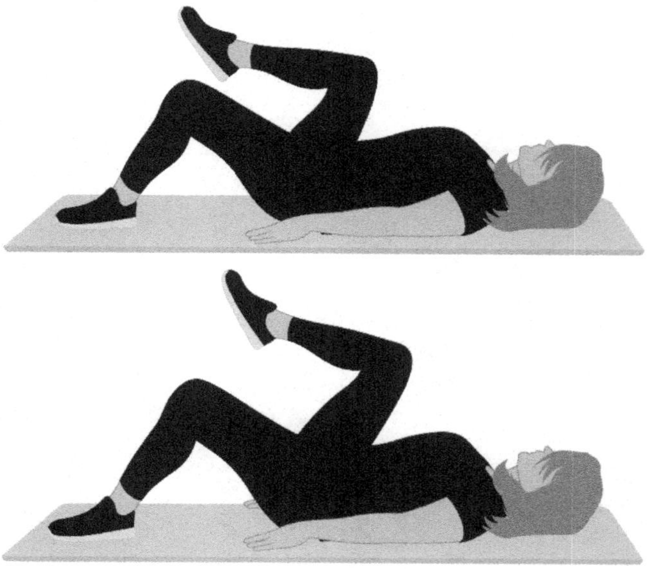

SCAN FOR VIDEO

Exercise #36 Marching in Place (Prone) with Leg Extension

This is a variation of the previous exercise (#36). Though the change is very small, the increase in difficulty is noticeable. That being said, it is still suitable for those with low mobility.

How to Perform:

1. Lie on your back with your knees bent and your feet flat on the floor. Place your arms by your sides with your hands resting on the floor.
2. Keeping your leg bent, raise your right leg off the floor towards your chest.
3. Pause, and then straighten your leg, pushing your heel upwards. It will now be at approximately a 45 degree angle.
4. Lower the leg to just above the floor and pause.
5. Bend your knee back, and then return your foot to the starting position.
6. Repeat with your left leg.

While you don't *need* an exercise mat for this exercise, it might be a good idea as it will keep you comfortable while performing it.

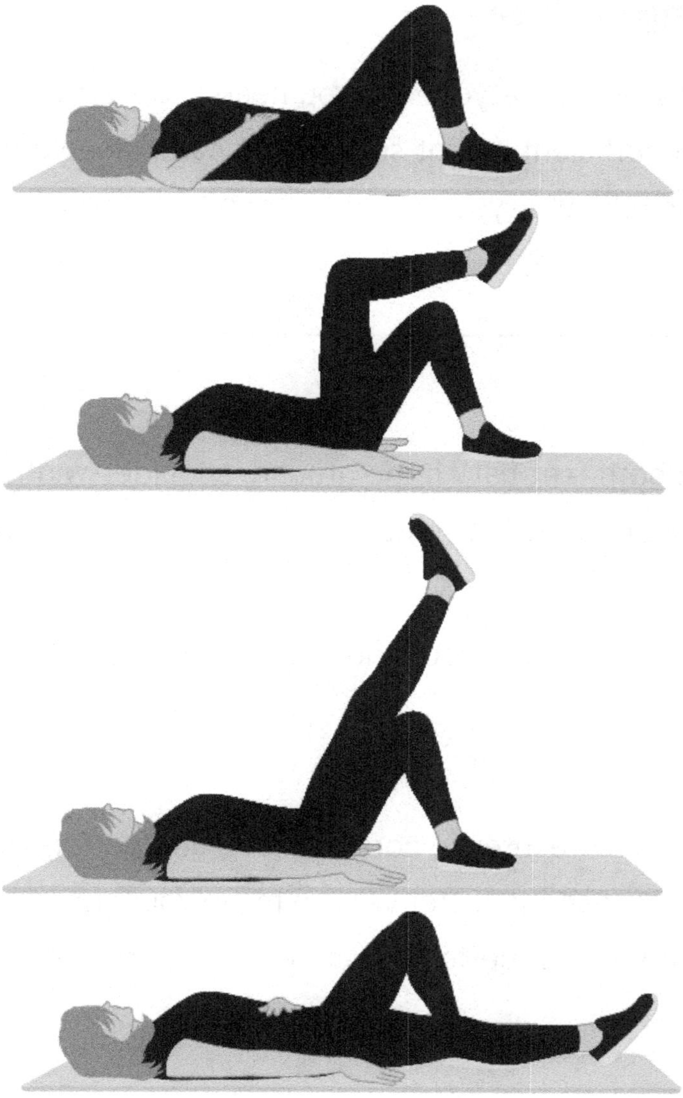

SCAN FOR VIDEO

Exercise #37 Seated Marching in Place

This is a fun exercise that is accessible to everyone. All you need is a sturdy chair. You also want to ensure that the chair is of sufficient height so that you can place your feet flat on the floor. If you want to increase the difficulty, you can add a set of ankle weights to increase resistance.

How to Perform:

1. Sit on the edge of a chair with both feet flat on the ground, shoulder-width apart. Push your chest out and pull your shoulders back to create a nice, straight back. Grip the edge of the seat with both hands.
2. Raise one of your feet up off the floor until your knee as high as possible, then lower it back down.
3. Repeat with the opposite foot.

Perform this exercise slowly for a more intense core workout, and perform it faster for a more cardio-based workout. If you choose the faster version move your arms back and forth as if marching outdoors. Of course you can perform it somewhere in between for a mix of cardio and core.

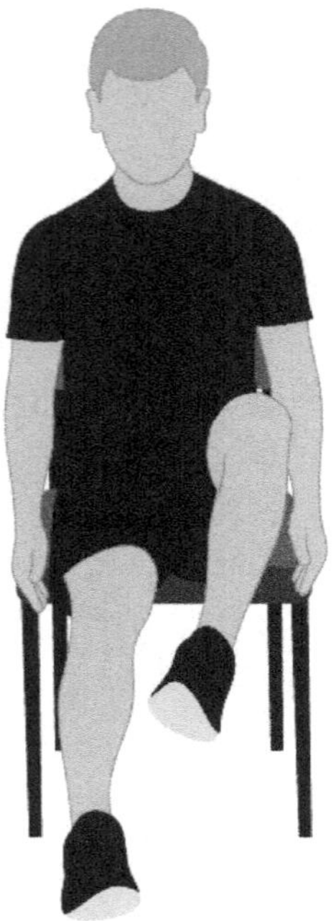

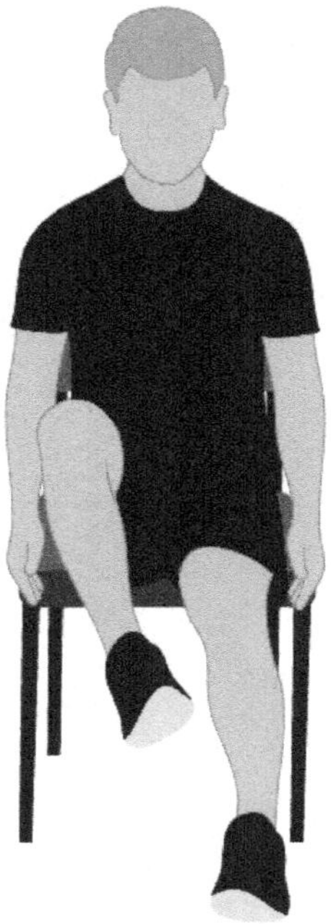

SCAN FOR VIDEO

Seated Marching in Place (Modified)

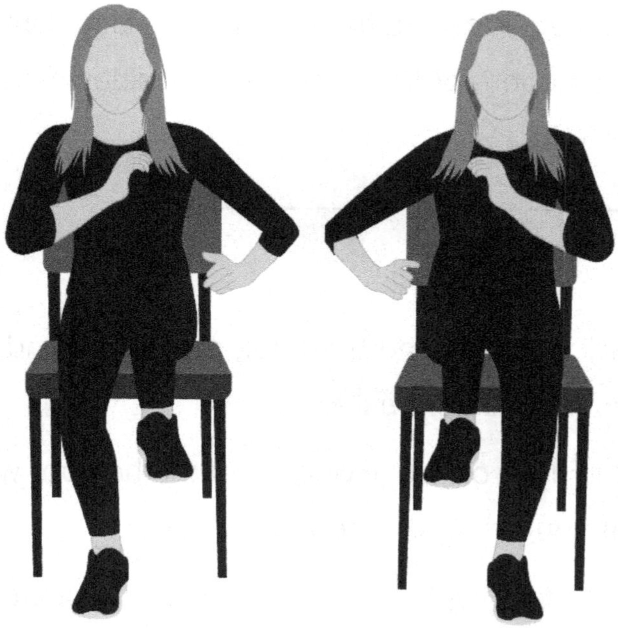

SCAN FOR VIDEO

Exercise #38 Seated Forward Bends

This exercise is similar to exercise #28 (seated forward roll-ups), but there are a couple of differences that you will notice once you have performed them both. This is a more dynamic movement, while the roll-ups are slower and contract the abdominal muscles more. A good program will have both of these exercises in it.

How to Perform:

1. Sit on a chair with your feet wide apart and touching the floor, rest your hands on your knees, push your chest out and pull your shoulders back.
2. Bend forward and bring your arms out in front of you, trying to touch the floor with them. Pause when you can go no lower (or if you manage to touch the floor).
3. Hold this position for five seconds, and then rise back up to the starting position.

Try not to pulse up and down when performing this exercise. This is often done subconsciously when trying to reach lower down than your body will allow. Just go as low as you can naturally. Don't try to force it.

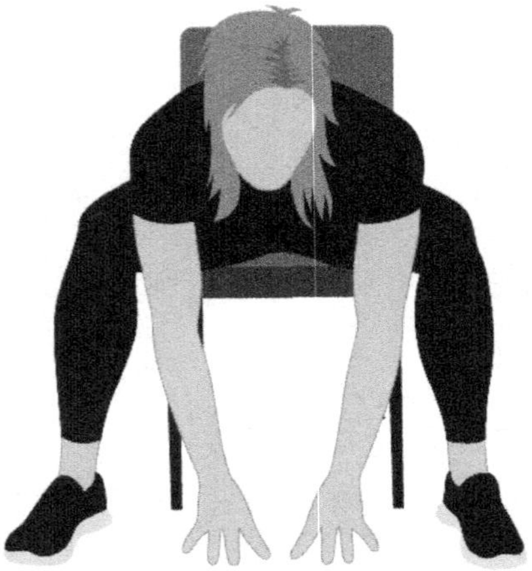

SCAN FOR VIDEO

CHAPTER 9

Intermediate Core Exercises

SCAN FOR AUDIO CHAPTER

In this chapter, we will be looking exclusively at core exercises that are suitable for intermediates. Remember, if any of the exercises feel too difficult, then just swap them for a beginner core exercise. If all of the exercises feel too difficult, then drop down to beginner and build a strong core to progress to this level.

Exercise #39 Plank (Push-Up Position)

The plank is perhaps the greatest core exercise you can perform, but it is also very difficult to master. Luckily, as the previous chapter showed us, there are many variations that you can use to progress towards a full plank. The push-up plank is the final progression before the full plank.

Despite the name, it does not involve any actual push-ups. You just perform a plank while in the traditional push-up position.

How to Perform:

1. Place your hands on the floor, shoulder-width apart
2. Place your feet on the floor, and raise your hips up until there is a straight line from your shoulders down to your heels.
3. Squeeze your abs tight, and squeeze your glutes
4. Hold this position for 30 seconds and then relax

Once you have mastered the push-up position plank, you can progress to the regular plank, which is an advanced exercise in this book. You can also combine the two movements to perform plank get-ups, a really effective core and cardiovascular exercise.

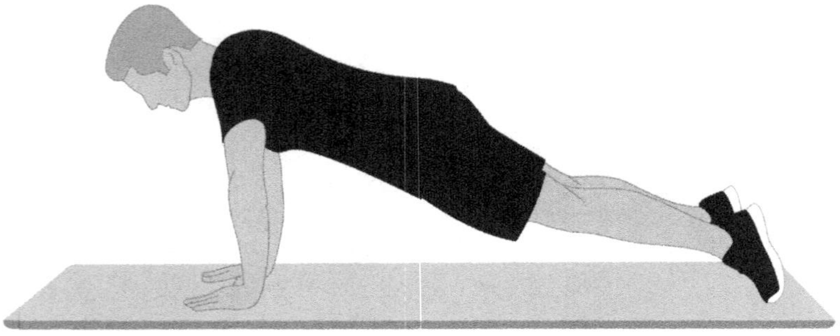

SCAN FOR VIDEO

Exercise #40 Heel Tap Exercise

This is an excellent abdominal exercise that is very intuitive. The only challenge is getting your feet in the right place to start. Once you have mastered this, you will find this exercise provides you with a top-quality core workout. Just make sure that you have an exercise mat or a comfortable bit of floor to lie on!

How to Perform:

1. Lie on your back with your arms raised straight above you. Bring your knees up in a right angle, as if you were resting your heels on an invisible chair.
2. Keeping the rest of your body still, lower your left heel down to the ground.
3. Pause, and then raise your left leg back up.
4. Repeat with your right heel to complete the rep.

For best results, you want to brace your abs. This means clenching as if someone was about to punch you in the stomach. It's a weird description, but from my experience by far the best way to teach someone how to brace their abs correctly.

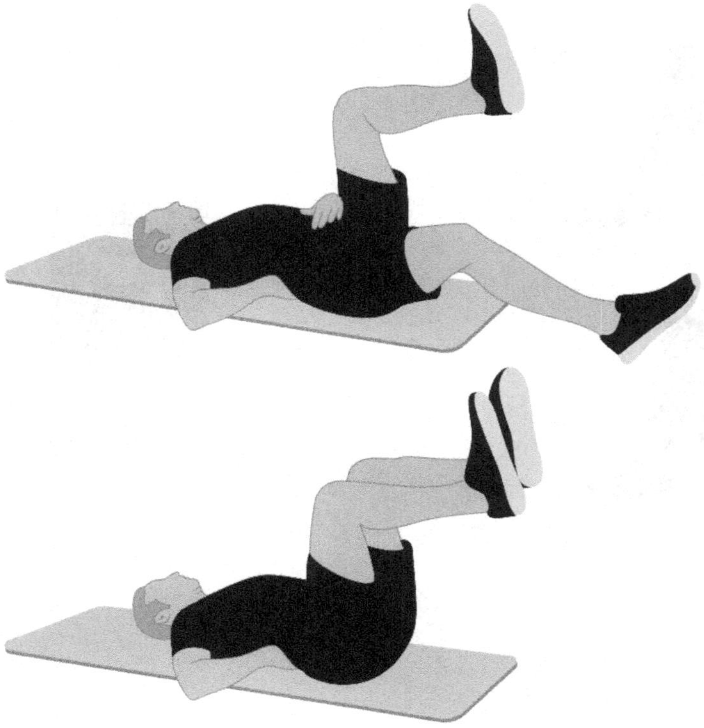

SCAN FOR VIDEO

Exercise #41 Abdominal Crunches

An absolute classic core exercise, the abdominal crunch is well-known, even in non-fitness circles, but it is also one of the most common

How to Perform:

1. Lie on your back with your feet flat on the ground and your knees bent. Place your hands lightly behind your ears with your elbows wide.
2. Brace your abs and then slowly curl your shoulders and upper torso off the floor.
3. Pause when you can curl no further, and then pause.
4. Slowly lower yourself back down to the starting position.

You really don't want to be dropping down after you've curled upwards. The slower that you travel down, the more your abdominal muscles will be worked. If you are struggling, then don't slow things down too much or you won't be able to perform more than a couple of reps.

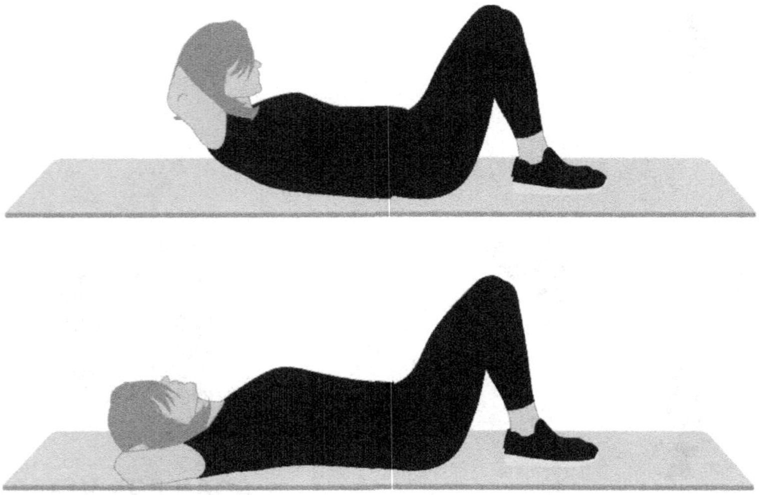

SCAN FOR VIDEO

Exercise #42 Foot-Raised Abdominal Crunches

This exercise is almost identical to the abdominal crunches (exercise #41) we looked at before. The only difference is that instead of having your feet flat on the ground, you have them raised up (similar to exercise #40). If you struggle to keep your feet up like this, then you can rest them on a chair, bench, or exercise box. However, it may make more sense just to perform abdominal crunches instead.

How to Perform:

1. Lie on your back with your feet flat on the ground and your knees bent. Place your hands lightly behind your ears with your elbows wide.
2. Bring your knees up at a right angle, as if you were resting your heels on an invisible chair.
3. Brace your abs and then slowly curl your shoulders and upper torso off the floor.
4. Briefly pause when you can curl no further.
5. Slowly lower yourself back down to the starting position.

Once you have mastered this exercise, you can learn many variations (which are in the advanced section). This will massively increase the variety of exercises that are available to you.

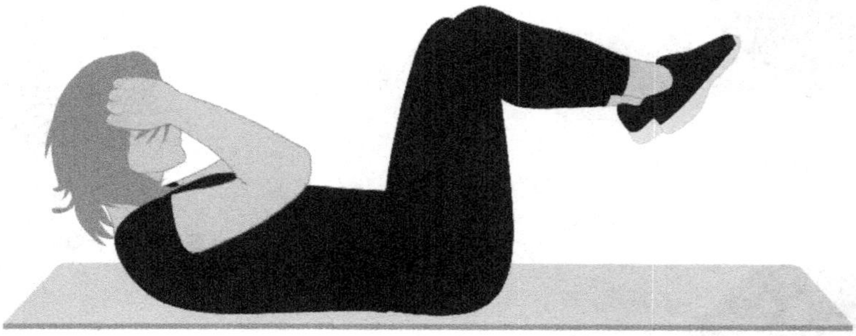

SCAN FOR VIDEO

Exercise #43 Long-Arm Crunches

The long-arm crunch is very similar to the abdominal crunch, but with your arms extended as if you were about to perform backstroke. Doing this changes the point of resistance, making the exercise more challenging to perform. Long-arm crunches are one of the best core exercises out there.

How to Perform:

1. Lie on your back with your feet flat on the ground and your knees bent. Place your arms above your head as if you are performing the backstroke in a swimming pool.
2. Brace your abs and then slowly curl your straightened arms and upper torso off the floor.
3. When you can curl no further pause briefly.
4. Slowly lower yourself back down to the starting position.

If you ever start to find this exercise easy, you can hold a weight or small exercise ball in your hands, which will really increase the resistance.

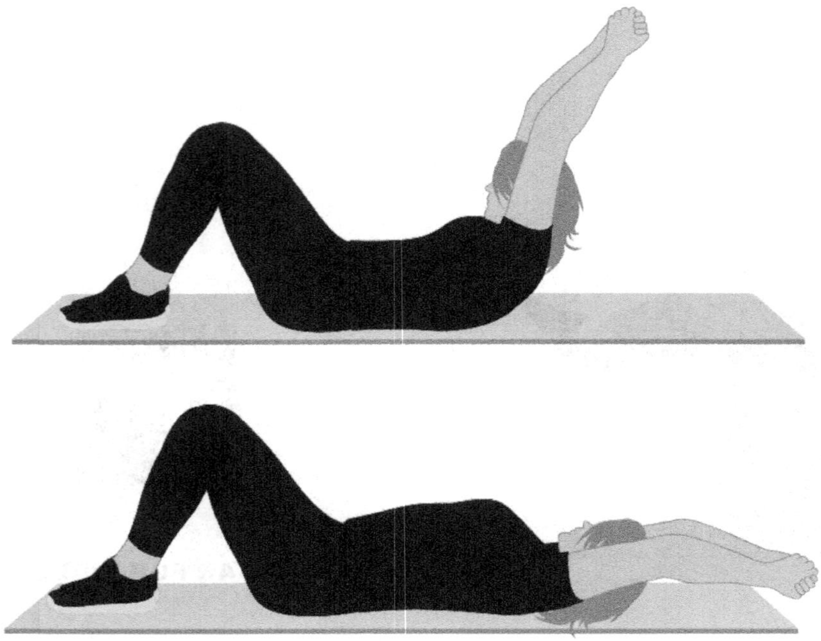

SCAN FOR VIDEO

Exercise #44 Single-Long-Arm Crunches

This exercise is identical to the previous exercise, but instead of having both arms in the air, you only have one. This means that you are slightly unbalanced, which brings your obliques into play.

How to Perform:

1. Lie on your back with your feet flat on the ground and your knees bent. Place one above your head and leave the other by your side as if you are performing the backstroke in a swimming pool.
2. Brace your abs and then slowly curl your straightened arm and upper torso off the floor.
3. Pause when you can curl no further, and hold that position briefly.
4. Slowly lower yourself back down to the starting position.
5. Once you have performed the required number of reps, you can swap arms.

While the name may be a bit of a mouthful, it really is a great core exercise. One thing to pay attention to is that you don't lean over too much to one side while performing each rep. A little bit of a lean is okay, but you'll know when you're going too far.

Exercise #45 Arm Over Crunches

This is a really enjoyable core exercise (at least I think so) that is similar to both the long-arm crunch and the abdominal crunch. The movement of the arms changes the resistance point as you crunch.

How to Perform:

1. Lie on your back with your feet flat on the ground and your knees bent. Place your arms above your head as if you are performing the backstroke in a swimming pool.
2. Brace your abs and then slowly curl your straightened arms and upper torso off the floor.
3. As you crunch up bring your arms over in an arc.
4. Pause when you can curl no further, with your arms resting near your feet.
5. Slowly lower yourself back down to the starting position bringing your arms back as you do.

As with the long-arm crunch, you can make this exercise harder by holding small weights in your hand. It also works with an exercise ball, but be careful as you bring the ball over your knees.

Exercise #46 Knee-to-Chest Crunches

This exercise is performed in a similar manner to abdominal crunches but reversed. Instead of bringing your upper chest up towards your knees, you are bringing your knees toward your chest. This is an easier exercise than the abdominal crunch, and therefore you can perform more reps.

How to Perform:

1. Lie on your back with your knees bent and your feet flat on the ground. Place your arms on either side of your body, flat on the ground.
2. Brace your abs (imagine you are about to get punched in the stomach).
3. Raise your feet off the ground, keep your knees bent, and bring them towards your chest.
4. Pause before your lower back rises off the ground, and then slowly lower your feet back down to the starting position.

This is a safe and easy-to-learn exercise that really works the lower abdominal muscles. You can increase the difficulty by really slowing down the lowering of your feet back to the ground.

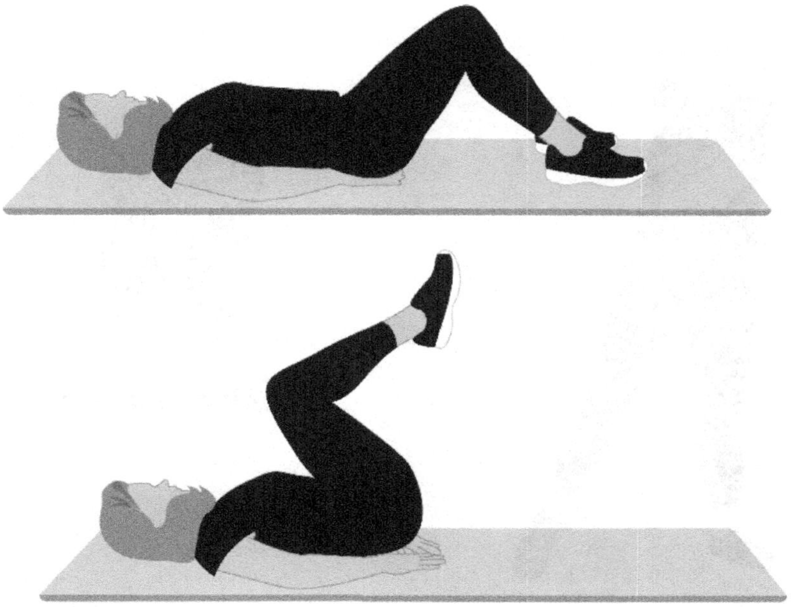

SCAN FOR VIDEO

Exercise #47 Wood Chops

The wood chop exercise is often performed with a dumbbell, resistance band, or cable station, but the bodyweight version is also highly effective. Once you have mastered the bodyweight wood chop you can increase the difficulty by adding some form of resistance (for example, holding a hand weight or dumbbell).

How to Perform:

1. Stand upright with feet shoulder-width apart
2. Hold your hands together, resting beside your left hip
3. Swing your arms across your body and upwards as if you were swinging an axe
4. Pause when your arms are raised above your right shoulder
5. Swing back to the starting position

The most common mistake with wood chops is to perform them too quickly, a nice steady rhythm will provide greater stimulation of the core muscles. It's also safer.

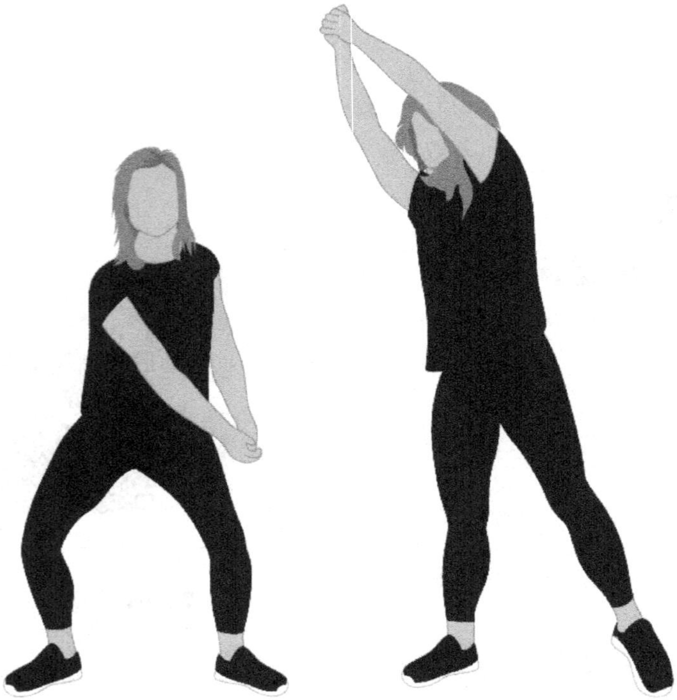

SCAN FOR VIDEO

Exercise #48 Seated Wood Chops

The seated wood chop is an easier version and one that is more suitable for people with mobility issues. However, it is still a formidable core exercise in its own right and should not be underestimated.

How to Perform:

1. Sit on a sturdy chair or box with your feet shoulder-width apart
2. Hold your hands together, resting beside your left hip
3. Swing your arms across your body and upwards as if you were swinging an axe
4. Pause when your arms are raised above your right shoulder
5. Swing back to the starting position

You can increase the difficulty of this exercise by holding a weight in both hands. A dumbbell works well, but you can use any form of weight to create some resistance and work the abs and obliques harder.

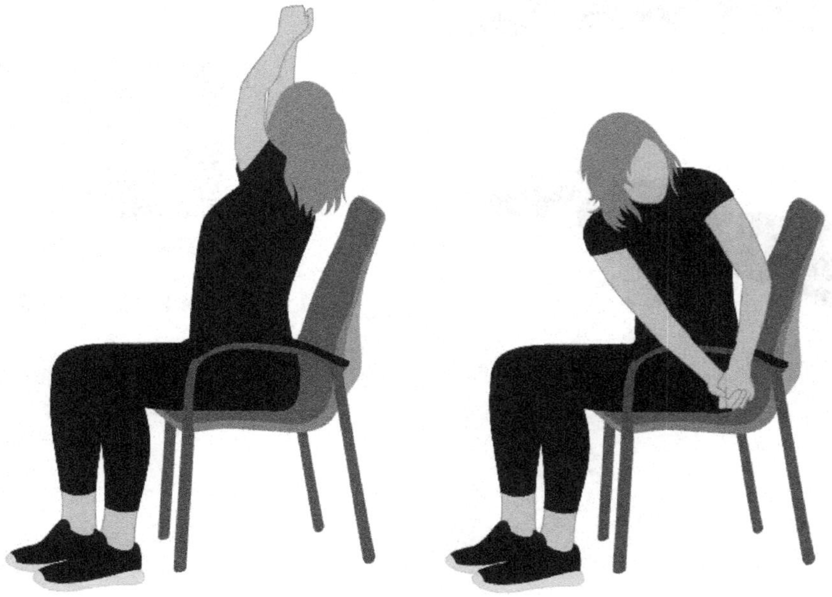

SCAN FOR VIDEO

Exercise #49 Superman

As you know, the core muscles include the muscles of the lower back and spine. But most core exercises focus on the abdominals. The Superman exercise is a fantastic bodyweight exercise that works the lower back while also working the abdominals (though not as much).

How to Perform:

1. Lie on your front with arms and legs straight
2. Raise your legs and arms up in the air, keeping them straight throughout. Your chest should also rise off the floor
3. Hold for a second or two, then lower your arms, chest, and legs back down

While this is not a glute exercise, you should pay attention to them while performing it. Squeeze them together, and the exercise will flow much more smoothly.

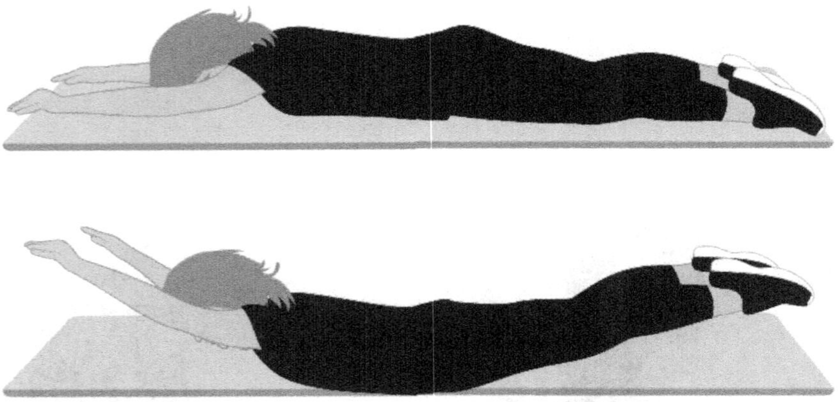

SCAN FOR VIDEO

Exercise #50 Mountain Climbers on Chair

Mountain climbers are one of the best cardio/core exercises out there, but they require a decent level of mobility to perform safely. Using a chair can make it a lot easier to perform them while still delivering superb results.

How to Perform:

1. Use a sturdy chair and place your hands on the seat (or to make it a little easier the chair back) so that you are facing the chair.
2. Push your chest out and pull your shoulders back so that you have a nice and straight posture.
3. Keep your torso still and bring one knee towards your chest.
4. Bring it back to the starting position, while doing so bring your opposite knee towards your chest.
5. Return the knee to starting position while simultaneously bringing the original knee forwards again.

Mountain climbers can be performed at fast and slow speeds. The slower you do them, the more emphasis is placed on core strength. The faster you perform them, the more emphasis is placed on cardio.

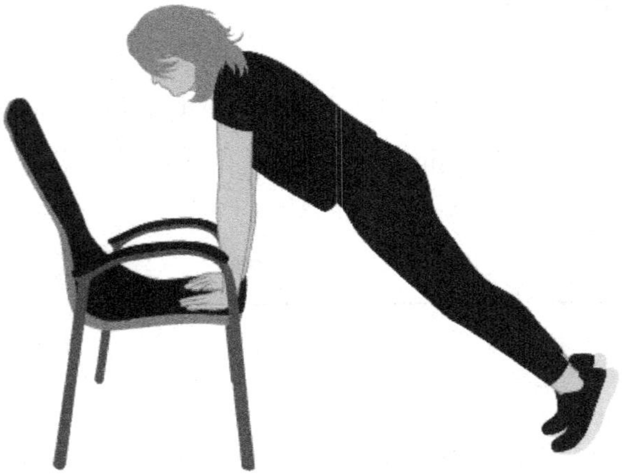

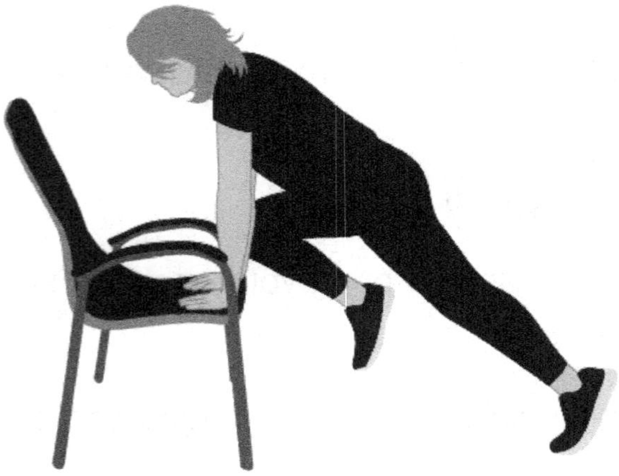

SCAN FOR VIDEO

Exercise #51 Dead Bugs

The dead bug exercise is a lot of fun and is ideally suited to someone with good but not great mobility. This exercise works all of the muscles in the core and is both safe and effective. It may take a few tries to coordinate the movement sequence.

How to Perform:

1. Lie on your back with your arms straight up in the air
2. Raise your feet up in the air with knees bent at a 90-degree angle
3. Lower your left arm to the floor (above your head)
4. At the same time, lower your right leg and straighten it
5. Stop both before they touch the ground and return them to the starting position
6. Switch arms and legs and repeat

This exercise is best performed slowly, even if you are tempted to rush things! Slow and smooth provide you with the best results.

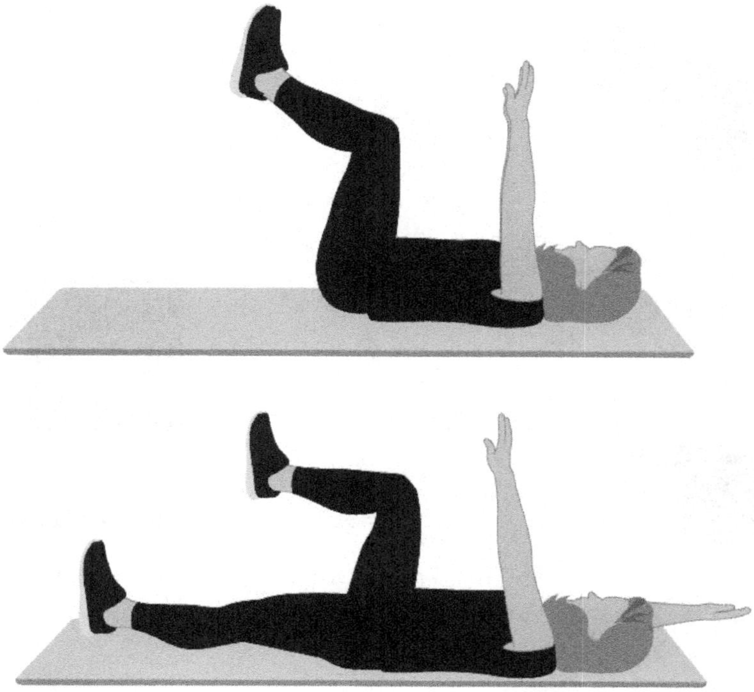

SCAN FOR VIDEO

Exercise #52 Bird Dog Exercise

The bird dog exercise is interesting because it is almost the reverse of the dead bug exercise (see exercise #51 above). Instead of lying on your back, you are on your knees, but the basic movement patterns are similar.

How to Perform:

1. Kneel on the floor and place your hands flat on the ground in front of you
2. Raise your right hand off the ground and extend it out in front of you
3. At the same time, raise your left leg off the floor and push it back behind you
4. Pause when both your arm and your leg are fully extended in the air
5. Now pull your arm and leg back in until your elbow touches your knee, then extend both again
6. Repeat for the correct number of reps and then swap to the opposite arm and leg

While this exercise is not difficult, it does require coordination, so take it slowly and focus on following the instructions.

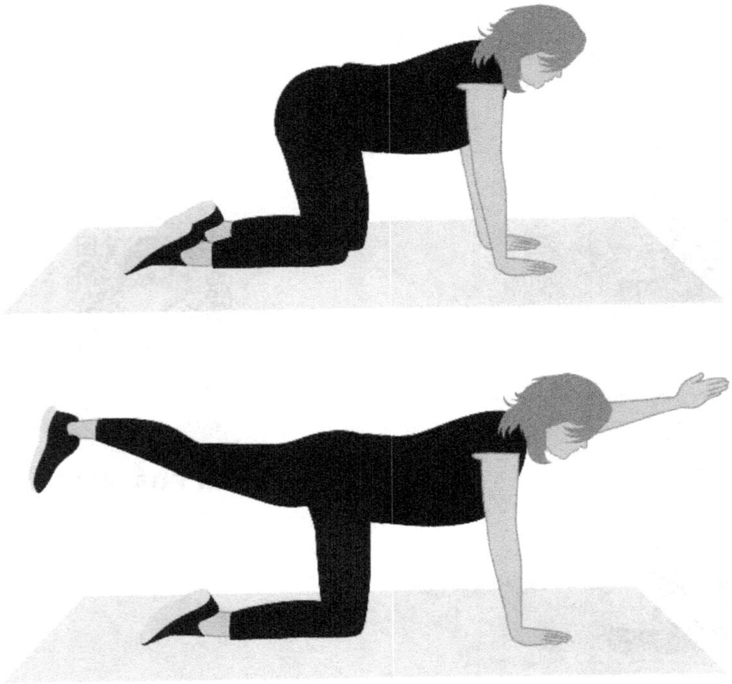

SCAN FOR VIDEO

Exercise #53 Seated Bicycle

The seated bicycle is an adaptation of the regular bicycle crunch that is performed while lying on your back. The seated bicycle is more accessible and more suitable to those with intermediate mobility. It's also a great exercise in its own right and should not be underestimated.

How to Perform:

1. Sit on the edge of a sturdy chair with your hands on your head and your elbows out wide. Have both feet shoulder-width apart.
2. Twisting your torso, bring your left elbow towards the centre of your body while simultaneously bringing your right knee up until both are touching.
3. Twist backwards and lower your right knee back down to the starting position.
4. Repeat with your opposite arm and leg.

This exercise is excellent when performed slowly. However, as you get stronger and more confident, you can increase the speed so that as you are bringing one foot down, your other foot is rising, twisting your torso faster to keep up. Only increase the speed when you have mastered the regular exercise, though.

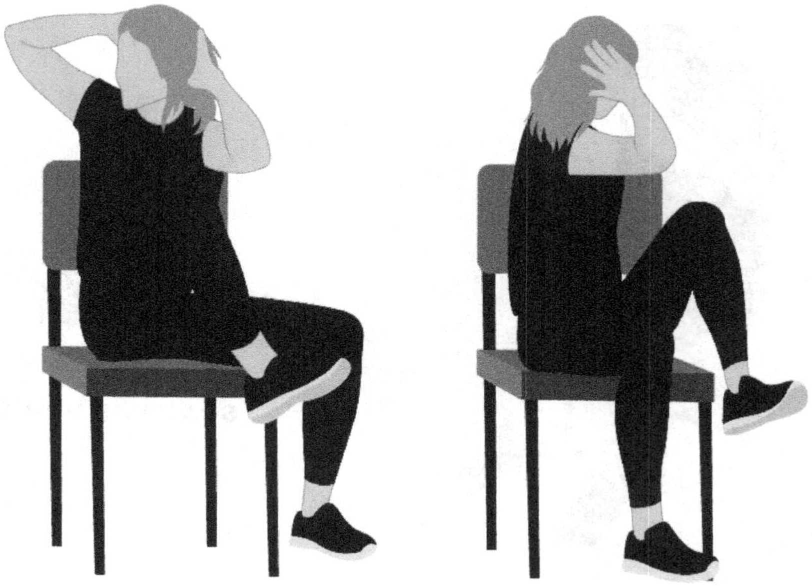

SCAN FOR VIDEO

Exercise #54 Seated Russian Twists (Chair)

This exercise sounds very easy on paper, but when you are performing it you will really feel it in your abs. The trick is to find a chair that allows you to lean back slightly. This is one exercise that you may find easier to perform on a bench or a plyometric box.

How to Perform:

1. Sit on the edge of a chair or box and clasp your hands together.
2. Lean back slightly with your feet flat on the floor. You should feel this in your abs already.
3. Pretend that you are grabbing a small box from your right-hand side and placing it on your left-hand side. Twist your torso as you do so, but ensure that you stay in a leaned-back position.
4. Repeat from left to right, right to left, and left to right for the required number of reps.

The progression for this exercise is to perform Russian twists on a mat, which is a lot more challenging and allows you to twist your torso significantly more. You can also hold a dumbbell to increase the difficulty further.

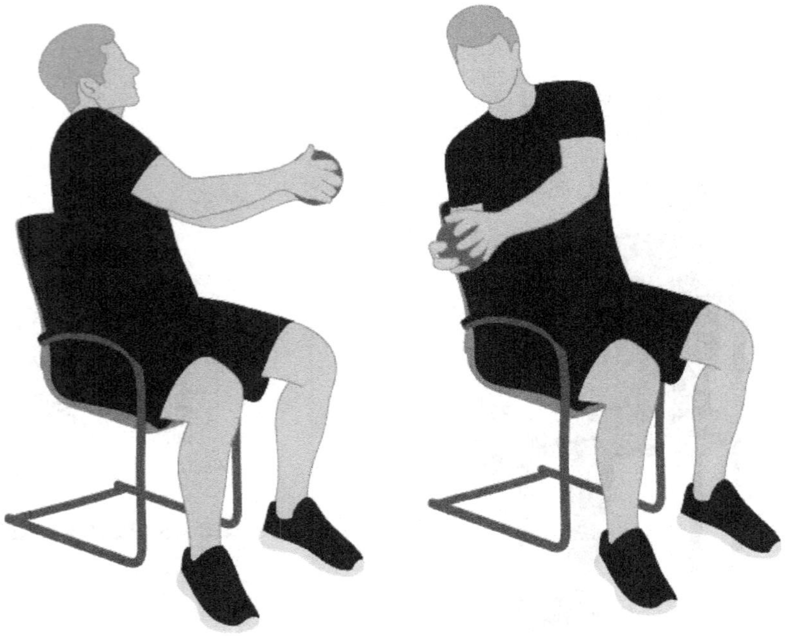

SCAN FOR VIDEO

CHAPTER 10

Advanced Core Exercises

SCAN FOR AUDIO CHAPTER

In this chapter, we will be taking a look at core exercises that are suitable for people with high mobility and high fitness levels. If you find that one or two of the exercises are too difficult, then just replace them with exercises from chapter nine.

However, if you are finding that the majority of exercises are too difficult, then you may not quite be ready for these exercises yet. Train hard using beginner or intermediate exercises, and you will soon be ready for chapter ten.

Exercise #55 Plank

This is the best core exercise around, and it is a real accomplishment if you can manage to perform this with good form. Focus on keeping your hips level, and if your forearms begin to hurt, you can change into the push-up plank position.

How to Perform:

1. Lie face down on the floor with your legs fully extended and your forearms supporting you. You want your forearms to be shoulder-width apart.
2. Raise your body off the floor and use your forearms to support you. Ensure that your hips are flat, not too high or too low.
3. Squeeze your glutes, hamstrings, and quadriceps, and brace your abdominals simultaneously.
4. Hold this position for the designated time (30 seconds, for example).

One mistake that is often made is trying to hold a plank for too long. What usually happens is that after a while, your form begins to wilt, and the contractions of your muscles become weaker. That is why performing the plank for shorter periods of time can actually yield greater results. Quality over quantity (or in this case time).

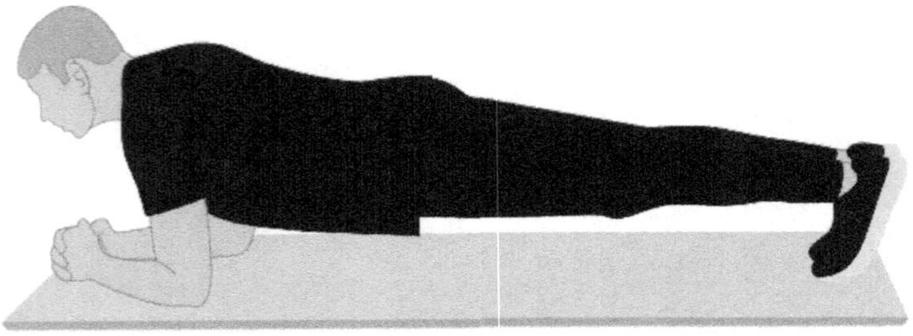

Exercise #56 Russian Twists

Russian twists are a great exercise for the obliques as well as the transverse abdominal muscles. We have already looked at a seated version of the Russian twist, which is substantially easier. Now we're looking at the original.

How to Perform:

1. Lie on your back with your feet flat (or heels) on the floor and your knees bent. Clasp both of your hands together and tuck your elbows into your sides.
2. Crunch up so that your head, shoulders, and chest are off the floor and hold this position.
3. With your hands clasped, bring your arms over to your right side, twisting your torso to do so.
4. Once you have turned as far as you can, pause and then rotate over to the other side. This is one rep.

While the twisting is difficult, the real challenge is maintaining your crunched position while performing the twists. For this reason, Russian twists are one of the few core exercises that can be performed quite fast.

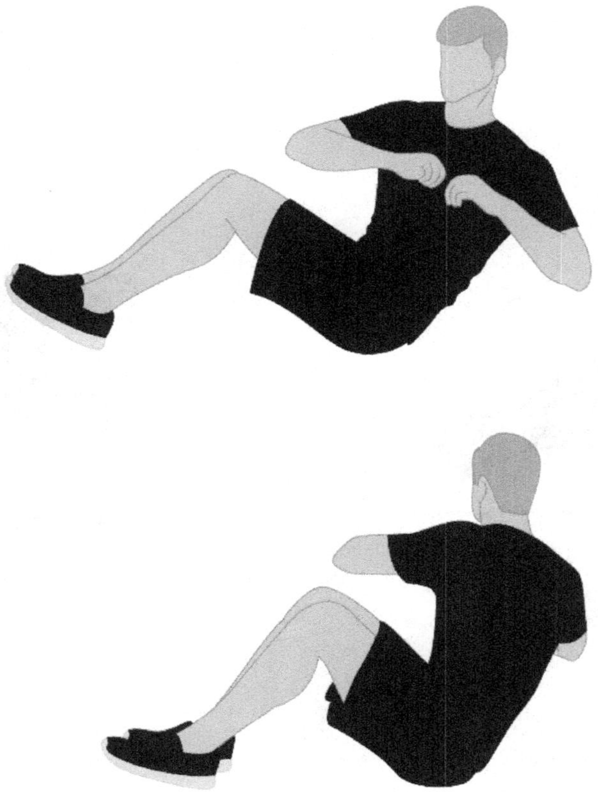

SCAN FOR VIDEO

Exercise #57 Forearm Side Plank

The forearm side plank is a very difficult exercise to master but well worth putting the effort in. If you struggle with it, try the standard side plank (exercise #58) instead.

How to Perform:

1. Lie on your right side with your legs straight and one foot resting on the other
2. Rest your right forearm on the ground straight out in front of you
3. Raise your right hip off the floor, resting your left hand on your left hip
4. Pause when your body is in a nice straight line
5. Hold for 30 seconds, then relax, swap sides and repeat

What you really want to focus on during this exercise is keeping your hips raised so that they don't droop. This is very common. If you cannot initially hold the plank for 30 seconds, hold only until you can no longer maintain your good posture.

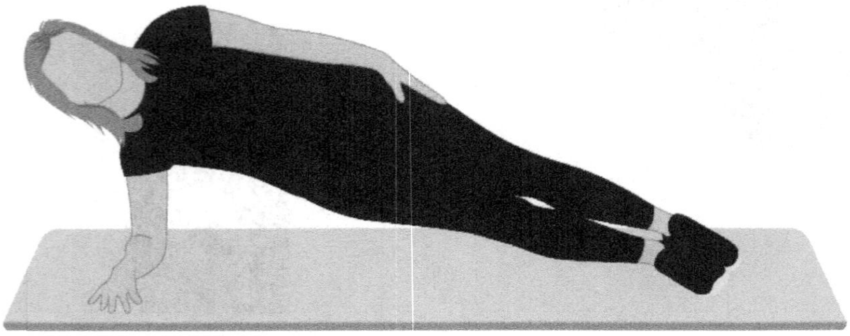

SCAN FOR VIDEO

Exercise #58 Standard Side Plank

This exercise is identical to the forearm side plank, except that instead of resting on your forearm, you rest on your hand. This means that your arm has to be straight rather than bent at the elbow. The exercise is more comfortable for some people but not necessarily easier. Therefore, it's a matter of personal preference which variation you perform.

How to Perform:

1. Lie on your right side with your legs straight and one foot resting on the other
2. Rest your right hand on the ground with your right arm straight.
3. Raise your right hip off the floor, resting your left hand on your left hip (or extend the arm straight up so your fingers are pointing towards the ceiling)
4. Pause when your body is in a nice straight line
5. Hold for 30 seconds, then relax, swap sides and repeat

If your wrists start to hurt while performing a standard side plank, then you may want to try to switch exercises to the forearm side plank. Alternatively, you can just perform a regular plank.

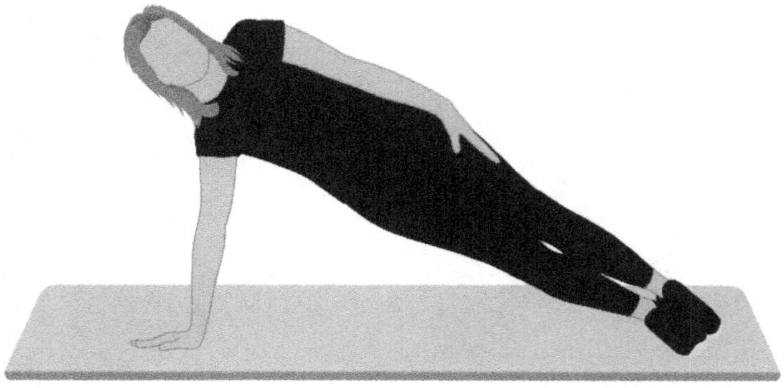

SCAN FOR VIDEO

Standard Side Plank (Modified)

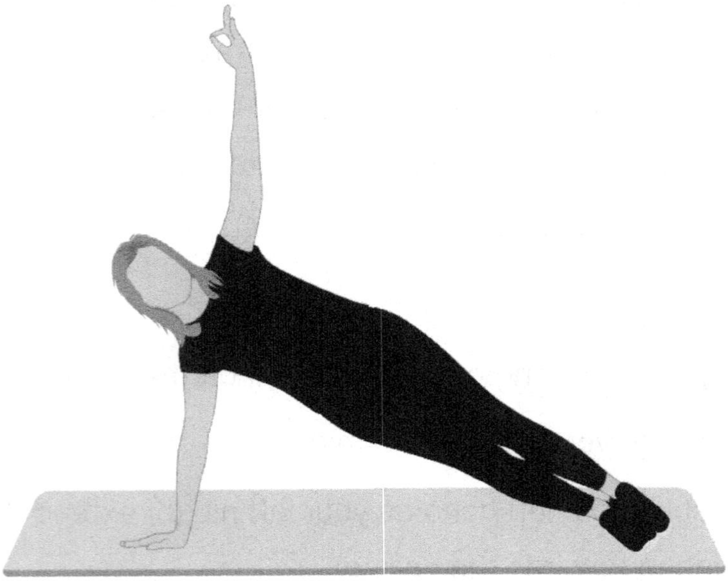

SCAN FOR VIDEO

Exercise #59 Feet Elevated Plank

This is an interesting plank variation and one that is quite a bit more challenging than a regular plank. To perform it, you will need something to elevate your feet on. A chair may be too high, so a bench or a step would be a better option.

How to Perform:

1. Lie face down on the floor with your legs fully extended and raised up on a step or bench. Your forearms should be on the floor, supporting you. You want your forearms to be shoulder-width apart.
2. Raise your body off the floor and use your forearms to support you. Ensure that your hips are flat, not too high or too low.
3. Squeeze your glutes, hamstrings, and quadriceps, and brace your abdominals simultaneously.
4. Hold this position for the designated time (30 seconds, for example).

As with all plank exercises, you want to ensure that your hips aren't sagging while performing the feet-elevated plank. However, it is even more important when your feet are elevated, so pay close attention.

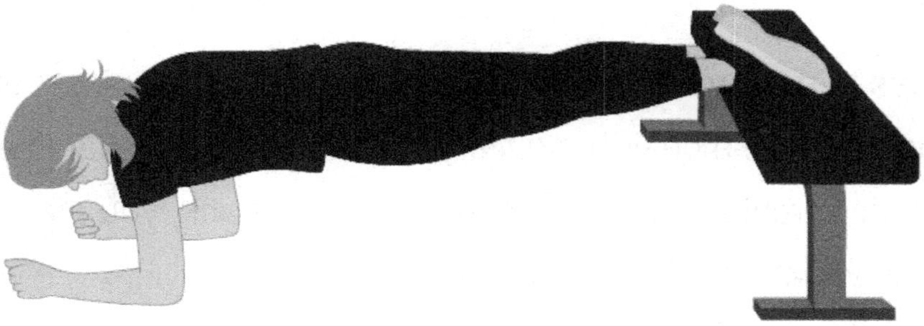

SCAN FOR VIDEO

Exercise #60 Mountain Climbers (Fast)

We have already looked at a chair-supported version of the mountain climber, and this variation is almost identical, except that instead of resting your arms and upper body on a chair, you rest your arms on the ground.

That does not mean that the exercise is more challenging, though! It just requires more mobility. Interestingly, you may find that you get a more intense workout from the chair-based version.

How to Perform:

1. Place your hands on the floor and get into the same position that a sprinter would before a 100-metre race. On tiptoes with one foot in front of the other and hands touching the ground.
2. Push your chest out and pull your shoulders back so that you have a nice and straight posture.
3. Keep your torso still and bring one knee towards your chest.
4. Bring it back to the starting position. While doing so bring your opposite knee towards your chest.
5. Return the knee to starting position while simultaneously bringing the original knee forwards again.
6. Perform this at a fast pace

There aren't any real advantages to performing mountain climbers on the floor instead of on a chair. Unless you don't happen to have a chair handy, if you're in a park for example, in which case the versatility is a benefit. Provided you can keep a straight back, you may see some more core activation with this variation.

If you are struggling to maintain your posture, though, just swap this exercise for the chair-based version, and you will still get a great workout.

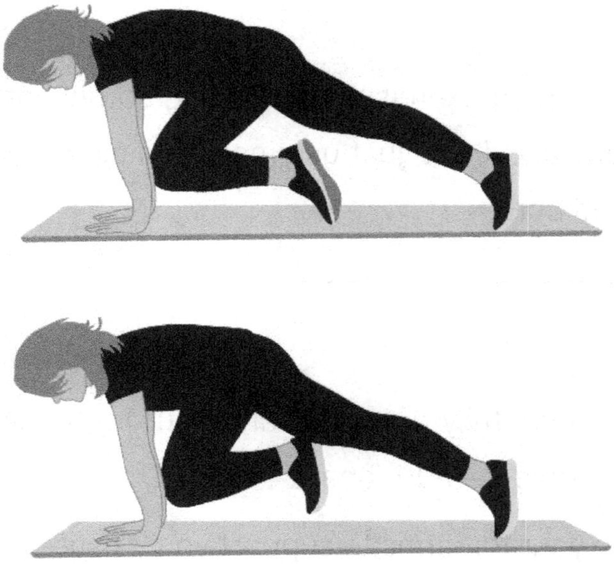

SCAN FOR VIDEO

Exercise #61 Plank Get-Ups

Plank get-ups are one of the most challenging exercises on this list, so only attempt them if you feel that you are able to do so sensibly. If not, just use mountain climbers instead, as they provide a similar blend of cardio and core.

How to Perform:

1. Lie face down on the floor with your legs fully extended and your forearms supporting you. You want your forearms to be shoulder-width apart.
2. Raise your body off the floor and use your forearms to support you. Ensure that your hips are flat, not too high or too low.
3. Squeeze your glutes, hamstrings, and quadriceps, and brace your abdominals simultaneously.
4. Raise your right forearm off the floor and place your right hand flat on the floor with your arm straight.
5. Raise your left forearm off the floor and place your left hand flat on the floor with your arm straight.
6. Lower your right forearm to the floor and then lower your left forearm to the floor until you are back to the starting position. This is one rep.

Plank get-ups are a fantastic core exercise and are perfect for anyone who finds regular planks a little dull. Start off slowly, but as you gain competence and confidence, you can speed them up and turn it into a cardio/core exercise.

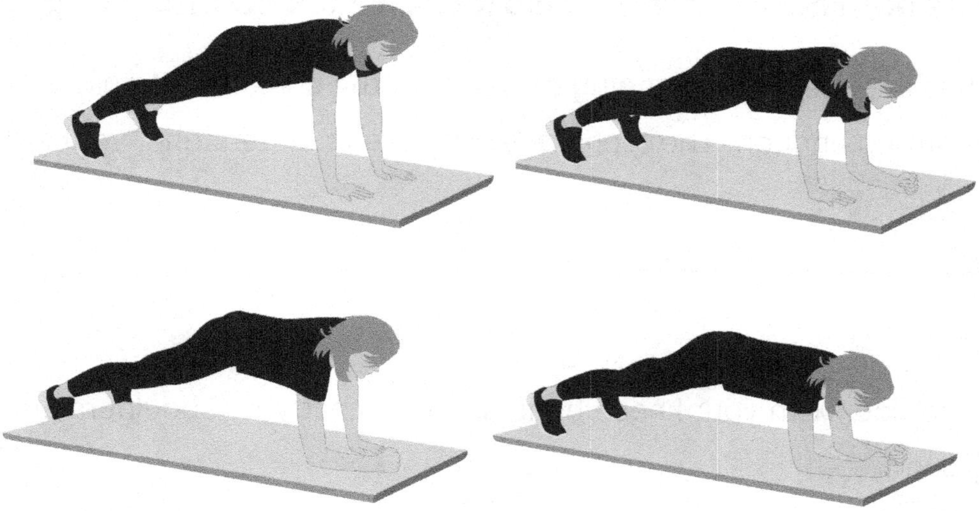

SCAN FOR VIDEO

Exercise #62 Negative Abdominal Crunches (also known as Eccentric Sit Up)

Negative abdominal crunches are a really challenging exercise for the core, and should only be attempted once you are strong enough. The technique is simple to understand, yet hard to master.

How to Perform:

1. Place your feet flat on the floor with your knees bent, sit up so that your shoulders and back are fully off the ground.
2. Brace your abs (yes you've guessed it) by imagining you are about to get punched in the stomach.
3. Lower your upper body down to the floor **as slowly as you can.** Squeeze your Abs tightly as you lower.
4. Pause, and then use your arms to help get your torso back to the starting position.

Negative crunches are basically sit-ups that only focus on the lowering part. It can be really hard to keep your feet flat on the ground while performing this, so either ask someone to hold your feet down or place them underneath a heavy object.

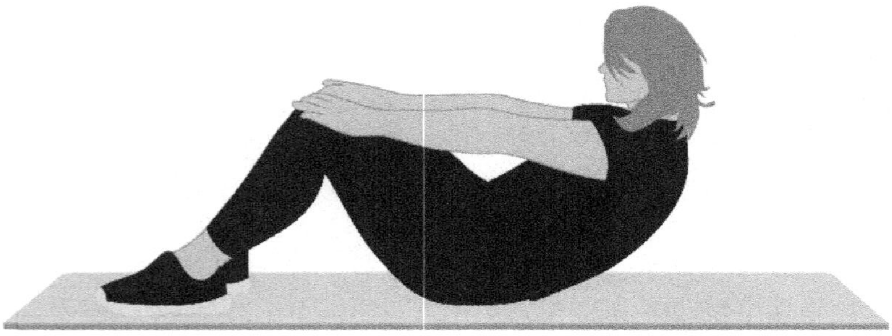

SCAN FOR VIDEO

Exercise #63 Knee-to-Chest Crunches with Leg Extension

This variation of the knee-to-chest crunch is a lot more challenging, allowing you to push your legs outwards which works your lower abdominals even more. If you find this exercise too hard, then just switch it out for the regular knee-to-chest crunches. On the other hand, if you are finding it too easy you can increase the difficulty by wearing ankle weights.

How to Perform:

1. Lie on your back with your knees bent and your feet flat on the ground. Place your arms on either side of your body, flat on the ground.
2. Brace your abs.
3. Raise your feet off the ground, keep your knees bent, and bring them towards your chest.
4. Stop before your lower back rises off the ground, and then kick both legs out in front of you until your legs are almost straight.
5. Bring your legs back in towards your chest.
6. Slowly lower your feet back down to the starting position.

For this exercise to be safe and effective you really need to brace your abs (step two). If you find that you are feeling the exercise in your lower back then swap the exercise back to regular knee-to-chest crunches.

The lower-back muscles form an integral part of your core, and while there are certain exercises that have targeted them in the compound section of your workout, it is a good idea to add in some lower-back exercises in this advanced core chapter that you can add in to your workout.

SCAN FOR VIDEO

Exercise #64 Bodyweight Good Mornings

The good morning is one of the best lower-back and core exercises, also working the hamstrings. There are a number of variations, you have the dumbbell, barbell, and bodyweight version. However, the dumbbell version is quite awkward, and the barbell version requires the use of a squat rack. Which leaves the bodyweight good morning as the best option for this book (though any of the three would work well if you have access to the equipment).

How to Perform:

1. Stand upright with feet shoulder width apart and hands resting behind your head with elbows out wide.
2. Bend your knees very slightly, push your chest out, and pull your shoulders back.
3. Keeping your chest pushed out, bend at the waist, pushing your hips back until your chest is almost parallel to the floor.
4. Pause, and then drive your chest back upwards until you reach the starting position.

Provided you perform this exercise with good form, you will not hurt yourself. It is really important to remember to keep that chest pushed out though. This helps to straighten your back, which is extra important during this type of movement as most people would subconsciously round their back while bending forward.

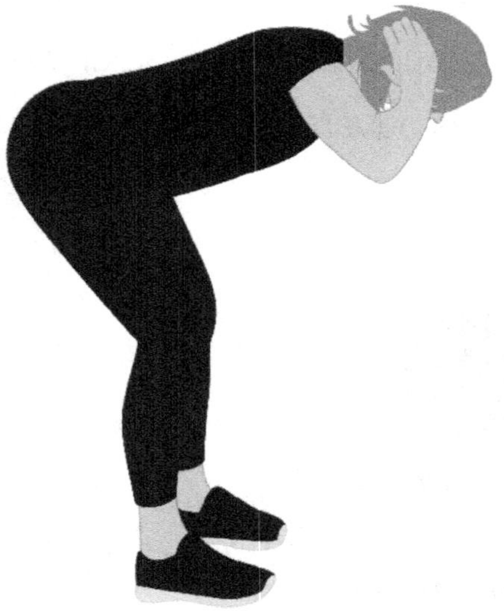

Exercise #65 Dumbbell Romanian Deadlifts

The Romanian deadlift is often thought of as a hamstring exercise, but the truth is that it works both the hamstrings and the lower back equally. Like the Good Morning, the Romanian deadlift is a perfect core exercise that is often underrated. While bodyweight versions of the Romanian deadlift exist, a dumbbell version is in many ways easier to learn.

How to Perform:

1. Stand with your feet facing forwards, slightly narrower than shoulder-width apart. Bend your knees slightly, push your chest out and pull your shoulders back.
2. Hold a dumbbell in each hand with palms facing your body (overhand grip).
3. Bow forwards until your chest is close to parallel with the floor. Keep your shoulders pulled back so that you have a nice and straight back. The dumbbells should travel down your shins in a straight line. Your hips will naturally push backwards as you do this.
4. Pause when you can't bring the dumbbells lower without bending your lower back, and then rise back to the starting position, driving your hips forwards as you do so.

The most important thing with this exercise is to keep your back flat. Repeat to yourself "chest out, shoulders back" while performing the movement. If you struggle, then don't bow as low. As your flexibility increases over time, your ability to bow lower will improve.

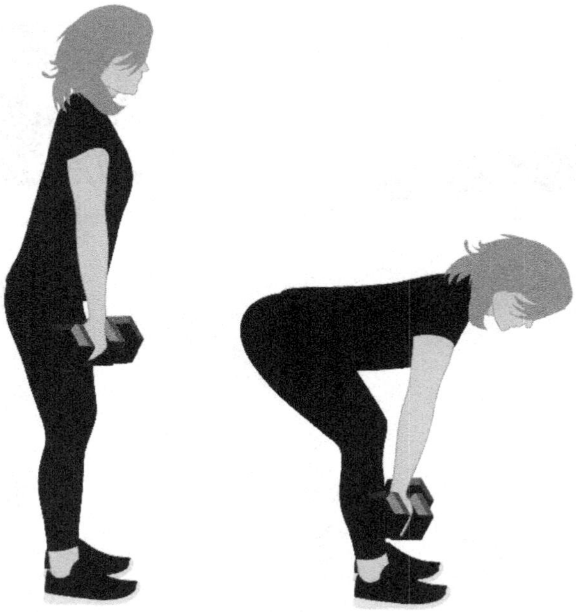

Exercise #66 Cobra Pose

This is a yoga pose that works the lower back and core muscles. It is very low impact and easy to learn.

How to Perform:

1. Lie on your front with your palms flat on the floor, directly beneath your shoulders. Your elbows should be bent, but also close to your body (rather than flared out). Your legs should be straight with feet close together.
2. Take a deep breath and then raise your shoulders and chest off the floor until you feel a nice stretch in your lower back. Squeeze your glutes throughout.
3. Pause, and then slowly lower your chest and shoulders back down to the starting position.

This is an exercise that really benefits from being performed slowly and in a relaxed manner. You are trying to strengthen your lower back and improve your mobility. Performing it quickly will offer no benefits, and will make the exercise a lot less safe.

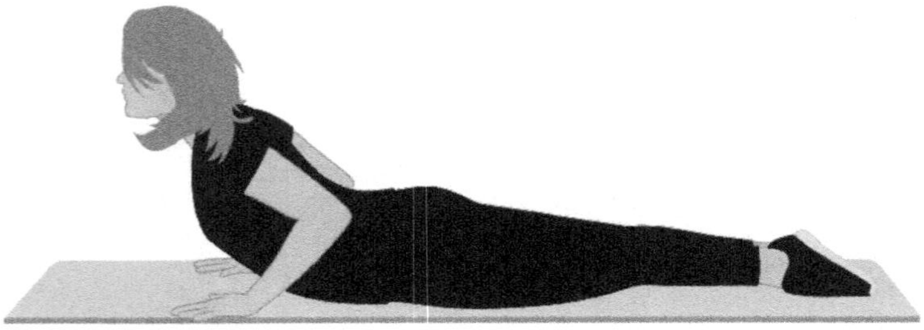

CHAPTER 11

Cardio for Core

SCAN FOR AUDIO CHAPTER

This will be a relatively short chapter, but it is important to separate it from the core exercises of the previous chapters. The first thing to address is whether cardiovascular exercises can also be described as core exercises.

The truth is that all exercises work the core to some extent. Any exercise that requires balance, strength, or agility, will use the core muscles. But that does not mean that they target the core muscles more than others.

A core exercise is one that focuses on the core muscles, and there are no core exercises that work the cardiovascular system particularly hard. Sports such as boxing are probably the closest, as there is so much movement of the torso.

The exercises in this chapter are not designed to improve your core strength, though a slight improvement may occur anyway. They are designed to help you improve your cardiovascular fitness and potentially drop a couple of lbs due to their calorie-burning potential.

Many of you may find that the workouts are challenging enough without the cardio, in which case feel free to avoid adding cardio exercises into your program. But if you want the best possible results, adding in 20 minutes or so of low-intensity cardio could make a significant difference.

Here are some examples of cardio that you can add to your training program:

- **Walking** – There is a distinction between regular walking and brisk walking. Regular walking has some health benefits but not many. Whereas brisk walking can be as beneficial as running or any other form of cardiovascular exercise. Brisk walking is where you can feel your heartbeat rise. The speed that achieves that is the correct speed for you.

- **Hiking** – Walking on uneven and challenging terrain. Due to the nature of hiking terrain, your speed will probably be slower than it would be for normal walking, but the challenge will be the same. This is an excellent form of cardio as it really works your core muscles too, however it is obviously not as accessible or easy to do as walking.
- **Cycling** – If you have a bicycle then using it for cardio is a great idea. Bikes are great even if you have low or medium mobility, and they are very safe to use provided you follow the rules.
- **Running** – If you are mobile enough to run, then this is an excellent way to improve your fitness and burn some extra calories. It is worth learning proper running technique if you have never run before, and a running coach or running club membership is a worthwhile investment. Please also ensure that you have good pair of running shoes.
- **Jogging** – Basically slow running, there has been a lot of debate about the merits of jogging, with some fitness experts looking down their noses at it. However, there are more benefits than negatives to frequent jogging. As with running, getting your technique analysed by a professional can be very useful.
- **Elliptical Machine/Cross Trainer** – An excellent cardio machine, particularly if you have mobility issues such as joint pain. Hold onto the handles to turn this into a full body cardio session.
- **Treadmill** – A great alternative to walking or running outside if you aren't a fan of the great outdoors. One of the most common mistakes that people make with treadmills is to overuse the incline setting. A small incline is more than enough to get a good workout from your treadmill, don't set it too high and definitely don't hold onto the handles if you do (otherwise, what's the point?).
- **Exercise Bike** – When setting up your exercise bike, make sure that the seat is at hip height (when standing beside it). This is usually, but not always, the perfect height for cycling. Set the seat too high or low and you are in for an uncomfortable ride. Exercise

bikes are great for long low-intensity rides, but are not great for faster and more intense cardio.

- **Rower** – One of the best full body cardio workouts you can get is from a rowing machine. The important thing is to get your technique and timing correct. Start with knees bent and hands holding the handle. Pull the handle towards your abdominals, straightening your knees before the handle passes over them. Once your legs are almost fully extended, bring the handles forwards and then bend your knees once the handle has already passed them.
- **Swimming** – A really effective form of cardio, albeit an awkward one to fit into a busy schedule. The benefits include it being fun, inexpensive, and easy on the joints. The downsides are that you need to live near a pool, know how to swim, and have the time to travel, change, swim, rechange, and travel back.
- **Sports** – No form of cardio is more enjoyable than sporting activities. You can find one that suits your desires and capabilities. With niche sports such as pickleball growing in popularity, the argument that "I'm too old" has never carried less weight!

So, there you have it, a quick breakdown of some of the more popular forms of cardiovascular exercises out there. Feel free to add some of them to your training program, or to perform them on "rest" days.

Remember to use the ratings of perceived exertion that we discussed earlier in the book, to ensure that you are training at the right intensity for your goals. If you pick an activity and find that you really struggle to enjoy it, then try a different one. It is really hard to stay motivated for cardio activities if you don't enjoy them, and there really is an activity out there for everyone.

CHAPTER 12

24 Weeks Core Training Program

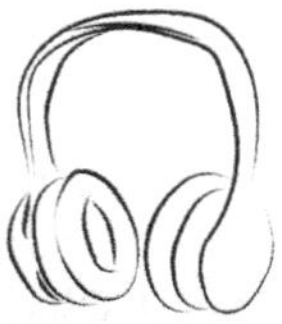

SCAN FOR AUDIO CHAPTER

Now that we have discussed the theory behind our training program, and instructed you in how to perform the many exercises contained within, we can now bring you your 24 week core training program. There are actually three programs in total. One designed for beginners, one for intermediates, and one for advanced users.

Don't try to force yourself into a group that is too challenging for you. If you are a beginner, then follow the beginner program. You can then move to the intermediate and then advanced programs in the future. In truth, if that were the case you would get the best value from this book as you get 72 weeks' worth of training program (3 × 24 week programs) to follow.

24 Week Beginner Workout

Warm Up

Exercise	Sets	Reps	Rest Between Sets
Gentle Cardio	1	5 minutes	n/a
Neck & Shoulder WU	1	5	n/a
Leg Warm-Up	1	5-10	n/a

Exercises

- Exercise #9 Box Squat
- Exercise #10 Squats while Holding Chair
- Exercise #11 Sumo Box Squat

- Exercise #12 Box Push-Ups
- Exercise #13 Seated Dumbbell Shoulder Press
- Exercise #14 Wall Push-Ups
- Exercise #27 Modified Plank
- Exercise #28 Seated Forward Roll-Ups
- Exercise #29 Seated Leg Extension
- Exercise #30 Seated Single-Leg Extension
- Exercise #31 Seated Side Bends
- Exercise #32 Bent Arm Seated Side Bends
- Exercise #33 Chair Planks
- Exercise #34 Seated Knee Lifts
- Exercise #35 Marching in Place
- Exercise #36 Marching in Place with Leg Extension
- Exercise #37 Seated Marching in Place
- Exercise #38 Seated Forward Bends

Week One

Exercise	Sets	Reps	Rest	Exercise Number
Warm Up Session				
Box Squat	3	10	45 secs	9
Squats while Holding Chair	3	10	45 secs	10
Box Push-Ups	3	10-15	45 secs	12
Seated Knee Lifts	3	10-15	45 secs	34
Seated Leg Extension	3	10-15	45 secs	29
Modified Plank	3	30 secs	45 secs	27

Exercise	Sets	Reps	Rest	Exercise Number
Warm Up Session				
Sumo Box Squat	3	10	45 secs	11
Squats while Holding Chair	3	10	45 secs	10
Marching in Place	3	45 secs	45 secs	35

Exercise	Sets	Reps	Rest	Exercise Number
Bent Arm Seated Side Bends	3	10 (each)	45 secs	32
Seated Leg Extension	3	10 (each)	45 secs	29
Chair Planks	3	30 secs	45 secs	33

Exercise	Sets	Reps	Rest	Exercise Number
Warm Up Session				
Wall Push Ups	3	10	45 secs	14
Seated Db Shoulder Press	3	10	45 secs	13
Seated Forward Roll Ups	3	10	45 secs	28
Seated Side Bends	3	10 (each)	45 secs	31
Marching in Place w/ Leg Ext	3	30 secs	45 secs	36
Seated Forward Bends	3	10	45 secs	38

Week Two

Exercise	Sets	Reps	Rest	Exercise Number
Warm Up Session				
Box Squat	3	10-15	45 secs	9
Squats while Holding Chair	3	10-15	45 secs	10
Box Push-Ups	3	11-15	45 secs	12
Seated Knee Lifts	3	11-15	45 secs	34
Seated Leg Extension	3	11-15	45 secs	29
Modified Plank	3	30 secs	45 secs	27

Exercise	Sets	Reps	Rest	Exercise Number
Warm Up Session				
Sumo Box Squat	3	10	45 secs	11
Squats while Holding Chair	3	10	45 secs	10
Marching in Place	3	45 secs	45 secs	35
Bent Arm Seated Side Bends	3	10 (each)	45 secs	32
Seated Leg Extension	3	10 (each)	45 secs	29
Chair Planks	3	30 secs	45 secs	33

Exercise	Sets	Reps	Rest	Exercise Number
Warm Up Session				
Wall Push Ups	3	10	45 secs	14
Seated Db Shoulder Press	3	10	45 secs	13
Seated Forward Roll Ups	3	10	45 secs	28
Seated Side Bends	3	10 (each)	45 secs	31
Marching in Place w/ Leg Ext	3	30 secs	45 secs	36
Seated Forward Bends	3	10	45 secs	38

Week Three

Exercise	Sets	Reps	Rest	Exercise Number
Warm Up Session				
Box Squat	3	10-15	45 secs	9
Squats while Holding Chair	3	10-15	45 secs	10
Box Push-Ups	3	11-16	45 secs	12
Seated Knee Lifts	3	11-16	45 secs	34
Seated Leg Extension	3	11-16	45 secs	29
Modified Plank	3	35 secs	45 secs	27

Exercise	Sets	Reps	Rest	Exercise Number
Warm Up Session				
Sumo Box Squat	3	10-15	45 secs	11
Squats while Holding Chair	3	10-15	45 secs	10
Marching in Place	3	45 secs	45 secs	35
Bent Arm Seated Side Bends	3	10 (each)	45 secs	32
Seated Leg Extension	3	10 (each)	45 secs	29
Chair Planks	3	35 secs	45 secs	33

Exercise	Sets	Reps	Rest	Exercise Number
Warm Up Session				
Wall Push Ups	3	10	45 secs	14
Seated Db Shoulder Press	3	10	45 secs	13
Seated Forward Roll Ups	3	10	45 secs	28

Exercise	Sets	Reps	Rest	Exercise Number
Seated Side Bends	3	10 (each)	45 secs	31
Marching in Place w/ Leg Ext	3	30 secs	45 secs	36
Seated Forward Bends	3	10	45 secs	38

Week Four

Exercise	Sets	Reps	Rest	Exercise Number
Warm Up Session				
Box Squat	3	10-15	45 secs	9
Squats while Holding Chair	3	10-15	45 secs	10
Box Push-Ups	3	11-16	45 secs	12
Seated Knee Lifts	3	11-16	45 secs	34
Seated Leg Extension	3	11-16	45 secs	29
Modified Plank	3	35 secs	45 secs	27

Exercise	Sets	Reps	Rest	Exercise Number
Warm Up Session				
Sumo Box Squat	3	10-15	45 secs	11
Squats while Holding Chair	3	10-15	45 secs	10
Marching in Place	3	45 secs	45 secs	35
Bent Arm Seated Side Bends	3	10 (each)	45 secs	32
Seated Leg Extension	3	10 (each)	45 secs	29
Chair Planks	3	35 secs	45 secs	33

Exercise	Sets	Reps	Rest	Exercise Number
Warm Up Session				
Wall Push Ups	3	10-12	45 secs	14
Seated Db Shoulder Press	3	10-12	45 secs	13
Seated Forward Roll Ups	3	10-12	45 secs	28
Seated Side Bends	3	12 (each)	45 secs	31
Marching in Place w/ Leg Ext	3	45 secs	45 secs	36
Seated Forward Bends	3	10-15	45 secs	38

Week Five

Exercise	Sets	Reps	Rest	Exercise Number
Warm Up Session				
Box Squat	3	11-16	45 secs	9
Squats while Holding Chair	3	11-16	45 secs	10
Box Push-Ups	3	12-17	45 secs	12
Seated Knee Lifts	3	12-17	45 secs	34
Seated Leg Extension	3	12-17	45 secs	29
Modified Plank	3	40 secs	45 secs	27

Exercise	Sets	Reps	Rest	Exercise Number
Warm Up Session				
Sumo Box Squat	3	10-15	45 secs	11
Squats while Holding Chair	3	10-15	45 secs	10
Marching in Place	3	45 secs	45 secs	35
Bent Arm Seated Side Bends	3	10 (each)	45 secs	32
Seated Leg Extension	3	10 (each)	45 secs	29
Chair Planks	3	40 secs	45 secs	33

Exercise	Sets	Reps	Rest	Exercise Number
Warm Up Session				
Wall Push Ups	3	10-12	45 secs	14
Seated Db Shoulder Press	3	10-12	45 secs	13
Seated Forward Roll Ups	3	10-12	45 secs	28
Seated Side Bends	3	12 (each)	45 secs	31
Marching in Place w/ Leg Ext	3	45 secs	45 secs	36
Seated Forward Bends	3	10-15	45 secs	38

Week Six

Exercise	Sets	Reps	Rest	Exercise Number
Warm Up Session				
Box Squat	3	11-16	45 secs	9
Squats while Holding Chair	3	11-16	45 secs	10

Exercise	Sets	Reps	Rest	Exercise Number
Box Push-Ups	3	12-17	45 secs	12
Seated Knee Lifts	3	12-17	45 secs	34
Seated Leg Extension	3	12-17	45 secs	29
Modified Plank	3	40 secs	45 secs	27

Exercise	Sets	Reps	Rest	Exercise Number
Warm Up Session				
Sumo Box Squat	3	12-15	45 secs	11
Squats while Holding Chair	3	12-15	45 secs	10
Marching in Place	3	60 secs	45 secs	35
Bent Arm Seated Side Bends	3	12 (each)	45 secs	32
Seated Leg Extension	3	12 (each)	45 secs	29
Chair Planks	3	40 secs	45 secs	33

Exercise	Sets	Reps	Rest	Exercise Number
Warm Up Session				
Wall Push Ups	3	10-12	45 secs	14
Seated Db Shoulder Press	3	10-12	45 secs	13
Seated Forward Roll Ups	3	10-12	45 secs	28
Seated Side Bends	3	12 (each)	45 secs	31
Marching in Place w/ Leg Ext	3	45 secs	45 secs	36
Seated Forward Bends	3	10-15	45 secs	38

Week Seven

Exercise	Sets	Reps	Rest	Exercise Number
Warm Up Session				
Box Squat	3	11-16	45 secs	9
Squats while Holding Chair	3	11-16	45 secs	10
Box Push-Ups	3	12-17	45 secs	12
Seated Knee Lifts	3	12-17	45 secs	34
Seated Leg Extension	3	12-17	45 secs	29
Modified Plank	3	45 secs	45 secs	27

Exercise	Sets	Reps	Rest	Exercise Number
Warm Up Session				
Sumo Box Squat	3	12-15	45 secs	11
Squats while Holding Chair	3	12-15	45 secs	10
Marching in Place	3	60 secs	45 secs	35
Bent Arm Seated Side Bends	3	12 (each)	45 secs	32
Seated Leg Extension	3	12 (each)	45 secs	29
Chair Planks	3	45 secs	45 secs	33

Exercise	Sets	Reps	Rest	Exercise Number
Warm Up Session				
Wall Push Ups	3	12-15	45 secs	14
Seated Db Shoulder Press	3	12-15	45 secs	13
Seated Forward Roll Ups	3	12-15	45 secs	28
Seated Side Bends	3	15 (each)	45 secs	31
Marching in Place w/ Leg Ext	3	45 secs	45 secs	36
Seated Forward Bends	3	12-15	45 secs	38

Week Eight

Exercise	Sets	Reps	Rest	Exercise Number
Warm Up Session				
Box Squat	3	11-16	45 secs	9
Squats while Holding Chair	3	11-16	45 secs	10
Box Push-Ups	3	12-17	45 secs	12
Seated Knee Lifts	3	12-17	45 secs	34
Seated Leg Extension	3	12-17	45 secs	29
Modified Plank	3	45 secs	45 secs	27

Exercise	Sets	Reps	Rest	Exercise Number
Warm Up Session				
Sumo Box Squat	3	12-15	45 secs	11
Squats while Holding Chair	3	12-15	45 secs	10
Marching in Place	3	60 secs	45 secs	35

Exercise	Sets	Reps	Rest	Exercise Number
Bent Arm Seated Side Bends	3	12 (each)	45 secs	32
Seated Leg Extension	3	12 (each)	45 secs	29
Chair Planks	3	45 secs	45 secs	33

Exercise	Sets	Reps	Rest	Exercise Number
Warm Up Session				
Wall Push Ups	3	12-15	45 secs	14
Seated Db Shoulder Press	3	12-15	45 secs	13
Seated Forward Roll Ups	3	12-15	45 secs	28
Seated Side Bends	3	15 (each)	45 secs	31
Marching in Place w/ Leg Ext	3	45 secs	45 secs	36
Seated Forward Bends	3	12-15	45 secs	38

Week Nine

Exercise	Sets	Reps	Rest	Exercise Number
Warm Up Session				
Box Squat	3	12-17	45 secs	9
Squats while Holding Chair	3	12-17	45 secs	10
Box Push-Ups	3	13-17	45 secs	12
Seated Knee Lifts	3	13-17	45 secs	34
Seated Leg Extension	3	13-17	45 secs	29
Modified Plank	3	50 secs	45 secs	27

Exercise	Sets	Reps	Rest	Exercise Number
Warm Up Session				
Sumo Box Squat	3	12-15	45 secs	11
Squats while Holding Chair	3	12-15	45 secs	10
Marching in Place	3	60 secs	45 secs	35
Bent Arm Seated Side Bends	3	12 (each)	45 secs	32
Seated Leg Extension	3	12 (each)	45 secs	29
Chair Planks	3	50 secs	45 secs	33

Exercise	Sets	Reps	Rest	Exercise Number
Warm Up Session				
Wall Push Ups	3	12-15	45 secs	14
Seated Db Shoulder Press	3	12-15	45 secs	13
Seated Forward Roll Ups	3	12-15	45 secs	28
Seated Side Bends	3	15 (each)	45 secs	31
Marching in Place w/ Leg Ext	3	45 secs	45 secs	36
Seated Forward Bends	3	12-15	45 secs	38

Week Ten

Exercise	Sets	Reps	Rest	Exercise Number
Warm Up Session				
Box Squat	3	12-17	45 secs	9
Squats while Holding Chair	3	12-17	45 secs	10

Exercise	Sets	Reps	Rest	Exercise Number
Box Push-Ups	3	13-17	45 secs	12
Seated Knee Lifts	3	13-17	45 secs	34
Seated Leg Extension	3	13-17	45 secs	29
Modified Plank	3	50 secs	45 secs	27

Exercise	Sets	Reps	Rest	Exercise Number
Warm Up Session				
Sumo Box Squat	3	15	45 secs	11
Squats while Holding Chair	3	15	45 secs	10
Marching in Place	3	60 secs	45 secs	35
Bent Arm Seated Side Bends	3	15 (each)	45 secs	32
Seated Leg Extension	3	15 (each)	45 secs	29
Chair Planks	3	50 secs	45 secs	33

Exercise	Sets	Reps	Rest	Exercise Number
Warm Up Session				
Wall Push Ups	3	12-15	45 secs	14
Seated Db Shoulder Press	3	12-15	45 secs	13
Seated Forward Roll Ups	3	12-15	45 secs	28
Seated Side Bends	3	15 (each)	45 secs	31
Marching in Place w/ Leg Ext	3	45 secs	45 secs	36
Seated Forward Bends	3	12-15	45 secs	38

Week Eleven

Exercise	Sets	Reps	Rest	Exercise Number
Warm Up Session				
Box Squat	3	12-17	45 secs	9
Squats while Holding Chair	3	12-17	45 secs	10
Box Push-Ups	3	13-17	45 secs	12
Seated Knee Lifts	3	13-17	45 secs	34
Seated Leg Extension	3	13-17	45 secs	29
Modified Plank	3	55 secs	45 secs	27

Exercise	Sets	Reps	Rest	Exercise Number
Warm Up Session				
Sumo Box Squat	3	15	45 secs	11
Squats while Holding Chair	3	15	45 secs	10
Marching in Place	3	60 secs	45 secs	35
Bent Arm Seated Side Bends	3	15 (each)	45 secs	32
Seated Leg Extension	3	15 (each)	45 secs	29
Chair Planks	3	55 secs	45 secs	33

Exercise	Sets	Reps	Rest	Exercise Number
Warm Up Session				
Wall Push Ups	3	15	45 secs	14
Seated Db Shoulder Press	3	15	45 secs	13
Seated Forward Roll Ups	3	15	45 secs	28
Seated Side Bends	3	20 (each)	45 secs	31
Marching in Place w/ Leg Ext	3	60 secs	45 secs	36
Seated Forward Bends	3	15	45 secs	38

Week Twelve

Exercise	Sets	Reps	Rest	Exercise Number
Warm Up Session				
Box Squat	3	12-17	45 secs	9
Squats while Holding Chair	3	12-17	45 secs	10
Box Push-Ups	3	13-17	45 secs	12
Seated Knee Lifts	3	13-17	45 secs	34
Seated Leg Extension	3	13-17	45 secs	29
Modified Plank	3	55 secs	45 secs	27

Exercise	Sets	Reps	Rest	Exercise Number
Warm Up Session				
Sumo Box Squat	3	15	45 secs	11
Squats while Holding Chair	3	15	45 secs	10
Marching in Place	3	60 secs	45 secs	35

Exercise	Sets	Reps	Rest	Exercise Number
Bent Arm Seated Side Bends	3	15 (each)	45 secs	32
Seated Leg Extension	3	15 (each)	45 secs	29
Chair Planks	3	55 secs	45 secs	33

Exercise	Sets	Reps	Rest	Exercise Number
Warm Up Session				
Wall Push Ups	3	15	45 secs	14
Seated Db Shoulder Press	3	15	45 secs	13
Seated Forward Roll Ups	3	15	45 secs	28
Seated Side Bends	3	20 (each)	45 secs	31
Marching in Place w/ Leg Ext	3	60 secs	45 secs	36
Seated Forward Bends	3	15	45 secs	38

Week Thirteen

Exercise	Sets	Reps	Rest	Exercise Number
Warm Up Session				
Box Squat	3	13-17	45 secs	9
Squats while Holding Chair	3	13-17	45 secs	10
Box Push-Ups	3	14-18	45 secs	12
Seated Knee Lifts	3	14-18	45 secs	34
Seated Leg Extension	3	14-18	45 secs	29
Modified Plank	3	60 secs	45 secs	27

Exercise	Sets	Reps	Rest	Exercise Number
Warm Up Session				
Sumo Box Squat	3	15	45 secs	11
Squats while Holding Chair	3	15	45 secs	10
Marching in Place	3	60 secs	45 secs	35
Bent Arm Seated Side Bends	3	15 (each)	45 secs	32
Seated Leg Extension	3	15 (each)	45 secs	29
Chair Planks	3	60 secs	45 secs	33

Exercise	Sets	Reps	Rest	Exercise Number
Warm Up Session				
Wall Push Ups	3	15	45 secs	14
Seated Db Shoulder Press	3	15	45 secs	13
Seated Forward Roll Ups	3	15	45 secs	28
Seated Side Bends	3	20 (each)	45 secs	31
Marching in Place w/ Leg Ext	3	60 secs	45 secs	36
Seated Forward Bends	3	15	45 secs	38

Week Fourteen

Exercise	Sets	Reps	Rest	Exercise Number
Warm Up Session				
Box Squat	3	14-18	45 secs	9
Squats while Holding Chair	3	14-18	45 secs	10
Box Push-Ups	3	14-18	45 secs	12
Seated Knee Lifts	3	14-18	45 secs	34
Seated Leg Extension	3	14-18	45 secs	29
Modified Plank	3	60 secs	45 secs	27

Exercise	Sets	Reps	Rest	Exercise Number
Warm Up Session				
Sumo Box Squat	3	15-20	45 secs	11
Squats while Holding Chair	3	15-20	45 secs	10
Marching in Place	3	60 secs	45 secs	35
Bent Arm Seated Side Bends	3	20 (each)	45 secs	32
Seated Leg Extension	3	20 (each)	45 secs	29
Chair Planks	3	60 secs	45 secs	33

Exercise	Sets	Reps	Rest	Exercise Number
Warm Up Session				
Wall Push Ups	3	15	45 secs	14
Seated Db Shoulder Press	3	15	45 secs	13
Seated Forward Roll Ups	3	15	45 secs	28

Exercise	Sets	Reps	Rest	Exercise Number
Seated Side Bends	3	20 (each)	45 secs	31
Marching in Place w/ Leg Ext	3	60 secs	45 secs	36
Seated Forward Bends	3	15	45 secs	38

Week Fifteen

Exercise	Sets	Reps	Rest	Exercise Number
Warm Up Session				
Box Squat	3	14-18	45 secs	9
Squats while Holding Chair	3	14-18	45 secs	10
Box Push-Ups	3	14-18	45 secs	12
Seated Knee Lifts	3	14-18	45 secs	34
Seated Leg Extension	3	14-18	45 secs	29
Modified Plank	3	60 secs	45 secs	27

Exercise	Sets	Reps	Rest	Exercise Number
Warm Up Session				
Sumo Box Squat	3	15-20	45 secs	11
Squats while Holding Chair	3	15-20	45 secs	10
Marching in Place	3	60 secs	45 secs	35
Bent Arm Seated Side Bends	3	20 (each)	45 secs	32
Seated Leg Extension	3	20 (each)	45 secs	29
Chair Planks	3	60 secs	45 secs	33

Exercise	Sets	Reps	Rest	Exercise Number
Warm Up Session				
Wall Push Ups	3	15	45 secs	14
Seated Db Shoulder Press	3	15	45 secs	13
Seated Forward Roll Ups	3	15	45 secs	28
Seated Side Bends	3	20 (each)	45 secs	31
Marching in Place w/ Leg Ext	3	60 secs	45 secs	36
Seated Forward Bends	3	15	45 secs	38

Week Sixteen

Exercise	Sets	Reps	Rest	Exercise Number
Warm Up Session				
Box Squat	3	14-18	45 secs	9
Squats while Holding Chair	3	14-18	45 secs	10
Box Push-Ups	3	15-19	45 secs	12
Seated Knee Lifts	3	15-19	45 secs	34
Seated Leg Extension	3	15-19	45 secs	29
Modified Plank	3	60 secs	45 secs	27

Exercise	Sets	Reps	Rest	Exercise Number
Warm Up Session				
Sumo Box Squat	3	15-20	45 secs	11
Squats while Holding Chair	3	15-20	45 secs	10
Marching in Place	3	60 secs	45 secs	35
Bent Arm Seated Side Bends	3	20 (each)	45 secs	32
Seated Leg Extension	3	20 (each)	45 secs	29
Chair Planks	3	60 secs	45 secs	33

Exercise	Sets	Reps	Rest	Exercise Number
Warm Up Session				
Wall Push Ups	3	15-20	45 secs	14
Seated Db Shoulder Press	3	15-20	45 secs	13
Seated Forward Roll Ups	3	15-20	45 secs	28
Seated Side Bends	3	20 (each)	45 secs	31
Marching in Place w/ Leg Ext	3	60 secs	45 secs	36
Seated Forward Bends	3	15-20	45 secs	38

Week Seventeen

Exercise	Sets	Reps	Rest	Exercise Number
Warm Up Session				
Box Squat	3	14-18	45 secs	9
Squats while Holding Chair	3	14-18	45 secs	10

Exercise	Sets	Reps	Rest	Exercise Number
Box Push-Ups	3	15-19	45 secs	12
Seated Knee Lifts	3	15-19	45 secs	34
Seated Leg Extension	3	15-19	45 secs	29
Modified Plank	3	60 secs	45 secs	27

Exercise	Sets	Reps	Rest	Exercise Number
Warm Up Session				
Sumo Box Squat	3	15-20	45 secs	11
Squats while Holding Chair	3	15-20	45 secs	10
Marching in Place	3	60 secs	45 secs	35
Bent Arm Seated Side Bends	3	20 (each)	45 secs	32
Seated Leg Extension	3	20 (each)	45 secs	29
Chair Planks	3	60 secs	45 secs	33

Exercise	Sets	Reps	Rest	Exercise Number
Warm Up Session				
Wall Push Ups	3	15-20	45 secs	14
Seated Db Shoulder Press	3	15-20	45 secs	13
Seated Forward Roll Ups	3	15-20	45 secs	28
Seated Side Bends	3	20 (each)	45 secs	31
Marching in Place w/ Leg Ext	3	60 secs	45 secs	36
Seated Forward Bends	3	15-20	45 secs	38

Week Eighteen

Exercise	Sets	Reps	Rest	Exercise Number
Warm Up Session				
Box Squat	3	15-19	45 secs	9
Squats while Holding Chair	3	15-19	45 secs	10
Box Push-Ups	3	15-19	45 secs	12
Seated Knee Lifts	3	15-19	45 secs	34
Seated Leg Extension	3	15-19	45 secs	29
Modified Plank	3	60 secs	45 secs	27

Exercise	Sets	Reps	Rest	Exercise Number
Warm Up Session				
Sumo Box Squat	3	15-20	45 secs	11
Squats while Holding Chair	3	15-20	45 secs	10
Marching in Place	3	60 secs	45 secs	35
Bent Arm Seated Side Bends	3	20 (each)	45 secs	32
Seated Leg Extension	3	20 (each)	45 secs	29
Chair Planks	3	60 secs	45 secs	33

Exercise	Sets	Reps	Rest	Exercise Number
Warm Up Session				
Wall Push Ups	3	15-20	45 secs	14
Seated Db Shoulder Press	3	15-20	45 secs	13
Seated Forward Roll Ups	3	15-20	45 secs	28
Seated Side Bends	3	20 (each)	45 secs	31
Marching in Place w/ Leg Ext	3	60 secs	45 secs	36
Seated Forward Bends	3	15-20	45 secs	38

Week Nineteen

Exercise	Sets	Reps	Rest	Exercise Number
Warm Up Session				
Box Squat	3	15-19	45 secs	9
Squats while Holding Chair	3	15-19	45 secs	10
Box Push-Ups	3	15-19	45 secs	12
Seated Knee Lifts	3	15-19	45 secs	34
Seated Leg Extension	3	15-19	45 secs	29
Modified Plank	3	60 secs	45 secs	27

Exercise	Sets	Reps	Rest	Exercise Number
Warm Up Session				
Sumo Box Squat	3	15-20	45 secs	11
Squats while Holding Chair	3	15-20	45 secs	10
Marching in Place	3	60 secs	45 secs	35

Exercise	Sets	Reps	Rest	Exercise Number
Bent Arm Seated Side Bends	3	20 (each)	45 secs	32
Seated Leg Extension	3	20 (each)	45 secs	29
Chair Planks	3	60 secs	45 secs	33

Exercise	Sets	Reps	Rest	Exercise Number
Warm Up Session				
Wall Push Ups	3	15-20	45 secs	14
Seated Db Shoulder Press	3	15-20	45 secs	13
Seated Forward Roll Ups	3	15-20	45 secs	28
Seated Side Bends	3	20 (each)	45 secs	31
Marching in Place w/ Leg Ext	3	60 secs	45 secs	36
Seated Forward Bends	3	15-20	45 secs	38

Week Twenty

Exercise	Sets	Reps	Rest	Exercise Number
Warm Up Session				
Box Squat	3	15-19	45 secs	9
Squats while Holding Chair	3	15-19	45 secs	10
Box Push-Ups	3	15-19	45 secs	12
Seated Knee Lifts	3	15-19	45 secs	34
Seated Leg Extension	3	15-19	45 secs	29
Modified Plank	3	60 secs	45 secs	27

Exercise	Sets	Reps	Rest	Exercise Number
Warm Up Session				
Sumo Box Squat	3	20	45 secs	11
Squats while Holding Chair	3	20	45 secs	10
Marching in Place	3	60 secs	45 secs	35
Bent Arm Seated Side Bends	3	20 (each)	45 secs	32
Seated Leg Extension	3	20 (each)	45 secs	29
Chair Planks	3	60 secs	45 secs	33

Exercise	Sets	Reps	Rest	Exercise Number
Warm Up Session				
Wall Push Ups	3	15-20	45 secs	14
Seated Db Shoulder Press	3	15-20	45 secs	13
Seated Forward Roll Ups	3	15-20	45 secs	28
Seated Side Bends	3	20 (each)	45 secs	31
Marching in Place w/ Leg Ext	3	60 secs	45 secs	36
Seated Forward Bends	3	15-20	45 secs	38

Week Twenty One

Exercise	Sets	Reps	Rest	Exercise Number
Warm Up Session				
Box Squat	3	15-19	45 secs	9
Squats while Holding Chair	3	15-19	45 secs	10
Box Push-Ups	3	15-20	45 secs	12
Seated Knee Lifts	3	15-20	45 secs	34
Seated Leg Extension	3	15-20	45 secs	29
Modified Plank	3	60 secs	45 secs	27

Exercise	Sets	Reps	Rest	Exercise Number
Warm Up Session				
Sumo Box Squat	3	20	45 secs	11
Squats while Holding Chair	3	20	45 secs	10
Marching in Place	3	60 secs	45 secs	35
Bent Arm Seated Side Bends	3	20 (each)	45 secs	32
Seated Leg Extension	3	20 (each)	45 secs	29
Chair Planks	3	60 secs	45 secs	33

Exercise	Sets	Reps	Rest	Exercise Number
Warm Up Session				
Wall Push Ups	3	15-20	45 secs	14
Seated Db Shoulder Press	3	15-20	45 secs	13
Seated Forward Roll Ups	3	15-20	45 secs	28

Exercise	Sets	Reps	Rest	Exercise Number
Seated Side Bends	3	20 (each)	45 secs	31
Marching in Place w/ Leg Ext	3	60 secs	45 secs	36
Seated Forward Bends	3	15-20	45 secs	38

Week Twenty Two

Exercise	Sets	Reps	Rest	Exercise Number
Warm Up Session				
Box Squat	3	15-19	45 secs	9
Squats while Holding Chair	3	15-19	45 secs	10
Box Push-Ups	3	15-20	45 secs	12
Seated Knee Lifts	3	15-20	45 secs	34
Seated Leg Extension	3	15-20	45 secs	29
Modified Plank	3	60 secs	45 secs	27

Exercise	Sets	Reps	Rest	Exercise Number
Warm Up Session				
Sumo Box Squat	3	20	45 secs	11
Squats while Holding Chair	3	20	45 secs	10
Marching in Place	3	60 secs	45 secs	35
Bent Arm Seated Side Bends	3	20 (each)	45 secs	32
Seated Leg Extension	3	20 (each)	45 secs	29
Chair Planks	3	60 secs	45 secs	33

Exercise	Sets	Reps	Rest	Exercise Number
Warm Up Session				
Wall Push Ups	3	20	45 secs	14
Seated Db Shoulder Press	3	20	45 secs	13
Seated Forward Roll Ups	3	20	45 secs	28
Seated Side Bends	3	20 (each)	45 secs	31
Marching in Place w/ Leg Ext	3	60 secs	45 secs	36
Seated Forward Bends	3	20	45 secs	38

Week Twenty Three

Exercise	Sets	Reps	Rest	Exercise Number
Warm Up Session				
Box Squat	3	15-20	45 secs	9
Squats while Holding Chair	3	15-20	45 secs	10
Box Push-Ups	3	15-20	45 secs	12
Seated Knee Lifts	3	15-20	45 secs	34
Seated Leg Extension	3	15-20	45 secs	29
Modified Plank	3	60 secs	45 secs	27

Exercise	Sets	Reps	Rest	Exercise Number
Warm Up Session				
Sumo Box Squat	3	20	45 secs	11
Squats while Holding Chair	3	20	45 secs	10
Marching in Place	3	60 secs	45 secs	35
Bent Arm Seated Side Bends	3	20 (each)	45 secs	32
Seated Leg Extension	3	20 (each)	45 secs	29
Chair Planks	3	60 secs	45 secs	33

Exercise	Sets	Reps	Rest	Exercise Number
Warm Up Session				
Wall Push Ups	3	20	45 secs	14
Seated Db Shoulder Press	3	20	45 secs	13
Seated Forward Roll Ups	3	20	45 secs	28
Seated Side Bends	3	20 (each)	45 secs	31
Marching in Place w/ Leg Ext	3	60 secs	45 secs	36
Seated Forward Bends	3	20	45 secs	38

Week Twenty Four

Exercise	Sets	Reps	Rest	Exercise Number
Warm Up Session				
Box Squat	3	15-20	45 secs	9
Squats while Holding Chair	3	15-20	45 secs	10
Box Push-Ups	3	15-20	45 secs	12
Seated Knee Lifts	3	15-20	45 secs	34
Seated Leg Extension	3	15-20	45 secs	29
Modified Plank	3	60 secs	45 secs	27

Exercise	Sets	Reps	Rest	Exercise Number
Warm Up Session				
Sumo Box Squat	3	20	45 secs	11
Squats while Holding Chair	3	20	45 secs	10
Marching in Place	3	60 secs	45 secs	35
Bent Arm Seated Side Bends	3	20 (each)	45 secs	32
Seated Leg Extension	3	20 (each)	45 secs	29
Chair Planks	3	60 secs	45 secs	33

Exercise	Sets	Reps	Rest	Exercise Number
Warm Up Session				
Wall Push Ups	3	20	45 secs	14
Seated Db Shoulder Press	3	20	45 secs	13
Seated Forward Roll Ups	3	20	45 secs	28
Seated Side Bends	3	20 (each)	45 secs	31
Marching in Place w/ Leg Ext	3	60 secs	45 secs	36
Seated Forward Bends	3	20	45 secs	38

Once you have finished this workout, you can repeat the fitness testing from earlier in the book. If your score has improved substantially, then you may be ready for the 24 week intermediate workout. If not, then repeat the beginner workout, with more focus on your form and perhaps slightly shorter rest periods.

24 Week Intermediate Workout

Warm Up

Exercise	Sets	Reps	Rest Between Sets
Gentle Cardio	1	5-7 minutes	n/a
Neck & Shoulder WU	1	10	n/a
Leg Warm-Up	1	10 (20 for calf raise)	n/a

Exercises

- Exercise #9 Box Squat
- Exercise #10 Squats while Holding Chair
- Exercise #11 Sumo Box Squat
- Exercise #12 Box Push-Ups
- Exercise #13 Seated Dumbbell Shoulder Press
- Exercise #14 Wall Push-Ups
- Exercise #15 Box Squat with Dumbbell
- Exercise #16 Box Squat into Shoulder Press (Dumbbells)
- Exercise #17 Single-Leg Romanian Deadlift (Chair)
- Exercise #18 Glute Bridges
- Exercise #19 Lateral Lunges
- Exercise #20 Knee Push-Ups
- Exercise #27 Modified Plank
- Exercise #28 Seated Forward Roll-Ups
- Exercise #29 Seated Leg Extension
- Exercise #30 Seated Single-Leg Extension
- Exercise #31 Seated Side Bends
- Exercise #32 Bent Arm Seated Side Bends
- Exercise #33 Chair Planks

- Exercise #34 Seated Knee Lifts
- Exercise #35 Marching in Place
- Exercise #36 Marching in Place with Leg Extension
- Exercise #37 Seated Marching in Place
- Exercise #38 Seated Forward Bends
- Exercise #39 Plank (Push-Up Position)
- Exercise #40 Heel Tap Exercise
- Exercise #41 Abdominal Crunches
- Exercise #42 Foot-Raised Abdominal Crunches
- Exercise #43 Long-Arm Crunches
- Exercise #44 Single-Long-Arm Crunches
- Exercise #45 Arm Over Crunches
- Exercise #46 Knee-to-Chest Crunches
- Exercise #47 Wood Chops
- Exercise #48 Seated Wood Chops
- Exercise #49 Superman
- Exercise #50 Mountain Climbers on Chair
- Exercise #51 Dead Bugs
- Exercise #52 Bird Dog Exercise
- Exercise #53 Seated Bicycle
- Exercise #54 Seated Russian Twists (Chair)

Week One

Exercise	Sets	Reps	Rest	Exercise Number
Warm Up Session				
Box Squat with Dumbbell	3	10	60 secs	15
Glute Bridges	3	10	60 secs	18
Single-Leg Rom Dead (Chair)	3	10 (each)	60 secs	17
Lateral Lunges	3	10 (each)	60 secs	19
Seated Knee Lifts	3	10	60 secs	34
Seated Marching in Place	3	30 secs	60 secs	37

Exercise	Sets	Reps	Rest	Exercise Number
Warm Up Session				
Knee Push-Ups	3	10	60 secs	20
Wall Push-Ups	3	20	60 secs	14
Box Push-Ups	3	10	60 secs	12
Bird Dog Exercise	3	10	60 secs	52
Wood Chops	3	10 (each)	60 secs	47
Knee-to-chest Crunches	3	10	60 secs	46

Exercise	Sets	Reps	Rest	Exercise Number
Warm Up Session				
Sumo Box Squat	3	10	60 secs	11
Box Squats into Press	3	10	60 secs	16
Glute Bridges	3	10	60 secs	18
Superman	3	10	60 secs	49
Seated Bicycle	3	10	60 secs	53
Plank Push-Up Position	3	30 secs	60 secs	39

Exercise	Sets	Reps	Rest	Exercise Number
Warm Up Session				
Box Squats into Press	3	10	60 secs	16
Knee Push-Ups	3	10	60 secs	20
Seated Dumbbell Press	3	10	60 secs	13

Exercise	Sets	Reps	Rest	Exercise Number
Seated Russian Twists (Chair)	3	10 (each)	60 secs	54
Arm Over Crunches	3	10	60 secs	45
Modified Plank	3	30 secs	60 secs	27

Week Two

Exercise	Sets	Reps	Rest	Exercise Number
Warm Up Session				
Knee Push-Ups	3	10	60 secs	20
Box Push-Ups	3	10	60 secs	12
Box Squats into Press	3	10	60 secs	16
Long Arm Crunches	3	10	60 secs	43
Single Long Arm Crunches	3	10 (each)	60 secs	44
Mountain Climbers on Chair	3	30 secs	60 secs	50

Exercise	Sets	Reps	Rest	Exercise Number
Warm Up Session				
Glute Bridges	3	10	60 secs	18
Box Squats	3	20	60 secs	9
Marching in Place	3	30 secs	60 secs	35
Foot Raised Abdominal Crunch	3	10	60 secs	42
Seated Wood Chops	3	10 (each)	60 secs	48
Dead Bugs	3	10	60 secs	51

Exercise	Sets	Reps	Rest	Exercise Number
Warm Up Session				
Wall Push-Ups	3	20	60 secs	14
Sumo Box Squat	3	10	60 secs	11
Squats While Holding Chair	3	20	60 secs	10
Abdominal Crunches	3	10	60 secs	41
Heel Taps	3	10 (each)	60 secs	40
Seated Marching in Place	3	30 secs	60 secs	37

Exercise	Sets	Reps	Rest	Exercise Number
Warm Up Session				
Knee Push-Ups	3	10	60 secs	20
Seated Dumbbell Press	3	10	60 secs	13
Box Push-Ups	3	10	60 secs	12
Seated Forward Bends	3	10	60 secs	38
Marching in Place w/ Leg Ext	3	30 secs	60 secs	36
Chair Planks	3	30 secs	60 secs	33

Week Three

Exercise	Sets	Reps	Rest	Exercise Number
Warm Up Session				
Box Squat with Dumbbell	3	10	60 secs	15
Glute Bridges	3	10	60 secs	18
Single-Leg Rom Dead (Chair)	3	10 (each)	60 secs	17
Lateral Lunges	3	10 (each)	60 secs	19
Seated Knee Lifts	3	10	60 secs	34
Seated Marching in Place	3	30 secs	60 secs	37

Exercise	Sets	Reps	Rest	Exercise Number
Warm Up Session				
Knee Push-Ups	3	10	60 secs	20
Wall Push-Ups	3	20	60 secs	14
Box Push-Ups	3	10	60 secs	12
Bird Dog Exercise	3	10	60 secs	52
Wood Chops	3	10 (each)	60 secs	47
Knee-to-chest Crunches	3	10	60 secs	46

Exercise	Sets	Reps	Rest	Exercise Number
Warm Up Session				
Sumo Box Squat	3	10	60 secs	11
Box Squats into Press	3	10	60 secs	16
Glute Bridges	3	10	60 secs	18
Superman	3	10	60 secs	49

Exercise	Sets	Reps	Rest	Exercise Number
Seated Bicycle	3	10	60 secs	53
Plank Push-Up Position	3	30 secs	60 secs	39

Exercise	Sets	Reps	Rest	Exercise Number
Warm Up Session				
Box Squats into Press	3	10	60 secs	16
Knee Push-Ups	3	10	60 secs	20
Seated Dumbbell Press	3	10	60 secs	13
Seated Russian Twists (Chair)	3	10 (each)	60 secs	54
Arm Over Crunches	3	10	60 secs	45
Modified Plank	3	30 secs	60 secs	27

Week Four

Exercise	Sets	Reps	Rest	Exercise Number
Warm Up Session				
Knee Push-Ups	3	10	60 secs	20
Box Push-Ups	3	10	60 secs	12
Box Squats into Press	3	10	60 secs	16
Long Arm Crunches	3	10	60 secs	43
Single Long Arm Crunches	3	10 (each)	60 secs	44
Mountain Climbers on Chair	3	30 secs	60 secs	50

Exercise	Sets	Reps	Rest	Exercise Number
Warm Up Session				
Glute Bridges	3	10	60 secs	18
Box Squats	3	20	60 secs	9
Marching in Place	3	30 secs	60 secs	35
Foot Raised Abdominal Crunch	3	10	60 secs	42
Seated Wood Chops	3	10 (each)	60 secs	48
Dead Bugs	3	10	60 secs	51

Exercise	Sets	Reps	Rest	Exercise Number
Warm Up Session				
Wall Push-Ups	3	20	60 secs	14

Exercise	Sets	Reps	Rest	Exercise Number
Sumo Box Squat	3	10	60 secs	11
Squats While Holding Chair	3	20	60 secs	10
Abdominal Crunches	3	10	60 secs	41
Heel Taps	3	10 (each)	60 secs	40
Seated Marching in Place	3	30 secs	60 secs	37

Exercise	Sets	Reps	Rest	Exercise Number
Warm Up Session				
Knee Push-Ups	3	10	60 secs	20
Seated Dumbbell Press	3	10	60 secs	13
Box Push-Ups	3	10	60 secs	12
Seated Forward Bends	3	10	60 secs	38
Marching in Place w/ Leg Ext	3	30 secs	60 secs	36
Chair Planks	3	30 secs	60 secs	33

Week Five

Exercise	Sets	Reps	Rest	Exercise Number
Warm Up Session				
Box Squat with Dumbbell	3	12	60 secs	15
Glute Bridges	3	12	60 secs	18
Single-Leg Rom Dead (Chair)	3	12 (each)	60 secs	17
Lateral Lunges	3	12 (each)	60 secs	19
Seated Knee Lifts	3	12	60 secs	34
Seated Marching in Place	3	40 secs	60 secs	37

Exercise	Sets	Reps	Rest	Exercise Number
Warm Up Session				
Knee Push-Ups	3	12	60 secs	20
Wall Push-Ups	3	20	60 secs	14
Box Push-Ups	3	12	60 secs	12
Bird Dog Exercise	3	12	60 secs	52
Wood Chops	3	12 (each)	60 secs	47
Knee-to-chest Crunches	3	12	60 secs	46

Exercise	Sets	Reps	Rest	Exercise Number
Warm Up Session				
Sumo Box Squat	3	12	60 secs	11
Box Squats into Press	3	12	60 secs	16
Glute Bridges	3	12	60 secs	18
Superman	3	12	60 secs	49
Seated Bicycle	3	12	60 secs	53
Plank Push-Up Position	3	40 secs	60 secs	39

Exercise	Sets	Reps	Rest	Exercise Number
Warm Up Session				
Box Squats into Press	3	12	60 secs	16
Knee Push-Ups	3	12	60 secs	20
Seated Dumbbell Press	3	12	60 secs	13
Seated Russian Twists (Chair)	3	12 (each)	60 secs	54
Arm Over Crunches	3	12	60 secs	45
Modified Plank	3	40 secs	60 secs	27

Week Six

Exercise	Sets	Reps	Rest	Exercise Number
Warm Up Session				
Knee Push-Ups	3	12	60 secs	20
Box Push-Ups	3	12	60 secs	12
Box Squats into Press	3	12	60 secs	16
Long Arm Crunches	3	12	60 secs	43
Single Long Arm Crunches	3	12 (each)	60 secs	44
Mountain Climbers on Chair	3	40 secs	60 secs	50

Exercise	Sets	Reps	Rest	Exercise Number
Warm Up Session				
Glute Bridges	3	12	60 secs	18
Box Squats	3	20	60 secs	9
Marching in Place	3	40 secs	60 secs	35
Foot Raised Abdominal Crunch	3	12	60 secs	42
Seated Wood Chops	3	12 (each)	60 secs	48
Dead Bugs	3	12	60 secs	51

Exercise	Sets	Reps	Rest	Exercise Number
Warm Up Session				
Wall Push-Ups	3	20	60 secs	14
Sumo Box Squat	3	12	60 secs	11
Squats While Holding Chair	3	20	60 secs	10
Abdominal Crunches	3	12	60 secs	41
Heel Taps	3	12 (each)	60 secs	40
Seated Marching in Place	3	40 secs	60 secs	37

Exercise	Sets	Reps	Rest	Exercise Number
Warm Up Session				
Knee Push-Ups	3	12	60 secs	20
Seated Dumbbell Press	3	12	60 secs	13
Box Push-Ups	3	12	60 secs	12
Seated Forward Bends	3	12	60 secs	38
Marching in Place w/ Leg Ext	3	40 secs	60 secs	36
Chair Planks	3	40 secs	60 secs	33

Week Seven

Exercise	Sets	Reps	Rest	Exercise Number
Warm Up Session				
Box Squat with Dumbbell	3	12	60 secs	15
Glute Bridges	3	12	60 secs	18
Single-Leg Rom Dead (Chair)	3	12 (each)	60 secs	17
Lateral Lunges	3	12 (each)	60 secs	19
Seated Knee Lifts	3	12	60 secs	34
Seated Marching in Place	3	40 secs	60 secs	37

Exercise	Sets	Reps	Rest	Exercise Number
Warm Up Session				
Knee Push-Ups	3	12	60 secs	20
Wall Push-Ups	3	20	60 secs	14
Box Push-Ups	3	12	60 secs	12

Exercise	Sets	Reps	Rest	Exercise Number
Bird Dog Exercise	3	12	60 secs	52
Wood Chops	3	12 (each)	60 secs	47
Knee-to-chest Crunches	3	12	60 secs	46

Exercise	Sets	Reps	Rest	Exercise Number
Warm Up Session				
Sumo Box Squat	3	12	60 secs	11
Box Squats into Press	3	12	60 secs	16
Glute Bridges	3	12	60 secs	18
Superman	3	12	60 secs	49
Seated Bicycle	3	12	60 secs	53
Plank Push-Up Position	3	40 secs	60 secs	39

Exercise	Sets	Reps	Rest	Exercise Number
Warm Up Session				
Box Squats into Press	3	12	60 secs	16
Knee Push-Ups	3	12	60 secs	20
Seated Dumbbell Press	3	12	60 secs	13
Seated Russian Twists (Chair)	3	12 (each)	60 secs	54
Arm Over Crunches	3	12	60 secs	45
Modified Plank	3	40 secs	60 secs	27

Week Eight

Exercise	Sets	Reps	Rest	Exercise Number
Warm Up Session				
Knee Push-Ups	3	12	60 secs	20
Box Push-Ups	3	12	60 secs	12
Box Squats into Press	3	12	60 secs	16
Long Arm Crunches	3	12	60 secs	43
Single Long Arm Crunches	3	12 (each)	60 secs	44
Mountain Climbers on Chair	3	40 secs	60 secs	50

Exercise	Sets	Reps	Rest	Exercise Number
Warm Up Session				
Glute Bridges	3	12	60 secs	18
Box Squats	3	20	60 secs	9
Marching in Place	3	40 secs	60 secs	35
Foot Raised Abdominal Crunch	3	12	60 secs	42
Seated Wood Chops	3	12 (each)	60 secs	48
Dead Bugs	3	12	60 secs	51

Exercise	Sets	Reps	Rest	Exercise Number
Warm Up Session				
Wall Push-Ups	3	20	60 secs	14
Sumo Box Squat	3	12	60 secs	11
Squats While Holding Chair	3	20	60 secs	10
Abdominal Crunches	3	12	60 secs	41
Heel Taps	3	12 (each)	60 secs	40
Seated Marching in Place	3	40 secs	60 secs	37

Exercise	Sets	Reps	Rest	Exercise Number
Warm Up Session				
Knee Push-Ups	3	12	60 secs	20
Seated Dumbbell Press	3	12	60 secs	13
Box Push-Ups	3	12	60 secs	12
Seated Forward Bends	3	12	60 secs	38
Marching in Place w/ Leg Ext	3	40 secs	60 secs	36
Chair Planks	3	40 secs	60 secs	33

Week Nine

Exercise	Sets	Reps	Rest	Exercise Number
Warm Up Session				
Box Squat with Dumbbell	3	12	60 secs	15
Glute Bridges	3	12	60 secs	18
Single-Leg Rom Dead (Chair)	3	12 (each)	60 secs	17
Lateral Lunges	3	12 (each)	60 secs	19

Exercise	Sets	Reps	Rest	Exercise Number
Seated Knee Lifts	3	12	60 secs	34
Seated Marching in Place	3	40 secs	60 secs	37

Exercise	Sets	Reps	Rest	Exercise Number
Warm Up Session				
Knee Push-Ups	3	12	60 secs	20
Wall Push-Ups	3	20	60 secs	14
Box Push-Ups	3	12	60 secs	12
Bird Dog Exercise	3	12	60 secs	52
Wood Chops	3	12 (each)	60 secs	47
Knee-to-chest Crunches	3	12	60 secs	46

Exercise	Sets	Reps	Rest	Exercise Number
Warm Up Session				
Sumo Box Squat	3	12	60 secs	11
Box Squats into Press	3	12	60 secs	16
Glute Bridges	3	12	60 secs	18
Superman	3	12	60 secs	49
Seated Bicycle	3	12	60 secs	53
Plank Push-Up Position	3	40 secs	60 secs	39

Exercise	Sets	Reps	Rest	Exercise Number
Warm Up Session				
Box Squats into Press	3	12	60 secs	16
Knee Push-Ups	3	12	60 secs	20
Seated Dumbbell Press	3	12	60 secs	13
Seated Russian Twists (Chair)	3	12 (each)	60 secs	54
Arm Over Crunches	3	12	60 secs	45
Modified Plank	3	40 secs	60 secs	27

Week Ten

Exercise	Sets	Reps	Rest	Exercise Number
Warm Up Session				
Knee Push-Ups	3	12	60 secs	20
Box Push-Ups	3	12	60 secs	12
Box Squats into Press	3	12	60 secs	16
Long Arm Crunches	3	12	60 secs	43
Single Long Arm Crunches	3	12 (each)	60 secs	44
Mountain Climbers on Chair	3	40 secs	60 secs	50

Exercise	Sets	Reps	Rest	Exercise Number
Warm Up Session				
Glute Bridges	3	12	60 secs	18
Box Squats	3	20	60 secs	9
Marching in Place	3	40 secs	60 secs	35
Foot Raised Abdominal Crunch	3	12	60 secs	42
Seated Wood Chops	3	12 (each)	60 secs	48
Dead Bugs	3	12	60 secs	51

Exercise	Sets	Reps	Rest	Exercise Number
Warm Up Session				
Wall Push-Ups	3	20	60 secs	14
Sumo Box Squat	3	12	60 secs	11
Squats While Holding Chair	3	20	60 secs	10
Abdominal Crunches	3	12	60 secs	41
Heel Taps	3	12 (each)	60 secs	40
Seated Marching in Place	3	40 secs	60 secs	37

Exercise	Sets	Reps	Rest	Exercise Number
Warm Up Session				
Knee Push-Ups	3	12	60 secs	20
Seated Dumbbell Press	3	12	60 secs	13
Box Push-Ups	3	12	60 secs	12
Seated Forward Bends	3	12	60 secs	38

Exercise	Sets	Reps	Rest	Exercise Number
Marching in Place w/ Leg Ext	3	40 secs	60 secs	36
Chair Planks	3	40 secs	60 secs	33

Week Eleven

Exercise	Sets	Reps	Rest	Exercise Number
Warm Up Session				
Box Squat with Dumbbell	3	12	60 secs	15
Glute Bridges	3	12-15	60 secs	18
Single-Leg Rom Dead (Chair)	3	12 (each)	60 secs	17
Lateral Lunges	3	12 (each)	60 secs	19
Seated Knee Lifts	3	12-15	60 secs	34
Seated Marching in Place	3	40 secs	60 secs	37

Exercise	Sets	Reps	Rest	Exercise Number
Warm Up Session				
Knee Push-Ups	3	12-15	60 secs	20
Wall Push-Ups	3	20	60 secs	14
Box Push-Ups	3	12-15	60 secs	12
Bird Dog Exercise	3	12-15	60 secs	52
Wood Chops	3	12 (each)	60 secs	47
Knee-to-chest Crunches	3	12-15	60 secs	46

Exercise	Sets	Reps	Rest	Exercise Number
Warm Up Session				
Sumo Box Squat	3	12-15	60 secs	11
Box Squats into Press	3	12-15	60 secs	16
Glute Bridges	3	12-15	60 secs	18
Superman	3	12-15	60 secs	49
Seated Bicycle	3	12-15	60 secs	53
Plank Push-Up Position	3	40 secs	60 secs	39

Exercise	Sets	Reps	Rest	Exercise Number
Warm Up Session				
Box Squats into Press	3	12-15	60 secs	16

Exercise	Sets	Reps	Rest	Exercise Number
Knee Push-Ups	3	12-15	60 secs	20
Seated Dumbbell Press	3	12-15	60 secs	13
Seated Russian Twists (Chair)	3	12 (each)	60 secs	54
Arm Over Crunches	3	12-15	60 secs	45
Modified Plank	3	40 secs	60 secs	27

Week Twelve

Exercise	Sets	Reps	Rest	Exercise Number
Warm Up Session				
Knee Push-Ups	3	12-15	60 secs	20
Box Push-Ups	3	12-15	60 secs	12
Box Squats into Press	3	12-15	60 secs	16
Long Arm Crunches	3	12-15	60 secs	43
Single Long Arm Crunches	3	12 (each)	60 secs	44
Mountain Climbers on Chair	3	40 secs	60 secs	50

Exercise	Sets	Reps	Rest	Exercise Number
Warm Up Session				
Glute Bridges	3	12-15	60 secs	18
Box Squats	3	20	60 secs	9
Marching in Place	3	40 secs	60 secs	35
Foot Raised Abdominal Crunch	3	12-15	60 secs	42
Seated Wood Chops	3	12 (each)	60 secs	48
Dead Bugs	3	12-15	60 secs	51

Exercise	Sets	Reps	Rest	Exercise Number
Warm Up Session				
Wall Push-Ups	3	20	60 secs	14
Sumo Box Squat	3	12-15	60 secs	11
Squats While Holding Chair	3	20	60 secs	10
Abdominal Crunches	3	12-15	60 secs	41
Heel Taps	3	12 (each)	60 secs	40
Seated Marching in Place	3	40 secs	60 secs	37

Exercise	Sets	Reps	Rest	Exercise Number
Warm Up Session				
Knee Push-Ups	3	12-15	60 secs	20
Seated Dumbbell Press	3	12-15	60 secs	13
Box Push-Ups	3	12-15	60 secs	12
Seated Forward Bends	3	12-15	60 secs	38
Marching in Place w/ Leg Ext	3	40 secs	60 secs	36
Chair Planks	3	40 secs	60 secs	33

Week Thirteen

Exercise	Sets	Reps	Rest	Exercise Number
Warm Up Session				
Box Squat with Dumbbell	3	12-15	60 secs	15
Glute Bridges	3	12-15	60 secs	18
Single-Leg Rom Dead (Chair)	3	12 (each)	60 secs	17
Lateral Lunges	3	12 (each)	60 secs	19
Seated Knee Lifts	3	12-15	60 secs	34
Seated Marching in Place	3	40 secs	60 secs	37

Exercise	Sets	Reps	Rest	Exercise Number
Warm Up Session				
Knee Push-Ups	3	12-15	60 secs	20
Wall Push-Ups	3	20	60 secs	14
Box Push-Ups	3	12-15	60 secs	12
Bird Dog Exercise	3	12-15	60 secs	52
Wood Chops	3	12 (each)	60 secs	47
Knee-to-chest Crunches	3	12-15	60 secs	46

Exercise	Sets	Reps	Rest	Exercise Number
Warm Up Session				
Sumo Box Squat	3	12-15	60 secs	11
Box Squats into Press	3	12-15	60 secs	16
Glute Bridges	3	12-15	60 secs	18
Superman	3	12-15	60 secs	49

Exercise	Sets	Reps	Rest	Exercise Number
Seated Bicycle	3	12-15	60 secs	53
Plank Push-Up Position	3	40 secs	60 secs	39

Exercise	Sets	Reps	Rest	Exercise Number
Warm Up Session				
Box Squats into Press	3	12-15	60 secs	16
Knee Push-Ups	3	12-15	60 secs	20
Seated Dumbbell Press	3	12-15	60 secs	13
Seated Russian Twists (Chair)	3	12 (each)	60 secs	54
Arm Over Crunches	3	12-15	60 secs	45
Modified Plank	3	40 secs	60 secs	27

Week Fourteen

Exercise	Sets	Reps	Rest	Exercise Number
Warm Up Session				
Knee Push-Ups	3	12-15	60 secs	20
Box Push-Ups	3	12-15	60 secs	12
Box Squats into Press	3	12-15	60 secs	16
Long Arm Crunches	3	12-15	60 secs	43
Single Long Arm Crunches	3	12 (each)	60 secs	44
Mountain Climbers on Chair	3	40 secs	60 secs	50

Exercise	Sets	Reps	Rest	Exercise Number
Warm Up Session				
Glute Bridges	3	12-15	60 secs	18
Box Squats	3	20	60 secs	9
Marching in Place	3	40 secs	60 secs	35
Foot Raised Abdominal Crunch	3	12-15	60 secs	42
Seated Wood Chops	3	12 (each)	60 secs	48
Dead Bugs	3	12-15	60 secs	51

Exercise	Sets	Reps	Rest	Exercise Number
Warm Up Session				
Wall Push-Ups	3	20	60 secs	14
Sumo Box Squat	3	12-15	60 secs	11

Exercise	Sets	Reps	Rest	Exercise Number
Squats While Holding Chair	3	20	60 secs	10
Abdominal Crunches	3	12-15	60 secs	41
Heel Taps	3	12 (each)	60 secs	40
Seated Marching in Place	3	40 secs	60 secs	37

Exercise	Sets	Reps	Rest	Exercise Number
Warm Up Session				
Knee Push-Ups	3	12-15	60 secs	20
Seated Dumbbell Press	3	12-15	60 secs	13
Box Push-Ups	3	12-15	60 secs	12
Seated Forward Bends	3	12-15	60 secs	38
Marching in Place w/ Leg Ext	3	40 secs	60 secs	36
Chair Planks	3	40 secs	60 secs	33

Week Fifteen

Exercise	Sets	Reps	Rest	Exercise Number
Warm Up Session				
Box Squat with Dumbbell	3	12-15	60 secs	15
Glute Bridges	3	12-15	60 secs	18
Single-Leg Rom Dead (Chair)	3	12 (each)	60 secs	17
Lateral Lunges	3	12 (each)	60 secs	19
Seated Knee Lifts	3	12-15	60 secs	34
Seated Marching in Place	3	40 secs	60 secs	37

Exercise	Sets	Reps	Rest	Exercise Number
Warm Up Session				
Knee Push-Ups	3	12-15	60 secs	20
Wall Push-Ups	3	20	60 secs	14
Box Push-Ups	3	12-15	60 secs	12
Bird Dog Exercise	3	12-15	60 secs	52
Wood Chops	3	12 (each)	60 secs	47
Knee-to-chest Crunches	3	12-15	60 secs	46

Exercise	Sets	Reps	Rest	Exercise Number
Warm Up Session				
Sumo Box Squat	3	12-15	60 secs	11
Box Squats into Press	3	12-15	60 secs	16
Glute Bridges	3	12-15	60 secs	18
Superman	3	12-15	60 secs	49
Seated Bicycle	3	12-15	60 secs	53
Plank Push-Up Position	3	40 secs	60 secs	39

Exercise	Sets	Reps	Rest	Exercise Number
Warm Up Session				
Box Squats into Press	3	12-15	60 secs	16
Knee Push-Ups	3	12-15	60 secs	20
Seated Dumbbell Press	3	12-15	60 secs	13
Seated Russian Twists (Chair)	3	12 (each)	60 secs	54
Arm Over Crunches	3	12-15	60 secs	45
Modified Plank	3	40 secs	60 secs	27

Week Sixteen

Exercise	Sets	Reps	Rest	Exercise Number
Warm Up Session				
Knee Push-Ups	3	12-15	60 secs	20
Box Push-Ups	3	12-15	60 secs	12
Box Squats into Press	3	12-15	60 secs	16
Long Arm Crunches	3	12-15	60 secs	43
Single Long Arm Crunches	3	12 (each)	60 secs	44
Mountain Climbers on Chair	3	40 secs	60 secs	50

Exercise	Sets	Reps	Rest	Exercise Number
Warm Up Session				
Glute Bridges	3	12-15	60 secs	18
Box Squats	3	20	60 secs	9
Marching in Place	3	40 secs	60 secs	35
Foot Raised Abdominal Crunch	3	12-15	60 secs	42
Seated Wood Chops	3	12 (each)	60 secs	48
Dead Bugs	3	12-15	60 secs	51

Exercise	Sets	Reps	Rest	Exercise Number
Warm Up Session				
Wall Push-Ups	3	20	60 secs	14
Sumo Box Squat	3	12-15	60 secs	11
Squats While Holding Chair	3	20	60 secs	10
Abdominal Crunches	3	12-15	60 secs	41
Heel Taps	3	12 (each)	60 secs	40
Seated Marching in Place	3	40 secs	60 secs	37

Exercise	Sets	Reps	Rest	Exercise Number
Warm Up Session				
Knee Push-Ups	3	12-15	60 secs	20
Seated Dumbbell Press	3	12-15	60 secs	13
Box Push-Ups	3	12-15	60 secs	12
Seated Forward Bends	3	12-15	60 secs	38
Marching in Place w/ Leg Ext	3	40 secs	60 secs	36
Chair Planks	3	40 secs	60 secs	33

Week Seventeen

Exercise	Sets	Reps	Rest	Exercise Number
Warm Up Session				
Box Squat with Dumbbell	3	15	60 secs	15
Glute Bridges	3	15	60 secs	18
Single-Leg Rom Dead (Chair)	3	15 (each)	60 secs	17
Lateral Lunges	3	15 (each)	60 secs	19
Seated Knee Lifts	3	15	60 secs	34
Seated Marching in Place	3	50 secs	60 secs	37

Exercise	Sets	Reps	Rest	Exercise Number
Warm Up Session				
Knee Push-Ups	3	15	60 secs	20
Wall Push-Ups	3	20	60 secs	14
Box Push-Ups	3	15	60 secs	12
Bird Dog Exercise	3	15	60 secs	52

Exercise	Sets	Reps	Rest	Exercise Number
Wood Chops	3	15 (each)	60 secs	47
Knee-to-chest Crunches	3	15	60 secs	46

Exercise	Sets	Reps	Rest	Exercise Number
Warm Up Session				
Sumo Box Squat	3	15	60 secs	11
Box Squats into Press	3	15	60 secs	16
Glute Bridges	3	15	60 secs	18
Superman	3	15	60 secs	49
Seated Bicycle	3	15	60 secs	53
Plank Push-Up Position	3	50 secs	60 secs	39

Exercise	Sets	Reps	Rest	Exercise Number
Warm Up Session				
Box Squats into Press	3	15	60 secs	16
Knee Push-Ups	3	15	60 secs	20
Seated Dumbbell Press	3	15	60 secs	13
Seated Russian Twists (Chair)	3	15 (each)	60 secs	54
Arm Over Crunches	3	15	60 secs	45
Modified Plank	3	50 secs	60 secs	27

Week Eighteen

Exercise	Sets	Reps	Rest	Exercise Number
Warm Up Session				
Knee Push-Ups	3	15	60 secs	20
Box Push-Ups	3	15	60 secs	12
Box Squats into Press	3	15	60 secs	16
Long Arm Crunches	3	15	60 secs	43
Single Long Arm Crunches	3	15 (each)	60 secs	44
Mountain Climbers on Chair	3	50 secs	60 secs	50

Exercise	Sets	Reps	Rest	Exercise Number
Warm Up Session				
Glute Bridges	3	15	60 secs	18

Exercise	Sets	Reps	Rest	Exercise Number
Box Squats	3	20	60 secs	9
Marching in Place	3	50 secs	60 secs	35
Foot Raised Abdominal Crunch	3	15	60 secs	42
Seated Wood Chops	3	15 (each)	60 secs	48
Dead Bugs	3	15	60 secs	51

Exercise	Sets	Reps	Rest	Exercise Number
Warm Up Session				
Wall Push-Ups	3	20	60 secs	14
Sumo Box Squat	3	15	60 secs	11
Squats While Holding Chair	3	20	60 secs	10
Abdominal Crunches	3	15	60 secs	41
Heel Taps	3	15 (each)	60 secs	40
Seated Marching in Place	3	50 secs	60 secs	37

Exercise	Sets	Reps	Rest	Exercise Number
Warm Up Session				
Knee Push-Ups	3	15	60 secs	20
Seated Dumbbell Press	3	15	60 secs	13
Box Push-Ups	3	15	60 secs	12
Seated Forward Bends	3	15	60 secs	38
Marching in Place w/ Leg Ext	3	50 secs	60 secs	36
Chair Planks	3	50 secs	60 secs	33

Week Nineteen

Exercise	Sets	Reps	Rest	Exercise Number
Warm Up Session				
Box Squat with Dumbbell	3	15	60 secs	15
Glute Bridges	3	15	60 secs	18
Single-Leg Rom Dead (Chair)	3	15 (each)	60 secs	17
Lateral Lunges	3	15 (each)	60 secs	19
Seated Knee Lifts	3	15	60 secs	34
Seated Marching in Place	3	50 secs	60 secs	37

Exercise	Sets	Reps	Rest	Exercise Number
Warm Up Session				
Knee Push-Ups	3	15	60 secs	20
Wall Push-Ups	3	20	60 secs	14
Box Push-Ups	3	15	60 secs	12
Bird Dog Exercise	3	15	60 secs	52
Wood Chops	3	15 (each)	60 secs	47
Knee-to-chest Crunches	3	15	60 secs	46

Exercise	Sets	Reps	Rest	Exercise Number
Warm Up Session				
Sumo Box Squat	3	15	60 secs	11
Box Squats into Press	3	15	60 secs	16
Glute Bridges	3	15	60 secs	18
Superman	3	15	60 secs	49
Seated Bicycle	3	15	60 secs	53
Plank Push-Up Position	3	50 secs	60 secs	39

Exercise	Sets	Reps	Rest	Exercise Number
Warm Up Session				
Box Squats into Press	3	15	60 secs	16
Knee Push-Ups	3	15	60 secs	20
Seated Dumbbell Press	3	15	60 secs	13
Seated Russian Twists (Chair)	3	15 (each)	60 secs	54

Exercise	Sets	Reps	Rest	Exercise Number
Arm Over Crunches	3	15	60 secs	45
Modified Plank	3	50 secs	60 secs	27

Week Twenty

Exercise	Sets	Reps	Rest	Exercise Number
Warm Up Session				
Knee Push-Ups	3	15	60 secs	20
Box Push-Ups	3	15	60 secs	12
Box Squats into Press	3	15	60 secs	16
Long Arm Crunches	3	15	60 secs	43
Single Long Arm Crunches	3	12 (each)	60 secs	44
Mountain Climbers on Chair	3	50 secs	60 secs	50

Exercise	Sets	Reps	Rest	Exercise Number
Warm Up Session				
Glute Bridges	3	15	60 secs	18
Box Squats	3	20	60 secs	9
Marching in Place	3	50 secs	60 secs	35
Foot Raised Abdominal Crunch	3	15	60 secs	42
Seated Wood Chops	3	15 (each)	60 secs	48
Dead Bugs	3	15	60 secs	51

Exercise	Sets	Reps	Rest	Exercise Number
Warm Up Session				
Wall Push-Ups	3	20	60 secs	14
Sumo Box Squat	3	15	60 secs	11
Squats While Holding Chair	3	20	60 secs	10
Abdominal Crunches	3	15	60 secs	41
Heel Taps	3	15 (each)	60 secs	40
Seated Marching in Place	3	50 secs	60 secs	37

Exercise	Sets	Reps	Rest	Exercise Number
Warm Up Session				
Knee Push-Ups	3	15	60 secs	20
Seated Dumbbell Press	3	15	60 secs	13

Exercise	Sets	Reps	Rest	Exercise Number
Box Push-Ups	3	15	60 secs	12
Seated Forward Bends	3	15	60 secs	38
Marching in Place w/ Leg Ext	3	50 secs	60 secs	36
Chair Planks	3	50 secs	60 secs	33

Week Twenty One

Exercise	Sets	Reps	Rest	Exercise Number
Warm Up Session				
Box Squat with Dumbbell	3	15	60 secs	15
Glute Bridges	3	15	60 secs	18
Single-Leg Rom Dead (Chair)	3	15 (each)	60 secs	17
Lateral Lunges	3	15 (each)	60 secs	19
Seated Knee Lifts	3	15	60 secs	34
Seated Marching in Place	3	50 secs	60 secs	37

Exercise	Sets	Reps	Rest	Exercise Number
Warm Up Session				
Knee Push-Ups	3	15	60 secs	20
Wall Push-Ups	3	20	60 secs	14
Box Push-Ups	3	15	60 secs	12
Bird Dog Exercise	3	15	60 secs	52
Wood Chops	3	15 (each)	60 secs	47
Knee-to-chest Crunches	3	15	60 secs	46

Exercise	Sets	Reps	Rest	Exercise Number
Warm Up Session				
Sumo Box Squat	3	15	60 secs	11
Box Squats into Press	3	15	60 secs	16
Glute Bridges	3	15	60 secs	18
Superman	3	15	60 secs	49
Seated Bicycle	3	15	60 secs	53
Plank Push-Up Position	3	50 secs	60 secs	39

Exercise	Sets	Reps	Rest	Exercise Number
Warm Up Session				
Box Squats into Press	3	15	60 secs	16
Knee Push-Ups	3	15	60 secs	20
Seated Dumbbell Press	3	15	60 secs	13
Seated Russian Twists (Chair)	3	15 (each)	60 secs	54
Arm Over Crunches	3	15	60 secs	45
Modified Plank	3	50 secs	60 secs	27

Week Twenty Two

Exercise	Sets	Reps	Rest	Exercise Number
Warm Up Session				
Knee Push-Ups	3	15	60 secs	20
Box Push-Ups	3	15	60 secs	12
Box Squats into Press	3	15	60 secs	16
Long Arm Crunches	3	15	60 secs	43
Single Long Arm Crunches	3	12 (each)	60 secs	44
Mountain Climbers on Chair	3	50 secs	60 secs	50

Exercise	Sets	Reps	Rest	Exercise Number
Warm Up Session				
Glute Bridges	3	15	60 secs	18
Box Squats	3	20	60 secs	9
Marching in Place	3	50 secs	60 secs	35
Foot Raised Abdominal Crunch	3	15	60 secs	42
Seated Wood Chops	3	15 (each)	60 secs	48
Dead Bugs	3	15	60 secs	51

Exercise	Sets	Reps	Rest	Exercise Number
Warm Up Session				
Wall Push-Ups	3	20	60 secs	14
Sumo Box Squat	3	15	60 secs	11
Squats While Holding Chair	3	20	60 secs	10
Abdominal Crunches	3	15	60 secs	41

Exercise	Sets	Reps	Rest	Exercise Number
Heel Taps	3	15 (each)	60 secs	40
Seated Marching in Place	3	50 secs	60 secs	37

Exercise	Sets	Reps	Rest	Exercise Number
Warm Up Session				
Knee Push-Ups	3	15	60 secs	20
Seated Dumbbell Press	3	15	60 secs	13
Box Push-Ups	3	15	60 secs	12
Seated Forward Bends	3	15	60 secs	38
Marching in Place w/ Leg Ext	3	50 secs	60 secs	36
Chair Planks	3	50 secs	60 secs	33

Week Twenty Three

Exercise	Sets	Reps	Rest	Exercise Number
Warm Up Session				
Box Squat with Dumbbell	3	15-20	60 secs	15
Glute Bridges	3	15-20	60 secs	18
Single-Leg Rom Dead (Chair)	3	15 (each)	60 secs	17
Lateral Lunges	3	15 (each)	60 secs	19
Seated Knee Lifts	3	15-20	60 secs	34
Seated Marching in Place	3	50 secs	60 secs	37

Exercise	Sets	Reps	Rest	Exercise Number
Warm Up Session				
Knee Push-Ups	3	15-20	60 secs	20
Wall Push-Ups	3	20	60 secs	14
Box Push-Ups	3	15-20	60 secs	12
Bird Dog Exercise	3	15-20	60 secs	52
Wood Chops	3	15 (each)	60 secs	47
Knee-to-chest Crunches	3	15-20	60 secs	46

Exercise	Sets	Reps	Rest	Exercise Number
Warm Up Session				
Sumo Box Squat	3	15-20	60 secs	11
Box Squats into Press	3	15-20	60 secs	16
Glute Bridges	3	15-20	60 secs	18
Superman	3	15-20	60 secs	49
Seated Bicycle	3	15-20	60 secs	53
Plank Push-Up Position	3	50 secs	60 secs	39

Exercise	Sets	Reps	Rest	Exercise Number
Warm Up Session				
Box Squats into Press	3	15-20	60 secs	16
Knee Push-Ups	3	15-20	60 secs	20
Seated Dumbbell Press	3	15-20	60 secs	13
Seated Russian Twists (Chair)	3	15 (each)	60 secs	54
Arm Over Crunches	3	15-20	60 secs	45
Modified Plank	3	50 secs	60 secs	27

Week Twenty Four

Exercise	Sets	Reps	Rest	Exercise Number
Warm Up Session				
Knee Push-Ups	3	15-20	60 secs	20
Box Push-Ups	3	15-20	60 secs	12
Box Squats into Press	3	15-20	60 secs	16
Long Arm Crunches	3	15-20	60 secs	43
Single Long Arm Crunches	3	12 (each)	60 secs	44
Mountain Climbers on Chair	3	50 secs	60 secs	50

Exercise	Sets	Reps	Rest	Exercise Number
Warm Up Session				
Glute Bridges	3	15-20	60 secs	18
Box Squats	3	20	60 secs	9
Marching in Place	3	50 secs	60 secs	35
Foot Raised Abdominal Crunch	3	15-20	60 secs	42
Seated Wood Chops	3	15 (each)	60 secs	48
Dead Bugs	3	15-20	60 secs	51

Exercise	Sets	Reps	Rest	Exercise Number
Warm Up Session				
Wall Push-Ups	3	20	60 secs	14
Sumo Box Squat	3	15-20	60 secs	11
Squats While Holding Chair	3	20	60 secs	10
Abdominal Crunches	3	15-20	60 secs	41
Heel Taps	3	15 (each)	60 secs	40
Seated Marching in Place	3	50 secs	60 secs	37

Exercise	Sets	Reps	Rest	Exercise Number
Warm Up Session				
Knee Push-Ups	3	15-20	60 secs	20
Seated Dumbbell Press	3	15-20	60 secs	13
Box Push-Ups	3	15-20	60 secs	12
Seated Forward Bends	3	15-20	60 secs	38
Marching in Place w/ Leg Ext	3	50 secs	60 secs	36
Chair Planks	3	50 secs	60 secs	33

24 Week Advanced Workout

Warm Up

Exercise	Sets	Reps	Rest Between Sets
Cardio	1	5-7 minutes	n/a
Deep Squats	1	8-10	n/a
Lateral Lunges	1 (each leg)	10	30 seconds
Gentle Burpees	1	10	n/a
Body Get Ups	2	5	30 seconds
Mountain Climbers	1	30-40 seconds	n/a

Exercises

- Exercise #9 Box Squat
- Exercise #10 Squats while Holding Chair
- Exercise #11 Sumo Box Squat
- Exercise #12 Box Push-Ups
- Exercise #13 Seated Dumbbell Shoulder Press
- Exercise #14 Wall Push-Ups
- Exercise #15 Box Squat with Dumbbell
- Exercise #16 Box Squat into Shoulder Press (Dumbbells)
- Exercise #17 Single-Leg Romanian Deadlift (Chair)
- Exercise #18 Glute Bridges
- Exercise #19 Lateral Lunges
- Exercise #20 Knee Push-Ups
- Exercise #21 Bodyweight Squats
- Exercise #22 Walking Lunges
- Exercise #23 Bodyweight Sumo Squats
- Exercise #24 Squats into Shoulder Press (Dumbbells)
- Exercise #25 Push-Ups

- Exercise #26 Dumbbell Shrugs
- Exercise #27 Modified Plank
- Exercise #28 Seated Forward Roll-Ups
- Exercise #29 Seated Leg Extension
- Exercise #30 Seated Single-Leg Extension
- Exercise #31 Seated Side Bends
- Exercise #32 Bent Arm Seated Side Bends
- Exercise #33 Chair Planks
- Exercise #34 Seated Knee Lifts
- Exercise #35 Marching in Place
- Exercise #36 Marching in Place with Leg Extension
- Exercise #37 Seated Marching in Place
- Exercise #38 Seated Forward Bends
- Exercise #39 Plank (Push-Up Position)
- Exercise #40 Heel Tap Exercise
- Exercise #41 Abdominal Crunches
- Exercise #42 Foot-Raised Abdominal Crunches
- Exercise #43 Long-Arm Crunches
- Exercise #44 Single-Long-Arm Crunches
- Exercise #45 Arm Over Crunches
- Exercise #46 Knee-to-Chest Crunches
- Exercise #47 Wood Chops
- Exercise #48 Seated Wood Chops
- Exercise #49 Superman
- Exercise #50 Mountain Climbers on Chair
- Exercise #51 Dead Bugs

- Exercise #52 Bird Dog Exercise
- Exercise #53 Seated Bicycle
- Exercise #54 Seated Russian Twists (Chair)
- Exercise #55 Plank
- Exercise #56 Russian Twists
- Exercise #57 Forearm Side Plank
- Exercise #58 Standard Side Plank
- Exercise #59 Feet Elevated Plank
- Exercise #60 Mountain Climbers (Fast)
- Exercise #61 Plank Get-Ups
- Exercise #62 Negative Abdominal Crunches
- Exercise #63 Knee-to-Chest Crunches with Leg Extension
- Exercise #64 Good Mornings
- Exercise #65 Dumbbell Romanian Deadlifts
- Exercise #66 Cobra Pose

Week One

Exercise	Sets	Reps	Rest	Exercise Number
Warm Up Session				
Box Squat	3	20	60 secs	9
Box Squat into Shoulder Press	3	10	60 secs	16
DB Romanian Deadlifts	3	10	60 secs	64
Push-Ups	3	1-10	60 secs	25
Modified Plank	3	30 secs	60 secs	27
Foot-Raised Ab Crunches	3	10	60 secs	42
Marching in Place	3	30 secs	60 secs	35

Exercise	Sets	Reps	Rest	Exercise Number
Warm Up Session				
Sumo Box Squat	3	15	60 secs	11
Walking Lunges	3	20	60 secs	22
Seated DB Shoulder Press	3	10	60 secs	13
Seated Side Bends	3	10 (each)	60 secs	31
Marching in Place (Leg Ext)	3	30 secs	60 secs	36
Abdominal Crunches	3	10	60 secs	41
Chair Plank	3	30 secs	60 secs	33

Exercise	Sets	Reps	Rest	Exercise Number
Warm Up Session				
Bodyweight Sumo Squats	3	10	60 secs	23
Good Mornings	3	10	60 secs	64
Glute Bridges	3	10	60 secs	18
Dumbbell Shrugs	3	10	60 secs	26
Seated Marching in Place	3	30 secs	60 secs	37
Long Arm Crunches	3	10	60 secs	43
Plank (Push-Up Position)	3	30 secs	60 secs	39

Exercise	Sets	Reps	Rest	Exercise Number
Warm Up Session				
Squats into Shoulder Press	3	10	60 secs	24
Lateral Lunges	3	10 (each)	60 secs	19
Cobra Pose	3	10	60 secs	66
Push-Ups	3	1-10	60 secs	25
Mountain Climbers on Chair	3	30 secs	60 secs	50
Seated Bicycle	3	10	60 secs	53
Plank	3	30 secs	60 secs	55

Week Two

Exercise	Sets	Reps	Rest	Exercise Number
Warm Up Session				
Bodyweight Squats	3	10	60 secs	21
Squats while Holding Chair	3	10	60 secs	10
S-L Romanian Dead (chair)	3	10 (each)	60 secs	17
Seated Russian Twists (chair)	3	10 (each)	60 secs	54
Wood Chops	3	10 (each)	60 secs	47
Mountain Climbers (Fast)	3	30 secs	60 secs	60
Forearm Side Plank	2 (each)	30 secs	60 secs	57

Exercise	Sets	Reps	Rest	Exercise Number
Warm Up Session				
Sumo Box Squat	3	10	60 secs	11
Box Squat with Dumbbells	3	10	60 secs	15
Push-Ups	3	1-10	60 secs	25
Negative Abdominal Crunches	3	5	60 secs	62
Knee-to-Chest Crunches w Leg	3	10	60 secs	63
Plank Get Ups	3	30 secs	60 secs	61
Standard Side Plank	2 (each)	30 secs	60 secs	58

Exercise	Sets	Reps	Rest	Exercise Number
Warm Up Session				
Squats into Shoulder Press	3	10	60 secs	24
DB Romanian Deadlifts	3	10	60 secs	64
Lateral Lunges	3	10 (each)	60 secs	19
Knee Push-Ups	3	10	60 secs	20
Russian Twists	3	10 (each)	60 secs	56
Marching in Place (Leg Ext)	3	30 secs	60 secs	36
Feet-Elevated Plank	3	30 secs	60 secs	59

Exercise	Sets	Reps	Rest	Exercise Number
Warm Up Session				
Glute Bridges	3	10	60 secs	18
Walking Lunges	3	20	60 secs	22
Box Push-Ups	3	10-15	60 secs	12
Superman	3	10	60 secs	49
Bird Dog Exercise	3	10	60 secs	52
Mountain Climbers (Fast)	3	30 secs	60 secs	60
Knee to Chest Crunches	3	10	60 secs	46

Week Three

Exercise	Sets	Reps	Rest	Exercise Number
Warm Up Session				
Box Squat	3	20	60 secs	9
Box Squat into Shoulder Press	3	10	60 secs	16
DB Romanian Deadlifts	3	10	60 secs	64
Push-Ups	3	1-10	60 secs	25
Modified Plank	3	30 secs	60 secs	27
Foot-Raised Ab Crunches	3	10	60 secs	42
Marching in Place	3	30 secs	60 secs	35

Exercise	Sets	Reps	Rest	Exercise Number
Warm Up Session				
Sumo Box Squat	3	15	60 secs	11

Exercise	Sets	Reps	Rest	Exercise Number
Walking Lunges	3	20	60 secs	22
Seated DB Shoulder Press	3	10	60 secs	13
Seated Side Bends	3	10 (each)	60 secs	31
Marching in Place (Leg Ext)	3	30 secs	60 secs	36
Abdominal Crunches	3	10	60 secs	41
Chair Plank	3	30 secs	60 secs	33

Exercise	Sets	Reps	Rest	Exercise Number
Warm Up Session				
Bodyweight Sumo Squats	3	10	60 secs	23
Good Mornings	3	10	60 secs	64
Glute Bridges	3	10	60 secs	18
Dumbbell Shrugs	3	10	60 secs	26
Seated Marching in Place	3	30 secs	60 secs	37
Long Arm Crunches	3	10	60 secs	43
Plank (Push-Up Position)	3	30 secs	60 secs	39

Exercise	Sets	Reps	Rest	Exercise Number
Warm Up Session				
Squats into Shoulder Press	3	10	60 secs	24
Lateral Lunges	3	10 (each)	60 secs	19
Cobra Pose	3	10	60 secs	66
Push-Ups	3	1-10	60 secs	25
Mountain Climbers on Chair	3	30 secs	60 secs	50
Seated Bicycle	3	10	60 secs	53
Plank	3	30 secs	60 secs	55

Week Four

Exercise	Sets	Reps	Rest	Exercise Number
Warm Up Session				
Bodyweight Squats	3	10	60 secs	21
Squats while Holding Chair	3	10	60 secs	10

Exercise	Sets	Reps	Rest	Exercise Number
S-L Romanian Dead (chair)	3	10 (each)	60 secs	17
Seated Russian Twists (chair)	3	10 (each)	60 secs	54
Wood Chops	3	10 (each)	60 secs	47
Mountain Climbers (Fast)	3	30 secs	60 secs	60
Forearm Side Plank	2 (each)	30 secs	60 secs	57

Exercise	Sets	Reps	Rest	Exercise Number
Warm Up Session				
Sumo Box Squat	3	10	60 secs	11
Box Squat with Dumbbells	3	10	60 secs	15
Push-Ups	3	1-10	60 secs	25
Negative Abdominal Crunches	3	5	60 secs	62
Knee-to-Chest Crunches w Leg	3	10	60 secs	63
Plank Get Ups	3	30 secs	60 secs	61
Standard Side Plank	2 (each)	30 secs	60 secs	58

Exercise	Sets	Reps	Rest	Exercise Number
Warm Up Session				
Squats into Shoulder Press	3	10	60 secs	24
DB Romanian Deadlifts	3	10	60 secs	64
Lateral Lunges	3	10 (each)	60 secs	19
Knee Push-Ups	3	10	60 secs	20
Russian Twists	3	10 (each)	60 secs	56
Marching in Place (Leg Ext)	3	30 secs	60 secs	36
Feet-Elevated Plank	3	30 secs	60 secs	59

Exercise	Sets	Reps	Rest	Exercise Number
Warm Up Session				
Glute Bridges	3	10	60 secs	18
Walking Lunges	3	20	60 secs	22
Box Push-Ups	3	10-15	60 secs	12
Superman	3	10	60 secs	49

Exercise	Sets	Reps	Rest	Exercise Number
Bird Dog Exercise	3	10	60 secs	52
Mountain Climbers (Fast)	3	30 secs	60 secs	60
Knee to Chest Crunches	3	10	60 secs	46

Week Five

Exercise	Sets	Reps	Rest	Exercise Number
Warm Up Session				
Box Squat	3	20	60 secs	9
Box Squat into Shoulder Press	3	10	60 secs	16
DB Romanian Deadlifts	3	10	60 secs	64
Push-Ups	3	1-10	60 secs	25
Modified Plank	3	30 secs	60 secs	27
Foot-Raised Ab Crunches	3	10	60 secs	42
Marching in Place	3	30 secs	60 secs	35

Exercise	Sets	Reps	Rest	Exercise Number
Warm Up Session				
Sumo Box Squat	3	15	60 secs	11
Walking Lunges	3	20	60 secs	22
Seated DB Shoulder Press	3	10	60 secs	13
Seated Side Bends	3	10 (each)	60 secs	31
Marching in Place (Leg Ext)	3	30 secs	60 secs	36
Abdominal Crunches	3	10	60 secs	41
Chair Plank	3	30 secs	60 secs	33

Exercise	Sets	Reps	Rest	Exercise Number
Warm Up Session				
Bodyweight Sumo Squats	3	10	60 secs	23
Good Mornings	3	10	60 secs	64
Glute Bridges	3	10	60 secs	18
Dumbbell Shrugs	3	10	60 secs	26
Seated Marching in Place	3	30 secs	60 secs	37

Exercise	Sets	Reps	Rest	Exercise Number
Long Arm Crunches	3	10	60 secs	43
Plank (Push-Up Position)	3	30 secs	60 secs	39

Exercise	Sets	Reps	Rest	Exercise Number
Warm Up Session				
Squats into Shoulder Press	3	10	60 secs	24
Lateral Lunges	3	10 (each)	60 secs	19
Cobra Pose	3	10	60 secs	66
Push-Ups	3	1-10	60 secs	25
Mountain Climbers on Chair	3	30 secs	60 secs	50
Seated Bicycle	3	10	60 secs	53
Plank	3	30 secs	60 secs	55

Week Six

Exercise	Sets	Reps	Rest	Exercise Number
Warm Up Session				
Bodyweight Squats	3	10	60 secs	21
Squats while Holding Chair	3	10	60 secs	10
S-L Romanian Dead (chair)	3	10 (each)	60 secs	17
Seated Russian Twists (chair)	3	10 (each)	60 secs	54
Wood Chops	3	10 (each)	60 secs	47
Mountain Climbers (Fast)	3	30 secs	60 secs	60
Forearm Side Plank	2 (each)	30 secs	60 secs	57

Exercise	Sets	Reps	Rest	Exercise Number
Warm Up Session				
Sumo Box Squat	3	10	60 secs	11
Box Squat with Dumbbells	3	10	60 secs	15
Push-Ups	3	1-10	60 secs	25
Negative Abdominal Crunches	3	5	60 secs	62
Knee-to-Chest Crunches w Leg	3	10	60 secs	63

Exercise	Sets	Reps	Rest	Exercise Number
Plank Get Ups	3	30 secs	60 secs	61
Standard Side Plank	2 (each)	30 secs	60 secs	58

Exercise	Sets	Reps	Rest	Exercise Number
Warm Up Session				
Squats into Shoulder Press	3	10	60 secs	24
DB Romanian Deadlifts	3	10	60 secs	64
Lateral Lunges	3	10 (each)	60 secs	19
Knee Push-Ups	3	10	60 secs	20
Russian Twists	3	10 (each)	60 secs	56
Marching in Place (Leg Ext)	3	30 secs	60 secs	36
Feet-Elevated Plank	3	30 secs	60 secs	59

Exercise	Sets	Reps	Rest	Exercise Number
Warm Up Session				
Glute Bridges	3	10	60 secs	18
Walking Lunges	3	20	60 secs	22
Box Push-Ups	3	10-15	60 secs	12
Superman	3	10	60 secs	49
Bird Dog Exercise	3	10	60 secs	52
Mountain Climbers (Fast)	3	30 secs	60 secs	60
Knee to Chest Crunches	3	10	60 secs	46

Week Seven

Exercise	Sets	Reps	Rest	Exercise Number
Warm Up Session				
Box Squat	3	20	60 secs	9
Box Squat into Shoulder Press	3	10-15	60 secs	16
DB Romanian Deadlifts	3	10-15	60 secs	64
Push-Ups	3	4-12	60 secs	25
Modified Plank	3	40 secs	60 secs	27
Foot-Raised Ab Crunches	3	10-15	60 secs	42
Marching in Place	3	40 secs	60 secs	35

Exercise	Sets	Reps	Rest	Exercise Number
Warm Up Session				
Sumo Box Squat	3	15	60 secs	11
Walking Lunges	3	20	60 secs	22
Seated DB Shoulder Press	3	10-15	60 secs	13
Seated Side Bends	3	12 (each)	60 secs	31
Marching in Place (Leg Ext)	3	40 secs	60 secs	36
Abdominal Crunches	3	10-15	60 secs	41
Chair Plank	3	40 secs	60 secs	33

Exercise	Sets	Reps	Rest	Exercise Number
Warm Up Session				
Bodyweight Sumo Squats	3	10-15	60 secs	23
Good Mornings	3	10-15	60 secs	64
Glute Bridges	3	10-15	60 secs	18
Dumbbell Shrugs	3	10-15	60 secs	26
Seated Marching in Place	3	40 secs	60 secs	37
Long Arm Crunches	3	10-15	60 secs	43
Plank (Push-Up Position)	3	40 secs	60 secs	39

Exercise	Sets	Reps	Rest	Exercise Number
Warm Up Session				
Squats into Shoulder Press	3	10-15	60 secs	24
Lateral Lunges	3	12 (each)	60 secs	19
Cobra Pose	3	10-15	60 secs	66
Push-Ups	3	4-12	60 secs	25
Mountain Climbers on Chair	3	40 secs	60 secs	50
Seated Bicycle	3	10-15	60 secs	53
Plank	3	40 secs	60 secs	55

Week Eight

Exercise	Sets	Reps	Rest	Exercise Number
Warm Up Session				
Bodyweight Squats	3	10-15	60 secs	21

Exercise	Sets	Reps	Rest	Exercise Number
Squats while Holding Chair	3	10-15	60 secs	10
S-L Romanian Dead (chair)	3	12 (each)	60 secs	17
Seated Russian Twists (chair)	3	12 (each)	60 secs	54
Wood Chops	3	12 (each)	60 secs	47
Mountain Climbers (Fast)	3	40 secs	60 secs	60
Forearm Side Plank	2 (each)	40 secs	60 secs	57

Exercise	Sets	Reps	Rest	Exercise Number
Warm Up Session				
Sumo Box Squat	3	10-15	60 secs	11
Box Squat with Dumbbells	3	10-15	60 secs	15
Push-Ups	3	1-10	60 secs	25
Negative Abdominal Crunches	3	5	60 secs	62
Knee-to-Chest Crunches w Leg	3	10-15	60 secs	63
Plank Get Ups	3	40 secs	60 secs	61
Standard Side Plank	2 (each)	40 secs	60 secs	58

Exercise	Sets	Reps	Rest	Exercise Number
Warm Up Session				
Squats into Shoulder Press	3	10-15	60 secs	24
DB Romanian Deadlifts	3	10-15	60 secs	64
Lateral Lunges	3	12 (each)	60 secs	19
Knee Push-Ups	3	10-15	60 secs	20
Russian Twists	3	12 (each)	60 secs	56
Marching in Place (Leg Ext)	3	40 secs	60 secs	36
Feet-Elevated Plank	3	40 secs	60 secs	59

Exercise	Sets	Reps	Rest	Exercise Number
Warm Up Session				
Glute Bridges	3	10-15	60 secs	18
Walking Lunges	3	20	60 secs	22
Box Push-Ups	3	15	60 secs	12

Exercise	Sets	Reps	Rest	Exercise Number
Superman	3	10-15	60 secs	49
Bird Dog Exercise	3	10-15	60 secs	52
Mountain Climbers (Fast)	3	40 secs	60 secs	60
Knee to Chest Crunches	3	10-15	60 secs	46

Week Nine

Exercise	Sets	Reps	Rest	Exercise Number
Warm Up Session				
Box Squat	3	20	60 secs	9
Box Squat into Shoulder Press	3	10-15	60 secs	16
DB Romanian Deadlifts	3	10-15	60 secs	64
Push-Ups	3	4-12	60 secs	25
Modified Plank	3	40 secs	60 secs	27
Foot-Raised Ab Crunches	3	10-15	60 secs	42
Marching in Place	3	40 secs	60 secs	35

Exercise	Sets	Reps	Rest	Exercise Number
Warm Up Session				
Sumo Box Squat	3	15	60 secs	11
Walking Lunges	3	20	60 secs	22
Seated DB Shoulder Press	3	10-15	60 secs	13
Seated Side Bends	3	12 (each)	60 secs	31
Marching in Place (Leg Ext)	3	40 secs	60 secs	36
Abdominal Crunches	3	10-15	60 secs	41
Chair Plank	3	40 secs	60 secs	33

Exercise	Sets	Reps	Rest	Exercise Number
Warm Up Session				
Bodyweight Sumo Squats	3	10-15	60 secs	23
Good Mornings	3	10-15	60 secs	64
Glute Bridges	3	10-15	60 secs	18
Dumbbell Shrugs	3	10-15	60 secs	26

Exercise	Sets	Reps	Rest	Exercise Number
Seated Marching in Place	3	40 secs	60 secs	37
Long Arm Crunches	3	10-15	60 secs	43
Plank (Push-Up Position)	3	40 secs	60 secs	39

Exercise	Sets	Reps	Rest	Exercise Number
Warm Up Session				
Squats into Shoulder Press	3	10-15	60 secs	24
Lateral Lunges	3	12 (each)	60 secs	19
Cobra Pose	3	10-15	60 secs	66
Push-Ups	3	4-12	60 secs	25
Mountain Climbers on Chair	3	40 secs	60 secs	50
Seated Bicycle	3	10-15	60 secs	53
Plank	3	40 secs	60 secs	55

Week Ten

Exercise	Sets	Reps	Rest	Exercise Number
Warm Up Session				
Bodyweight Squats	3	10-15	60 secs	21
Squats while Holding Chair	3	10-15	60 secs	10
S-L Romanian Dead (chair)	3	12 (each)	60 secs	17
Seated Russian Twists (chair)	3	12 (each)	60 secs	54
Wood Chops	3	12 (each)	60 secs	47
Mountain Climbers (Fast)	3	40 secs	60 secs	60
Forearm Side Plank	2 (each)	40 secs	60 secs	57

Exercise	Sets	Reps	Rest	Exercise Number
Warm Up Session				
Sumo Box Squat	3	10-15	60 secs	11
Box Squat with Dumbbells	3	10-15	60 secs	15
Push-Ups	3	1-10	60 secs	25
Negative Abdominal Crunches	3	5	60 secs	62

Exercise	Sets	Reps	Rest	Exercise Number
Knee-to-Chest Crunches w Leg	3	10-15	60 secs	63
Plank Get Ups	3	40 secs	60 secs	61
Standard Side Plank	2 (each)	40 secs	60 secs	58

Exercise	Sets	Reps	Rest	Exercise Number
Warm Up Session				
Squats into Shoulder Press	3	10-15	60 secs	24
DB Romanian Deadlifts	3	10-15	60 secs	64
Lateral Lunges	3	12 (each)	60 secs	19
Knee Push-Ups	3	10-15	60 secs	20
Russian Twists	3	12 (each)	60 secs	56
Marching in Place (Leg Ext)	3	40 secs	60 secs	36
Feet-Elevated Plank	3	40 secs	60 secs	59

Exercise	Sets	Reps	Rest	Exercise Number
Warm Up Session				
Glute Bridges	3	10-15	60 secs	18
Walking Lunges	3	20	60 secs	22
Box Push-Ups	3	15	60 secs	12
Superman	3	10-15	60 secs	49
Bird Dog Exercise	3	10-15	60 secs	52
Mountain Climbers (Fast)	3	40 secs	60 secs	60
Knee to Chest Crunches	3	10-15	60 secs	46

Week Eleven

Exercise	Sets	Reps	Rest	Exercise Number
Warm Up Session				
Box Squat	3	20	60 secs	9
Box Squat into Shoulder Press	3	10-15	60 secs	16
DB Romanian Deadlifts	3	10-15	60 secs	64
Push-Ups	3	4-12	60 secs	25
Modified Plank	3	40 secs	60 secs	27

Exercise	Sets	Reps	Rest	Exercise Number
Foot-Raised Ab Crunches	3	10-15	60 secs	42
Marching in Place	3	40 secs	60 secs	35

Exercise	Sets	Reps	Rest	Exercise Number
Warm Up Session				
Sumo Box Squat	3	15	60 secs	11
Walking Lunges	3	20	60 secs	22
Seated DB Shoulder Press	3	10-15	60 secs	13
Seated Side Bends	3	12 (each)	60 secs	31
Marching in Place (Leg Ext)	3	40 secs	60 secs	36
Abdominal Crunches	3	10-15	60 secs	41
Chair Plank	3	40 secs	60 secs	33

Exercise	Sets	Reps	Rest	Exercise Number
Warm Up Session				
Bodyweight Sumo Squats	3	10-15	60 secs	23
Good Mornings	3	10-15	60 secs	64
Glute Bridges	3	10-15	60 secs	18
Dumbbell Shrugs	3	10-15	60 secs	26
Seated Marching in Place	3	40 secs	60 secs	37
Long Arm Crunches	3	10-15	60 secs	43
Plank (Push-Up Position)	3	40 secs	60 secs	39

Exercise	Sets	Reps	Rest	Exercise Number
Warm Up Session				
Squats into Shoulder Press	3	10-15	60 secs	24
Lateral Lunges	3	12 (each)	60 secs	19
Cobra Pose	3	10-15	60 secs	66
Push-Ups	3	4-12	60 secs	25
Mountain Climbers on Chair	3	40 secs	60 secs	50
Seated Bicycle	3	10-15	60 secs	53
Plank	3	40 secs	60 secs	55

Week Twelve

Exercise	Sets	Reps	Rest	Exercise Number
Warm Up Session				
Bodyweight Squats	3	10-15	60 secs	21
Squats while Holding Chair	3	10-15	60 secs	10
S-L Romanian Dead (chair)	3	12 (each)	60 secs	17
Seated Russian Twists (chair)	3	12 (each)	60 secs	54
Wood Chops	3	12 (each)	60 secs	47
Mountain Climbers (Fast)	3	40 secs	60 secs	60
Forearm Side Plank	2 (each)	40 secs	60 secs	57

Exercise	Sets	Reps	Rest	Exercise Number
Warm Up Session				
Sumo Box Squat	3	10-15	60 secs	11
Box Squat with Dumbbells	3	10-15	60 secs	15
Push-Ups	3	1-10	60 secs	25
Negative Abdominal Crunches	3	5	60 secs	62
Knee-to-Chest Crunches w Leg	3	10-15	60 secs	63
Plank Get Ups	3	40 secs	60 secs	61
Standard Side Plank	2 (each)	40 secs	60 secs	58

Exercise	Sets	Reps	Rest	Exercise Number
Warm Up Session				
Squats into Shoulder Press	3	10-15	60 secs	24
DB Romanian Deadlifts	3	10-15	60 secs	64
Lateral Lunges	3	12 (each)	60 secs	19
Knee Push-Ups	3	10-15	60 secs	20
Russian Twists	3	12 (each)	60 secs	56
Marching in Place (Leg Ext)	3	40 secs	60 secs	36
Feet-Elevated Plank	3	40 secs	60 secs	59

Exercise	Sets	Reps	Rest	Exercise Number
Warm Up Session				
Glute Bridges	3	10-15	60 secs	18
Walking Lunges	3	20	60 secs	22
Box Push-Ups	3	15	60 secs	12
Superman	3	10-15	60 secs	49
Bird Dog Exercise	3	10-15	60 secs	52
Mountain Climbers (Fast)	3	40 secs	60 secs	60
Knee to Chest Crunches	3	10-15	60 secs	46

Week Thirteen

Exercise	Sets	Reps	Rest	Exercise Number
Warm Up Session				
Box Squat	3	20	60 secs	9
Box Squat into Shoulder Press	3	15	60 secs	16
DB Romanian Deadlifts	3	15	60 secs	64
Push-Ups	3	6-15	60 secs	25
Modified Plank	3	50 secs	60 secs	27
Foot-Raised Ab Crunches	3	15	60 secs	42
Marching in Place	3	50 secs	60 secs	35

Exercise	Sets	Reps	Rest	Exercise Number
Warm Up Session				
Sumo Box Squat	3	15	60 secs	11
Walking Lunges	3	20	60 secs	22
Seated DB Shoulder Press	3	15	60 secs	13
Seated Side Bends	3	15 (each)	60 secs	31
Marching in Place (Leg Ext)	3	50 secs	60 secs	36
Abdominal Crunches	3	15	60 secs	41
Chair Plank	3	50 secs	60 secs	33

Exercise	Sets	Reps	Rest	Exercise Number
Warm Up Session				
Bodyweight Sumo Squats	3	15	60 secs	23

Exercise	Sets	Reps	Rest	Exercise Number
Good Mornings	3	15	60 secs	64
Glute Bridges	3	15	60 secs	18
Dumbbell Shrugs	3	15	60 secs	26
Seated Marching in Place	3	50 secs	60 secs	37
Long Arm Crunches	3	15	60 secs	43
Plank (Push-Up Position)	3	50 secs	60 secs	39

Exercise	Sets	Reps	Rest	Exercise Number
Warm Up Session				
Squats into Shoulder Press	3	15	60 secs	24
Lateral Lunges	3	15 (each)	60 secs	19
Cobra Pose	3	15	60 secs	66
Push-Ups	3	4-12	60 secs	25
Mountain Climbers on Chair	3	50 secs	60 secs	50
Seated Bicycle	3	15	60 secs	53
Plank	3	50 secs	60 secs	55

Week Fourteen

Exercise	Sets	Reps	Rest	Exercise Number
Warm Up Session				
Bodyweight Squats	3	15	60 secs	21
Squats while Holding Chair	3	15	60 secs	10
S-L Romanian Dead (chair)	3	12 (each)	60 secs	17
Seated Russian Twists (chair)	3	12 (each)	60 secs	54
Wood Chops	3	12 (each)	60 secs	47
Mountain Climbers (Fast)	3	50 secs	60 secs	60
Forearm Side Plank	2 (each)	50 secs	60 secs	57

Exercise	Sets	Reps	Rest	Exercise Number
Warm Up Session				
Sumo Box Squat	3	15	60 secs	11
Box Squat with Dumbbells	3	15	60 secs	15

Exercise	Sets	Reps	Rest	Exercise Number
Push-Ups	3	1-15	60 secs	25
Negative Abdominal Crunches	3	5	60 secs	62
Knee-to-Chest Crunches w Leg	3	15	60 secs	63
Plank Get Ups	3	50 secs	60 secs	61
Standard Side Plank	2 (each)	50 secs	60 secs	58

Exercise	Sets	Reps	Rest	Exercise Number
Warm Up Session				
Squats into Shoulder Press	3	15	60 secs	24
DB Romanian Deadlifts	3	15	60 secs	64
Lateral Lunges	3	15 (each)	60 secs	19
Knee Push-Ups	3	15	60 secs	20
Russian Twists	3	15 (each)	60 secs	56
Marching in Place (Leg Ext)	3	50 secs	60 secs	36
Feet-Elevated Plank	3	50 secs	60 secs	59

Exercise	Sets	Reps	Rest	Exercise Number
Warm Up Session				
Glute Bridges	3	15	60 secs	18
Walking Lunges	3	20	60 secs	22
Box Push-Ups	3	15	60 secs	12
Superman	3	15	60 secs	49
Bird Dog Exercise	3	15	60 secs	52
Mountain Climbers (Fast)	3	50 secs	60 secs	60
Knee to Chest Crunches	3	15	60 secs	46

Week Fifteen

Exercise	Sets	Reps	Rest	Exercise Number
Warm Up Session				
Box Squat	3	20	60 secs	9
Box Squat into Shoulder Press	3	15	60 secs	16
DB Romanian Deadlifts	3	15	60 secs	64

Exercise	Sets	Reps	Rest	Exercise Number
Push-Ups	3	6-15	60 secs	25
Modified Plank	3	50 secs	60 secs	27
Foot-Raised Ab Crunches	3	15	60 secs	42
Marching in Place	3	50 secs	60 secs	35

Exercise	Sets	Reps	Rest	Exercise Number
Warm Up Session				
Sumo Box Squat	3	15	60 secs	11
Walking Lunges	3	20	60 secs	22
Seated DB Shoulder Press	3	15	60 secs	13
Seated Side Bends	3	15 (each)	60 secs	31
Marching in Place (Leg Ext)	3	50 secs	60 secs	36
Abdominal Crunches	3	15	60 secs	41
Chair Plank	3	50 secs	60 secs	33

Exercise	Sets	Reps	Rest	Exercise Number
Warm Up Session				
Bodyweight Sumo Squats	3	15	60 secs	23
Good Mornings	3	15	60 secs	64
Glute Bridges	3	15	60 secs	18
Dumbbell Shrugs	3	15	60 secs	26
Seated Marching in Place	3	50 secs	60 secs	37
Long Arm Crunches	3	15	60 secs	43
Plank (Push-Up Position)	3	50 secs	60 secs	39

Exercise	Sets	Reps	Rest	Exercise Number
Warm Up Session				
Squats into Shoulder Press	3	15	60 secs	24
Lateral Lunges	3	15 (each)	60 secs	19
Cobra Pose	3	15	60 secs	66
Push-Ups	3	4-12	60 secs	25
Mountain Climbers on Chair	3	50 secs	60 secs	50
Seated Bicycle	3	15	60 secs	53
Plank	3	50 secs	60 secs	55

Week Sixteen

Exercise	Sets	Reps	Rest	Exercise Number
Warm Up Session				
Bodyweight Squats	3	15	60 secs	21
Squats while Holding Chair	3	15	60 secs	10
S-L Romanian Dead (chair)	3	12 (each)	60 secs	17
Seated Russian Twists (chair)	3	12 (each)	60 secs	54
Wood Chops	3	12 (each)	60 secs	47
Mountain Climbers (Fast)	3	50 secs	60 secs	60
Forearm Side Plank	2 (each)	50 secs	60 secs	57

Exercise	Sets	Reps	Rest	Exercise Number
Warm Up Session				
Sumo Box Squat	3	15	60 secs	11
Box Squat with Dumbbells	3	15	60 secs	15
Push-Ups	3	1-15	60 secs	25
Negative Abdominal Crunches	3	5	60 secs	62
Knee-to-Chest Crunches w Leg	3	15	60 secs	63
Plank Get Ups	3	50 secs	60 secs	61
Standard Side Plank	2 (each)	50 secs	60 secs	58

Exercise	Sets	Reps	Rest	Exercise Number
Warm Up Session				
Squats into Shoulder Press	3	15	60 secs	24
DB Romanian Deadlifts	3	15	60 secs	64
Lateral Lunges	3	15 (each)	60 secs	19
Knee Push-Ups	3	15	60 secs	20
Russian Twists	3	15 (each)	60 secs	56
Marching in Place (Leg Ext)	3	50 secs	60 secs	36
Feet-Elevated Plank	3	50 secs	60 secs	59

Exercise	Sets	Reps	Rest	Exercise Number
Warm Up Session				
Glute Bridges	3	15	60 secs	18
Walking Lunges	3	20	60 secs	22
Box Push-Ups	3	15	60 secs	12
Superman	3	15	60 secs	49
Bird Dog Exercise	3	15	60 secs	52
Mountain Climbers (Fast)	3	50 secs	60 secs	60
Knee to Chest Crunches	3	15	60 secs	46

Week Seventeen

Exercise	Sets	Reps	Rest	Exercise Number
Warm Up Session				
Box Squat	3	20	60 secs	9
Box Squat into Shoulder Press	3	15	60 secs	16
DB Romanian Deadlifts	3	15	60 secs	64
Push-Ups	3	6-15	60 secs	25
Modified Plank	3	50 secs	60 secs	27
Foot-Raised Ab Crunches	3	15	60 secs	42
Marching in Place	3	50 secs	60 secs	35

Exercise	Sets	Reps	Rest	Exercise Number
Warm Up Session				
Sumo Box Squat	3	15	60 secs	11
Walking Lunges	3	20	60 secs	22
Seated DB Shoulder Press	3	15	60 secs	13
Seated Side Bends	3	15 (each)	60 secs	31
Marching in Place (Leg Ext)	3	50 secs	60 secs	36
Abdominal Crunches	3	15	60 secs	41
Chair Plank	3	50 secs	60 secs	33

Exercise	Sets	Reps	Rest	Exercise Number
Warm Up Session				
Bodyweight Sumo Squats	3	15	60 secs	23

Exercise	Sets	Reps	Rest	Exercise Number
Good Mornings	3	15	60 secs	64
Glute Bridges	3	15	60 secs	18
Dumbbell Shrugs	3	15	60 secs	26
Seated Marching in Place	3	50 secs	60 secs	37
Long Arm Crunches	3	15	60 secs	43
Plank (Push-Up Position)	3	50 secs	60 secs	39

Exercise	Sets	Reps	Rest	Exercise Number
Warm Up Session				
Squats into Shoulder Press	3	15	60 secs	24
Lateral Lunges	3	15 (each)	60 secs	19
Cobra Pose	3	15	60 secs	66
Push-Ups	3	4-12	60 secs	25
Mountain Climbers on Chair	3	50 secs	60 secs	50
Seated Bicycle	3	15	60 secs	53
Plank	3	50 secs	60 secs	55

Week Eighteen

Exercise	Sets	Reps	Rest	Exercise Number
Warm Up Session				
Bodyweight Squats	3	15	60 secs	21
Squats while Holding Chair	3	15	60 secs	10
S-L Romanian Dead (chair)	3	15 (each)	60 secs	17
Seated Russian Twists (chair)	3	15 (each)	60 secs	54
Wood Chops	3	15 (each)	60 secs	47
Mountain Climbers (Fast)	3	60 secs	60 secs	60
Forearm Side Plank	2 (each)	60 secs	60 secs	57

Exercise	Sets	Reps	Rest	Exercise Number
Warm Up Session				
Sumo Box Squat	3	15	60 secs	11
Box Squat with Dumbbells	3	15	60 secs	15

Exercise	Sets	Reps	Rest	Exercise Number
Push-Ups	3	1-15	60 secs	25
Negative Abdominal Crunches	3	5	60 secs	62
Knee-to-Chest Crunches w Leg	3	15	60 secs	63
Plank Get Ups	3	60 secs	60 secs	61
Standard Side Plank	2 (each)	60 secs	60 secs	58

Exercise	Sets	Reps	Rest	Exercise Number
Warm Up Session				
Squats into Shoulder Press	3	15	60 secs	24
DB Romanian Deadlifts	3	15	60 secs	64
Lateral Lunges	3	15 (each)	60 secs	19
Knee Push-Ups	3	15	60 secs	20
Russian Twists	3	15 (each)	60 secs	56
Marching in Place (Leg Ext)	3	60 secs	60 secs	36
Feet-Elevated Plank	3	60 secs	60 secs	59

Exercise	Sets	Reps	Rest	Exercise Number
Warm Up Session				
Glute Bridges	3	15	60 secs	18
Walking Lunges	3	20	60 secs	22
Box Push-Ups	3	15	60 secs	12
Superman	3	15	60 secs	49
Bird Dog Exercise	3	15	60 secs	52
Mountain Climbers (Fast)	3	60 secs	60 secs	60
Knee to Chest Crunches	3	15	60 secs	46

Week Nineteen

Exercise	Sets	Reps	Rest	Exercise Number
Warm Up Session				
Bodyweight Squats	3	15-20	60 secs	21
Squats while Holding Chair	3	15-20	60 secs	10
S-L Romanian Dead (chair)	3	15 (each)	60 secs	17

Exercise	Sets	Reps	Rest	Exercise Number
Seated Russian Twists (chair)	3	15 (each)	60 secs	54
Wood Chops	3	15 (each)	60 secs	47
Mountain Climbers (Fast)	3	60 secs	60 secs	60
Forearm Side Plank	2 (each)	60 secs	60 secs	57

Exercise	Sets	Reps	Rest	Exercise Number
Warm Up Session				
Sumo Box Squat	3	15-20	60 secs	11
Box Squat with Dumbbells	3	15-20	60 secs	15
Push-Ups	3	1-15	60 secs	25
Negative Abdominal Crunches	3	5	60 secs	62
Knee-to-Chest Crunches w Leg	3	15-20	60 secs	63
Plank Get Ups	3	60 secs	60 secs	61
Standard Side Plank	2 (each)	60 secs	60 secs	58

Exercise	Sets	Reps	Rest	Exercise Number
Warm Up Session				
Squats into Shoulder Press	3	15-20	60 secs	24
DB Romanian Deadlifts	3	15-20	60 secs	64
Lateral Lunges	3	15 (each)	60 secs	19
Knee Push-Ups	3	15	60 secs	20
Russian Twists	3	15 (each)	60 secs	56
Marching in Place (Leg Ext)	3	60 secs	60 secs	36
Feet-Elevated Plank	3	60 secs	60 secs	59

Exercise	Sets	Reps	Rest	Exercise Number
Warm Up Session				
Glute Bridges	3	15-20	60 secs	18
Walking Lunges	3	20	60 secs	22
Box Push-Ups	3	15-20	60 secs	12
Superman	3	15-20	60 secs	49
Bird Dog Exercise	3	15-20	60 secs	52

Exercise	Sets	Reps	Rest	Exercise Number
Mountain Climbers (Fast)	3	60 secs	60 secs	60
Knee to Chest Crunches	3	15-20	60 secs	46

Week Twenty

Exercise	Sets	Reps	Rest	Exercise Number
Warm Up Session				
Bodyweight Squats	3	15-20	60 secs	21
Squats while Holding Chair	3	15-20	60 secs	10
S-L Romanian Dead (chair)	3	15 (each)	60 secs	17
Seated Russian Twists (chair)	3	15 (each)	60 secs	54
Wood Chops	3	15 (each)	60 secs	47
Mountain Climbers (Fast)	3	60 secs	60 secs	60
Forearm Side Plank	2 (each)	60 secs	60 secs	57

Exercise	Sets	Reps	Rest	Exercise Number
Warm Up Session				
Sumo Box Squat	3	15-20	60 secs	11
Box Squat with Dumbbells	3	15-20	60 secs	15
Push-Ups	3	1-15	60 secs	25
Negative Abdominal Crunches	3	5	60 secs	62
Knee-to-Chest Crunches w Leg	3	15-20	60 secs	63
Plank Get Ups	3	60 secs	60 secs	61
Standard Side Plank	2 (each)	60 secs	60 secs	58

Exercise	Sets	Reps	Rest	Exercise Number
Warm Up Session				
Squats into Shoulder Press	3	15-20	60 secs	24
DB Romanian Deadlifts	3	15-20	60 secs	64
Lateral Lunges	3	15 (each)	60 secs	19
Knee Push-Ups	3	15	60 secs	20
Russian Twists	3	15 (each)	60 secs	56

Exercise	Sets	Reps	Rest	Exercise Number
Marching in Place (Leg Ext)	3	60 secs	60 secs	36
Feet-Elevated Plank	3	60 secs	60 secs	59

Exercise	Sets	Reps	Rest	Exercise Number
Warm Up Session				
Glute Bridges	3	15-20	60 secs	18
Walking Lunges	3	20	60 secs	22
Box Push-Ups	3	15-20	60 secs	12
Superman	3	15-20	60 secs	49
Bird Dog Exercise	3	15-20	60 secs	52
Mountain Climbers (Fast)	3	60 secs	60 secs	60
Knee to Chest Crunches	3	15-20	60 secs	46

Week Twenty One

Exercise	Sets	Reps	Rest	Exercise Number
Warm Up Session				
Bodyweight Squats	3	15-20	60 secs	21
Squats while Holding Chair	3	15-20	60 secs	10
S-L Romanian Dead (chair)	3	15 (each)	60 secs	17
Seated Russian Twists (chair)	3	15 (each)	60 secs	54
Wood Chops	3	15 (each)	60 secs	47
Mountain Climbers (Fast)	3	60 secs	60 secs	60
Forearm Side Plank	2 (each)	60 secs	60 secs	57

Exercise	Sets	Reps	Rest	Exercise Number
Warm Up Session				
Sumo Box Squat	3	15-20	60 secs	11
Box Squat with Dumbbells	3	15-20	60 secs	15
Push-Ups	3	1-15	60 secs	25
Negative Abdominal Crunches	3	5	60 secs	62
Knee-to-Chest Crunches w Leg	3	15-20	60 secs	63

Exercise	Sets	Reps	Rest	Exercise Number
Plank Get Ups	3	60 secs	60 secs	61
Standard Side Plank	2 (each)	60 secs	60 secs	58

Exercise	Sets	Reps	Rest	Exercise Number
Warm Up Session				
Squats into Shoulder Press	3	15-20	60 secs	24
DB Romanian Deadlifts	3	15-20	60 secs	64
Lateral Lunges	3	15 (each)	60 secs	19
Knee Push-Ups	3	15	60 secs	20
Russian Twists	3	15 (each)	60 secs	56
Marching in Place (Leg Ext)	3	60 secs	60 secs	36
Feet-Elevated Plank	3	60 secs	60 secs	59

Exercise	Sets	Reps	Rest	Exercise Number
Warm Up Session				
Glute Bridges	3	15-20	60 secs	18
Walking Lunges	3	20	60 secs	22
Box Push-Ups	3	15-20	60 secs	12
Superman	3	15-20	60 secs	49
Bird Dog Exercise	3	15-20	60 secs	52
Mountain Climbers (Fast)	3	60 secs	60 secs	60
Knee to Chest Crunches	3	15-20	60 secs	46

Week Twenty Two

Exercise	Sets	Reps	Rest	Exercise Number
Warm Up Session				
Bodyweight Squats	3	15-20	60 secs	21
Squats while Holding Chair	3	15-20	60 secs	10
S-L Romanian Dead (chair)	3	15 (each)	60 secs	17
Seated Russian Twists (chair)	3	15 (each)	60 secs	54
Wood Chops	3	15 (each)	60 secs	47
Mountain Climbers (Fast)	3	60 secs	60 secs	60
Forearm Side Plank	2 (each)	60 secs	60 secs	57

Exercise	Sets	Reps	Rest	Exercise Number
Warm Up Session				
Sumo Box Squat	3	15-20	60 secs	11
Box Squat with Dumbbells	3	15-20	60 secs	15
Push-Ups	3	1-15	60 secs	25
Negative Abdominal Crunches	3	5	60 secs	62
Knee-to-Chest Crunches w Leg	3	15-20	60 secs	63
Plank Get Ups	3	60 secs	60 secs	61
Standard Side Plank	2 (each)	60 secs	60 secs	58

Exercise	Sets	Reps	Rest	Exercise Number
Warm Up Session				
Squats into Shoulder Press	3	15-20	60 secs	24
DB Romanian Deadlifts	3	15-20	60 secs	64
Lateral Lunges	3	15 (each)	60 secs	19
Knee Push-Ups	3	15	60 secs	20
Russian Twists	3	15 (each)	60 secs	56
Marching in Place (Leg Ext)	3	60 secs	60 secs	36
Feet-Elevated Plank	3	60 secs	60 secs	59

Exercise	Sets	Reps	Rest	Exercise Number
Warm Up Session				
Glute Bridges	3	15-20	60 secs	18
Walking Lunges	3	20	60 secs	22
Box Push-Ups	3	15-20	60 secs	12
Superman	3	15-20	60 secs	49
Bird Dog Exercise	3	15-20	60 secs	52
Mountain Climbers (Fast)	3	60 secs	60 secs	60
Knee to Chest Crunches	3	15-20	60 secs	46

Week Twenty Three

Exercise	Sets	Reps	Rest	Exercise Number
Warm Up Session				
Bodyweight Squats	3	15-20	60 secs	21
Squats while Holding Chair	3	15-20	60 secs	10
S-L Romanian Dead (chair)	3	15 (each)	60 secs	17
Seated Russian Twists (chair)	3	15 (each)	60 secs	54
Wood Chops	3	15 (each)	60 secs	47
Mountain Climbers (Fast)	3	60 secs	60 secs	60
Forearm Side Plank	2 (each)	60 secs	60 secs	57

Exercise	Sets	Reps	Rest	Exercise Number
Warm Up Session				
Sumo Box Squat	3	15-20	60 secs	11
Box Squat with Dumbbells	3	15-20	60 secs	15
Push-Ups	3	1-15	60 secs	25
Negative Abdominal Crunches	3	5	60 secs	62
Knee-to-Chest Crunches w Leg	3	15-20	60 secs	63
Plank Get Ups	3	60 secs	60 secs	61
Standard Side Plank	2 (each)	60 secs	60 secs	58

Exercise	Sets	Reps	Rest	Exercise Number
Warm Up Session				
Squats into Shoulder Press	3	15-20	60 secs	24
DB Romanian Deadlifts	3	15-20	60 secs	64
Lateral Lunges	3	15 (each)	60 secs	19
Knee Push-Ups	3	15	60 secs	20
Russian Twists	3	15 (each)	60 secs	56
Marching in Place (Leg Ext)	3	60 secs	60 secs	36
Feet-Elevated Plank	3	60 secs	60 secs	59

Exercise	Sets	Reps	Rest	Exercise Number
Warm Up Session				
Glute Bridges	3	15-20	60 secs	18
Walking Lunges	3	20	60 secs	22
Box Push-Ups	3	15-20	60 secs	12
Superman	3	15-20	60 secs	49
Bird Dog Exercise	3	15-20	60 secs	52
Mountain Climbers (Fast)	3	60 secs	60 secs	60
Knee to Chest Crunches	3	15-20	60 secs	46

Week Twenty Four

Exercise	Sets	Reps	Rest	Exercise Number
Warm Up Session				
Bodyweight Squats	3	15-20	60 secs	21
Squats while Holding Chair	3	15-20	60 secs	10
S-L Romanian Dead (chair)	3	15 (each)	60 secs	17
Seated Russian Twists (chair)	3	15 (each)	60 secs	54
Wood Chops	3	15 (each)	60 secs	47
Mountain Climbers (Fast)	3	60 secs	60 secs	60
Forearm Side Plank	2 (each)	60 secs	60 secs	57

Exercise	Sets	Reps	Rest	Exercise Number
Warm Up Session				
Sumo Box Squat	3	15-20	60 secs	11
Box Squat with Dumbbells	3	15-20	60 secs	15
Push-Ups	3	1-15	60 secs	25
Negative Abdominal Crunches	3	5	60 secs	62
Knee-to-Chest Crunches w Leg	3	15-20	60 secs	63
Plank Get Ups	3	60 secs	60 secs	61
Standard Side Plank	2 (each)	60 secs	60 secs	58

Exercise	Sets	Reps	Rest	Exercise Number
Warm Up Session				
Squats into Shoulder Press	3	15-20	60 secs	24
DB Romanian Deadlifts	3	15-20	60 secs	64
Lateral Lunges	3	15 (each)	60 secs	19
Knee Push-Ups	3	15	60 secs	20
Russian Twists	3	15 (each)	60 secs	56
Marching in Place (Leg Ext)	3	60 secs	60 secs	36
Feet-Elevated Plank	3	60 secs	60 secs	59

Exercise	Sets	Reps	Rest	Exercise Number
Warm Up Session				
Glute Bridges	3	15-20	60 secs	18
Walking Lunges	3	20	60 secs	22
Box Push-Ups	3	15-20	60 secs	12
Superman	3	15-20	60 secs	49
Bird Dog Exercise	3	15-20	60 secs	52
Mountain Climbers (Fast)	3	60 secs	60 secs	60
Knee to Chest Crunches	3	15-20	60 secs	46

CHAPTER 13

Frequently Asked Questions

SCAN FOR AUDIO CHAPTER

My muscles ache, should I still train?

Muscle soreness is a normal part of training, particularly during the first few weeks of a training program. Whether you train or rest an extra day will depend on how debilitating the pain feels. Some of you may find that your muscles ache too much for exercise to be comfortable, while others will barely notice the difference.

How can I reduce pain from muscle soreness?

Pain killers, muscle pain relieving gels, hot baths with Epsom salts, a good night's sleep, and some gentle exercise (walking, yoga, stretching etc). Time is the greatest healer when it comes to muscle soreness.

The rest periods feel too long, can I shorten them?

The rest periods have been designed for people who are aged between 50 and 100, so you may find that the rest period is a little longer than you need. If this is the case, then you can shorten your rest periods. However, if you are not feeling tired after a set, then you may need to ascertain whether you are training hard enough.

I feel pain in X when I perform Y exercise, what should I do?

There are many reasons why you may be feeling pain during an exercise. 1) You may be performing the exercise incorrectly, 2) Your muscle may be aching from overuse, 3) the specific movement may not be a good fit for your body, or 4) You may have an underlying injury that is only exposed when your body is in certain positions. The easiest reason to address is #1, as you can study the exercise more carefully and check your form. For any other reason, talk to a physiotherapist.

Should I eat more protein if I am working out regularly?

If you are over 60, then you should be increasing your protein intake anyway. As very few people over 60 get enough protein in their diets. But yes, regular exercise requires more protein. Finding high-protein foods or purchasing a protein supplement is a very good idea.

I can't hit the rep target for an exercise in the program, what should I do?

Don't try and force it, just perform as many reps as you can with good form. If you aren't even close (say that the target is 10 reps and you can only perform 1) then swap in an easier exercise. Or just perform that one rep focusing on ensuring the exercise is performed correctly and build from there.

Do I need to complete every exercise in a workout session?

You will get the best results that way, but no you do not need to perform every exercise. Provided you are working hard and feel fatigued at the end of each session, you will do well.

CHAPTER 14

Conclusion

SCAN FOR AUDIO CHAPTER

'Take pride in how far you've come. Have faith in how far you can go. But don't forget to enjoy the journey'.

Michael Josephson

So, there you have it. Three 24-week training programs that can help you to build a stronger and more robust core. This will help to improve your lifestyle, give you more confidence and competence in everyday life, and may well improve your independence as you age.

Remember to always talk to a doctor before embarking on a new training program, and study each exercise description and illustration carefully before performing them for the first time. Do that and you can expect incredible results in just 6 months.

Good luck!

Spread the Word

If you enjoyed this book as much as I have enjoyed writing it, and if you feel (as I surely hope) that the core exercises and workouts that you've received here provide benefits that improve your health and fitness please tell others.

Spread the word by referrals to friends, family, and other seniors (and soon-to-be seniors) whom you know, and who you think can benefit.

Our Community:

To be one of the first people to receive notification of future books in the series *"For Seniors 50, 60 and Beyond"* when they are released join our community. I'll personally notify you as soon the next book in the series is available. Our monthly newsletter also contains tip, tricks and advice to help you on your fitness journey.

As a member you have access to the exercise videos directly from our website ***www.iaa.pub***, without the need to scan individual QR codes within the book.

Finally, I wish to thank you so much for reading *Core Training for Seniors 50, 60 and Beyond*. It was written to provide exercises for seniors of all current fitness and mobility levels. If you follow the appropriate 24 week core training program (beginner, intermediate or advanced) you will add a crucial component to your fitness training and be amazed by the results you'll achieve!

I Have A Favor To Ask:

Would you please take a couple of minutes to write a review of this book on Amazon? I'll be checking the reviews personally and your honest feedback will help me better help other seniors achieve their goals.

Reviews are the life blood of indie authors trying to compete with the large advertising budgets of established publishers. Every review means so much and is greatly appreciated.

Thank you in advance!

To Leave A Review:

You can either:

- Scan the QR Code on your mobile

or

- ***Use this Amazon link:*** https://Amazon.com/review/create-review?&asin=B0CCSHL8Z1

Thank you very much, and I look forward to reading your comments!

David O'Connor

For Seniors 50, 60 and Beyond

BOOK SERIES

Book 1: **Fitness For Seniors 50, 60 and Beyond**

It's never too early to improve your fitness and definitely never to late to start. Consider this a fitness guide book, dip into to its sections as and when required.

Book 2: **Resistance Bands For Seniors 50, 60 and Beyond**

Strength and flexibility training without the need to purchase expensive weights and with less risk of injury, or a gym membership.

Book 3: **Balance Exercise For Seniors 50, 60 and Beyond**

Improve your balance to significantly reduce the risk and overcome the fear of falling. Live an active life in your golden years with increased self-confidence.

Book 4: **Chair Yoga For Seniors 50, 60 and Beyond**

All the benefits of yoga achievable while sitting or using a chair for additional support. Chair yoga offers variations that are perfect for seniors, even for those with limited mobility.

Book 5: **Stretches For Seniors 50, 60 and Beyond**

Stretches to improve flexibility, balance, mobility and reduce muscle pain for beginner through to advanced practitioners. Stretching helps release muscle tension, soreness and reduces the risk of injury.

Book 6: **Core Training For Seniors 50, 60 and Beyond**

A strong core stabilizes your entire body, providing better balance and posture. Core strength is essential at any age but especially as you get older and your risk of falling increases.

An overview of the For Seniors 50, 60 and Beyond book series is available at www.iaa.pub or scan the QR code.

SCAN FOR BOOK INFORMATION

References

[1] Gremaud, A. L., Carr, L. J., Simmering, J. E., Evans, N. J., Cremer, J. F., Segre, A. M., Polgreen, L. A., & Polgreen, P. M. (2018). Gamifying Accelerometer Use Increases Physical Activity Levels of Sedentary Office Workers. *Journal of the American Heart Association*, 7(13). https://doi.org/10.1161/jaha.117.007735

[2] Barber, S.E./A. Forster/K.M. Birch (2015): Levels and Patterns of Daily Physical Activity and Sedentary Behavior Measured Objectively in Older Care Home Residents in the United Kingdom, in: *Journal of Aging and Physical Activity,* Human Kinetics, vol. 23, no. 1, pp. 133–143, [online] doi:10.1123/japa.2013-0091

[3] Bhore, Prachiti Rajan/Khushboo Bathia/Smita Kanase/Amrutkuvar Jadhav (2019): Prevalence of Core Weakness in Bank Employees, in: *Journal of Clinical and Diagnostic Research, JCDR* Research and Publications, [online] doi:10.7860/jcdr/2019/40155.12697.

[4] Langhammer, Birgitta/Astrid Bergland/Elisabeth Rydwik (2018): The Importance of Physical Activity Exercise among Older People, in: *BioMed Research International*, Hindawi Publishing Corporation, vol. 2018, pp. 1–3, [online] doi:10.1155/2018/7856823.

[5] Fujita, Satoshi/Elena Volpi (2006): Amino Acids and Muscle Loss with Aging, in: *The Journal of Nutrition*, Elsevier BV, vol. 136, no. 1, pp. S277–S280, [online] doi:10.1093/jn/136.1.277s.

[6] Walston, Jeremy D. (2012): Sarcopenia in older adults, in: *Current Opinion in Rheumatology*, Ovid Technologies (Wolters Kluwer Health), vol. 24, no. 6, pp. 623–627, [online] doi:10.1097/bor.0b013e328358d59b.

[7] Yoo, Su-Zi/Mi-Hyun No/Jun-Won Heo/Dong-Ho Park/Ju-Hee Kang/So Hun Kim/Hyo-Bum Kwak (2018): Role of exercise in age-related sarcopenia, in: *Journal of Exercise Rehabilitation*, Korean Society of Exercise Rehabilitation, vol. 14, no. 4, pp. 551–558, [online] doi:10.12965/jer.1836268.134.

[8] HÄGGMARK, T./A. THORSTENSSON (1979): Fibre types in human abdominal muscles, in: *Acta Physiologica Scandinavica*, Wiley, vol. 107, no. 4, pp. 319–325, [online] doi:10.1111/j.1748-1716.1979.tb06482.x.

[9] De Salles, B. F., Simão, R., Miranda, F., Da Silva Novaes, J., Lemos, A., & Willardson, J. M. (2009). Rest Interval between Sets in Strength Training. *Sports Medicine*, 39(9), 765–777. https://doi.org/10.2165/11315230-000000000-00000

[10] Lemmink, K. A., Han, K., De Greef, M. H. G., Rispens, P., & Stevens, M. (2001). Reliability of the Groningen Fitness Test for the Elderly. *Journal of Aging and Physical Activity*, 9(2), 194–212. https://doi.org/10.1123/japa.9.2.194

[11] Rikli, R. E., & Jones, C. J. (2002). Senior fitness test manual. *Choice Reviews Online*, 39(06), 39–3447. https://doi.org/10.5860/choice.39-3447

[12] MACKENZIE, B. (2002) Core Muscle Strength and Stability Test [WWW] Available from: *https://www.brianmac.co.uk/coretest.htm* [Accessed 18/3/2023]

Exercise Index

Made in United States
North Haven, CT
10 November 2026

22100370R00213